MCQs for FRCOphth Part 2

MCQs for FRCOphth Part 2

Edited by

Darren S. J. Ting, MBChB, PgCertHPE, DRCOphth, FRCOphth
(Recipient of FRCOphth Crombie Medal and DRCOphth Cornwall Prize)
Fight for Sight/John Lee, Royal College of Ophthalmologists (RCOphth)
Primer Fellow
Academic Ophthalmology
University of Nottingham
Nottingham, UK

David H. W. Steel, MBBS, MD, FRCOphth
Consultant Ophthalmologist,
Sunderland Eye Infirmary
Sunderland, UK; and
Honorary Professor of Retinal Surgery,
Newcastle University
Newcastle upon Tyne, UK

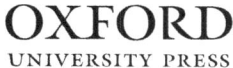

OXFORD
UNIVERSITY PRESS

Great Clarendon Street, Oxford, OX2 6DP,
United Kingdom

Oxford University Press is a department of the University of Oxford.
It furthers the University's objective of excellence in research, scholarship,
and education by publishing worldwide. Oxford is a registered trade mark of
Oxford University Press in the UK and in certain other countries

© Oxford University Press 2020

The moral rights of the authors have been asserted

First Edition published in 2020

All rights reserved. No part of this publication may be reproduced, stored in
a retrieval system, or transmitted, in any form or by any means, without the
prior permission in writing of Oxford University Press, or as expressly permitted
by law, by licence or under terms agreed with the appropriate reprographics
rights organization. Enquiries concerning reproduction outside the scope of the
above should be sent to the Rights Department, Oxford University Press, at the
address above

You must not circulate this work in any other form
and you must impose this same condition on any acquirer

Published in the United States of America by Oxford University Press
198 Madison Avenue, New York, NY 10016, United States of America

British Library Cataloguing in Publication Data
Data available

Library of Congress Control Number: 2019957201

ISBN 978–0–19–882576–0

Oxford University Press makes no representation, express or implied, that the
drug dosages in this book are correct. Readers must therefore always check
the product information and clinical procedures with the most up-to-date
published product information and data sheets provided by the manufacturers
and the most recent codes of conduct and safety regulations. The authors and
the publishers do not accept responsibility or legal liability for any errors in the
text or for the misuse or misapplication of material in this work. Except where
otherwise stated, drug dosages and recommendations are for the non-pregnant
adult who is not breast-feeding

Links to third party websites are provided by Oxford in good faith and
for information only. Oxford disclaims any responsibility for the materials
contained in any third party website referenced in this work.

DEDICATION

'To my wife, Jiani, and my family for their unconditional support and love; and to my trainers, colleagues, and friends in the North East Deanery for the amazing time and memories during my ophthalmology training.'

Darren S. J. Ting

'To the many ophthalmic trainees at Sunderland Eye Infirmary and the North East Deanery that I have had the pleasure of working with.'

David H. W. Steel

FOREWORD

Test yourself and teach yourself. To do both at the same time: read this book, study it, and learn from it. The format and content are unique compared to other MCQ books that I read in my long gone days as a trainee, or have seen in recent times. The questions are standard, testing factual knowledge and the application of knowledge in clinical settings. The big selling point of this book is in the answer section. The authors have provided elaborate explanations for the answers, which enhance the learning experience and the retention of knowledge. At times, getting an answer correct can still leave a gap in one's knowledge as MCQs do not test the depth of understanding an individual may or may not have of the subject. But for this book, the answers and the explanations go that extra step to fill any gaps that might have existed. It actually makes the test an enjoyable experience and by the time the fun is over, you will be well prepared for the actual examination, which hopefully will no longer be a daunting experience.

Reading this book is also a great way for those who have passed all their examinations to refresh their knowledge.

Harminder S Dua, CBE
MBBS, DO, DO (London), MS, MNAMS, FRCS (Edinburgh), FEBO (EU), FRCOphth,
FRCP (Edinburgh, Honorary), FCOptom. (UK, Honorary), FRCOphth (UK, Honorary), MD, PhD

(Former President of Royal College of Ophthalmologists 2011–2014)
Chair and Professor of Ophthalmology
University of Nottingham
Queen's Medical Centre
Nottingham
United Kingdom

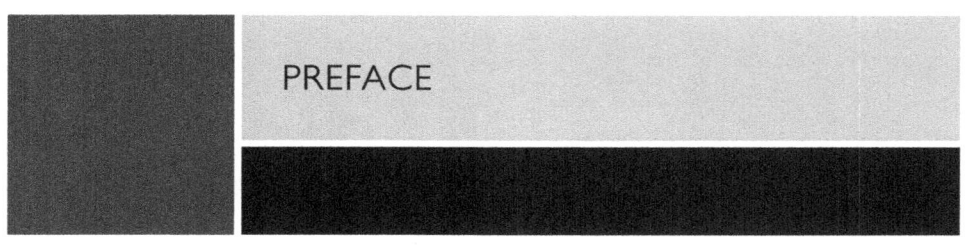

PREFACE

'Too much to do, too little time'—a common notion that probably describes the life of most trainees, including me.

As a clinical and research fellow who had just recently passed the Fellowship of the Royal College of Ophthalmologists (FRCOphth) final exam, I realize that we, as trainees, often have limited time to prepare and revise for the 'test' while trying to juggle so many things in our work and home lives simultaneously. For the preparation of my FRCOphth written exam (see Table P.1), I relied on several different revision materials and question banks; however, many of these were either outdated, associated with expensive subscription fees, or orientated to US practice, which often differs from that in the UK. In addition, few questions covered recent landmark studies and the Royal College of Ophthalmologists (RCOphth) curriculum, including relevant GMC/NICE/RCOphth/Good Medical Practice guidelines, all of which are frequently tested in both the written and oral parts of the exam.

This book aims to provide up-to-date revision material specifically targeting the FRCOphth Part 2 multiple choice questions (MCQs) exam. It places more emphasis on areas that are not well covered in other revision materials, including the GMC/RCOphth guidelines, professional guidance, and the choice and rationale for clinical investigations and management. The questions are organised into five sections reflecting the subdivisions of the MCQ exam, and one mock exam containing an additional 90 questions. All 360 MCQs are provided with a detailed explanation and referenced. The questions are accurately mapped against the RCOphth curriculum and we therefore hope it will help not only in the MCQs, but also in the other parts of the exam.

We are extremely grateful to the expert clinicians who have contributed questions from their own subspecialist areas. The book could not have been completed without their expertise and help. As editors we have tried to ensure a consistent style and approach throughout the book to ease the learning process. We hope that this book will help you on your path to success in the FRCOphth Part 2 exam.

Good luck!

Darren S. J. Ting and David H. W. Steel

CONTENTS

Abbreviations xiii
Contributors xix
Structure of the FRCOphth Part 2 Written Exam xxi

1 Clinical Ophthalmology 1
Questions 1
Answers 15

2 Clinical Ophthalmology 2
Questions 35
Answers 54

3 Clinical Ophthalmology 3
Questions 77
Answers 92

4 Pharmacology, Therapeutics, and Investigations
Questions 115
Answers 125

5 Basic Science and Miscellaneous
Questions 137
Answers 145

6 Mock Exam
Questions 157
Answers 177

Index 205

ABBREVIATIONS

A&E	accident and emergency
AC	anterior chamber
ACE	angiotensin-converting enzyme
AChR	antiacetylcholine receptors
AF	atrial fibrillation
AGIS	Advanced Glaucoma Intervention Study
AIDS	acquired immune deficiency syndrome
AK	acanthamoeba keratitis
AMD	age-related macular degeneration
ANA	antinuclear antibody
ANCA	antineutrophilic cytoplasmic antibody
APMPPE	acute posterior multifocal placoid pigment epitheliopathy
ARC	abnormal retinal correspondence
AREDS	Age-related Eye Disease Study
ARN	acute retinal necrosis
ASCRS	American Society of Cataract and Refractive Surgery
ASRS	American Society of Retina Specialists
AU	anterior uveitis
BCC	basal cell carcinoma
BCG	bacillus Calmette–Guérin
BCVA	best corrected visual acuity
BD	twice a day
BE	Basic exotropia
BETT	Birmingham Eye Trauma Terminology
BHL	bilateral hilar lymphadenopathy
BM	Bruch's membrane
BMI	body mass index
BNF	British National Formulary
BPES	blepharophimosis, ptosis, and epicanthus inversus syndrome
BSV	binocular single vision
CAI	carbonic anhydrase inhibitor

CAR	cancer-associated retinopathy
CCF	carotico-cavernous fistula
CCTS	Collaborative Corneal Transplant Studies
CFEOM	congenital fibrosis of extraocular muscles
CH	cluster headache
CI	convergence insufficiency
CJD	Creutzfeldt–Jakob disease
CL	contact lens
CMO	cystoid macular oedema
CMT	central macular thickness
CNS	central nervous system
CNTGS	Collaborative Normal Tension Glaucoma Study
CNVM	choroidal neovascular membrane
COAG	chronic open angle glaucoma
COG	Children's Oncology Group
COMS	Collaborative Ocular Melanoma Study
COPD	chronic obstructive pulmonary disease
CPEO	chronic progressive external ophthalmoplegia
CRAO	central retinal artery occlusion
CRP	C-reactive protein
CRT	central retinal thickness
CSCR	central serous chorioretinopathy
CSF	cerebrospinal fluid
CSS	Churg–Strauss syndrome
CT	computed tomography
CTA	computed tomography angiogram
CTG	cytosine-thymine-guanine
CZS	congenital Zika syndrome
DALK	deep anterior lamellar keratoplasty
DCCT	Diabetes Control and Complications Trial
DE	distance exotropia
DEXA	dual energy X-ray absorptiometry
DMARD	disease-modifying antirheumatic drug
DMO	diabetic macular oedema
DON	dysthyroid optic neuropathy
DREAM	DRy Eye Amniotic Membrane
DRS	Diabetic Retinopathy Study
DRVS	Diabetic Retinopathy Vitrectomy Study
DS	Duane syndrome

DSG	dacryoscintigram
DVLA	Driver and Vehicle Licensing Agency
EGF	epidermal growth factor
EGFR	epidermal growth factor receptor
EMGS	Early Manifest Glaucoma Study
ENT	ear, nose, and throat
EON	ethambutol optic neuropathy
ESCRS	European Society of Cataract & Refractive Surgeons
ESR	erythrocyte sedimentation rate
ETDRS	Early Treatment for Diabetic Retinopathy Study
ETROP	Early Treatment of Retinopathy of Prematurity
EUGOGO	European Group on Graves' orbitopathy
EVS	Endophthalmitis Vitrectomy Study
FA	fluocinolone acetonide
FAF	fundus autofluorescence
FBC	full blood count
FDA	Food and Drug Administration
FDT	forced duction test
FFA	fundus fluorescein angiography
FHC	Fuchs' heterochromic cyclitis
FLACS	femtosecond laser-assisted cataract surgery
FLAIR	fluid attenuated inversion recovery
G6PD	glucose-6-phosphate dehydrogenase
GA	gyrate atrophy
GABA	gamma-aminobutyric acid
GCA	giant cell arteritis
GMC	General Medical Council
GON	glaucomatous optic neuropathy
GP	general practitioner
H&E	haematoxylin & eosin
HEDS	Herpetic Eye Disease Study
HIV	human immunodeficiency virus
HLA	human leukocyte antigen
HORV	haemorrhagic occlusive retinal vasculitis
HSK	herpes simplex keratitis
HSV	herpes simplex virus
HZO	herpes zoster ophthalmicus
ICG	indocyanine green
ICGA	indocyanine green angiography

IDEX	Intermittent distance exotropia
IFIS	intraoperative floppy iris syndrome
IIH	idiopathic intracranial hypertension
IIHTT	IIH treatment trial
ILM	internal limiting membrane
INO	internuclear ophthalmoplegia
IOP	intraocular pressure
IPD	interpupillary distance
IR	inferior rectus
ISCEV	International Society for Clinical Electrophysiology of Vision
ITC	iridotrabecular contact
JIA	juvenile idiopathic arthritis
KF	Kayser–Fleischer
KSS	Kearns–Sayers syndrome
LFT	liver function test
LHON	Leber's hereditary optic neuropathy
LIO	left inferior oblique
LR	lateral rectus
LSCD	limbal stem cell deficiency
LSR	left superior rectus
MAR	melanoma-associated retinopathy
MCQ	multiple-choice question
MD	myotonic dystrophy
MED	monocular elevation deficiency
MG	myasthenia gravis
MGJWS	Marcus-Gunn jaw winking syndrome
MLD	maximum linear diameter
MLF	medial longitudinal fasciculus
MOA	mechanisms of action
MR	medial rectus
MRA	magnetic resonance angiography
MRI	magnetic resonance imaging
MRSE	mean refractive spherical equivalent
MuSK	muscle-specific kinase
NASCET	North American Symptomatic Carotid Endarterectomy Trial
NDESP	NHS Diabetic Eye Screening Programme
NFAT	nuclear factor of activated T cells
NICE	National Institute for Health and Care Excellence
NNT	numbers need to treat

NOG	National Osteoporosis Guideline Group
NPL	non-perceptive to light
OCP	ocular cicatricial pemphigoid
OCT	optical coherence tomography
OD	left eye
OHTS	Ocular Hypertension Study
OID	orbital inflammatory disease
ONTT	Optic Neuritis Treatment Trial
OS	right eye
OSSN	ocular surface squamous neoplasia
OTS	ocular trauma score
PACG	primary angle closure glaucoma
PACS	primary angle closure suspect
PAM	primary acquired melanosis
PAS	peripheral anterior synechiae
PAT	prism adaptation test
PCG	primary congenital glaucoma
PCMO	post-cataract surgery macular oedema
PCO	posterior capsular opacification
PD	prism dioptres
PDR	proliferative diabetic retinopathy
PDS	pigment dispersion syndrome
PED	pigment epithelial detachments
PEDF	Pigment epithelium derived factor
PGA	prostaglandin analogues
PHN	post-herpetic neuralgia
PIC	punctate inner choroidopathy
PK	penetrating keratoplasty
PlGF	placental growth factor
PMD	pellucid marginal degeneration
POGS	Parinaud's oculo-glandular syndrome
POHS	presumed ocular histoplasmosis syndrome
POT	parietal-occipital-temporal
PPCD	posterior polymorphous corneal dystrophy
PPD	plasma protein derivative
PPRF	paramedian pontine reticular formation
PRN	*pro re nata*
PSS	primary Sjogren's syndrome
PUK	peripheral ulcerative keratitis

QALY	quality-adjusted life year or quality-adjusted-life-year
QID	four times a day
RAM	retinal arterial macroaneurysm
RAPD	relative afferent pupillary defect
RD	retinal detachment
RIO	right inferior oblique
RLR	right lateral rectus
RP	retinitis pigmentosa
RPE	retinal pigment epithelium
RSR	right superior rectus
RVO	retinal vein occlusions
SCC	squamous cell carcinoma
SJS	Steven–Johnson syndrome
SLT	selective laser trabeculoplasty
SO	superior oblique (also Sympathetic ophthalmia)
SOD	septo-optic dysplasia
SOF	superior orbital fissure
SOM	superior oblique myokymia
SR	superior rectus
SSS	silent sinus syndrome
SUN	Standardization of Uveitis Nomenclature
TED	thyroid eye disease
TIA	transient ischaemic attack
TON	traumatic optic neuropathy
TPMT	thiopurine methyltransferase
TVT	Tube Versus Trabeculectomy
U&E	urea and electrolytes test
UBM	ultrasound biomicroscopy
UC	ulcerative colitis
UZS	Urrets–Zavalia syndrome
VEGF	vascular endothelial growth factor
VEP	visual evoked potential
VHL	Von Hippel Lindau
VKH	Vogt–Koyanagi–Harada
VR	vitreo-retinal
WD	Wilson's disease
WHO	World Health Organization
XLOA	X-linked ocular albinism
XLRS	X-linked recessive juvenile retinoschisis

CONTRIBUTORS

Wendy Adams Consultant Ophthalmologist (Neuro-Ophthalmology), Sunderland Eye Infirmary, Sunderland, UK

Lucy Clarke Consultant Ophthalmologist (Oculoplastic, Orbit and Emergency Eye Care), Newcastle Eye Centre, Royal Victoria Infirmary, Newcastle upon Tyne, UK

Lawrence Gnanaraj Consultant Ophthalmologist (Paediatric Ophthalmology and Strabismus), Sunderland Eye Infirmary, Sunderland, UK

William Innes Consultant Medical Ophthalmologist, Newcastle Eye Centre, Royal Victoria Infirmary, Newcastle upon Tyne, UK

David L. Lunt Consultant Ophthalmologist (Glaucoma), Department of Ophthalmology, South Tees Hospitals NHS Foundation Trust, Middlesbrough, UK

Philip Severn Consultant Ophthalmologist (Medical Retina) and Clinical Director, Department of Ophthalmology, South Tees Hospital NHS Foundation Trust, Middlesbrough, UK

Jonathan Smith Consultant Ophthalmologist (Medical and Surgical Retina), Sunderland Eye Infirmary, Sunderland, UK

Laura Steeples Consultant Ophthalmologist (Uveitis), Manchester Royal Eye Hospital, Manchester, UK

Shi Zhuan Tan Vitreoretinal Fellow, Guys' and St Thomas Hospital, London, UK

Darren S. J. Ting Fight for Sight/John Lee, Royal College of Ophthalmologists (RCOphth) Primer Fellow, Academic Ophthalmology, University of Nottingham, Nottingham, UK

STRUCTURE OF THE FRCOphth PART 2 WRITTEN EXAM

Table P.1 Structure of the FRCOphth part 2 written exam

Clinical ophthalmology	**128**
Cornea and external eye	20
Glaucoma	10
Cataract and lens	10
Retina	10
Neurology and pupil	16
Medicine	10
Strabismus and paediatrics	16
Trauma	4
Oculoplastic and orbit	10
Uveitis and oncology	12
Pharmacology and therapeutics	**12**
Investigations	**16**
Ophthalmic	9
Orthoptic	3
Neuroimaging	3
Other	1
Basic science	**8**
Anatomy/Physiology	2
Pathology	2
Genetics	3
Optics	1
Miscellaneous	**16**
Statistics/Epidemiology	3
Research/EBM	3
Nutrition	1
Ethics/Driving	4
Economics	1
Guidelines/Standards	4

Reproduced with the kind permission of The Royal College of Ophthalmologists.
https://www.rcophth.ac.uk/wp-content/uploads/2019/03/Part-2-FRCOphth-Written-Notes-for-Candidates-Updated-March-2019.pdf

chapter 1

CLINICAL OPHTHALMOLOGY 1

QUESTIONS

1. A 35-year-old man presented with a 2-day history of right painful red eye. Examination revealed dendritic ulcer with no stromal vascularization/oedema or keratic precipitates. Anterior chamber is deep and quiet. He had two similar episodes of dendritic keratitis in the past year. What is the best management plan for this patient?
   A. Topical aciclovir 3% 5×/day for 2 weeks +/− epithelial debridement
   B. Topical aciclovir 3% 5×/day for 2 weeks + topical prednisolone 1% QID for 2 weeks
   C. Topical aciclovir 3% 5×/day for 2 weeks + oral aciclovir 400 mg BD for at least 6 months
   D. Topical aciclovir 3% 5×/day for 2 weeks + oral aciclovir 400 mg 5×/day for 2 weeks then BD for at least 6 months

2. Which of the following statements about ocular cicatricial pemphigoid (OCP) is correct?
   A. Identification of linear deposition of immunoglobulin G (IgG), IgE, and C3 complement factors at the epithelial basement membrane zone using direct immunofluorescence (DIF) test is diagnostic of OCP
   B. Negative immunofluorescent test of conjunctival biopsy excludes the diagnosis of OCP
   C. To achieve best diagnostic yield of OCP, it is best to obtain the conjunctival biopsy from less inflamed areas
   D. Conjunctival sample should be transported in a sterile pot containing formalin solution for immunohistochemical analysis

3. Which of the following histopathological stains is **MOST** useful in the diagnosis of Avellino corneal dystrophy?
   A. Alcian blue stain
   B. Congo red stain
   C. Haematoxylin & eosin (H&E stain)
   D. Oil-red-O stain

4. In addition to limbal ischaemia, which of the following signs has been shown to have a poor prognostic value in chemical eye injury?
   A. More than 2+ cells in anterior chamber
   B. Central epithelial defect of > 80%
   C. Raised intraocular pressure (IOP) of 28 mmHg or more
   D. Severe conjunctival involvement of > 80%

5. Which of the following statements regarding ocular surface squamous neoplasia (OSSN) is correct?
   A. Patients presenting with OSSN should always be screened for human immunodeficiency virus (HIV) and acquired immune deficiency syndrome (AIDS)
   B. The incidence of OSSN has been estimated at around 1–2 per 10 000/year in Caucasian populations
   C. OSSN usually presents as a unilateral vascularized mass at the inferior fornix area
   D. Bowen's disease is a type of OSSN that affects the conjunctival basement membrane

6. Which of the following organisms has the potential to penetrate an intact corneal epithelium?
   A. *Corynebacterium diphtheriae*
   B. Group A streptococcus
   C. *Moraxella lacunata*
   D. *Pseudomonas aeruginosa*

7. A 24-year-old patient presents to the eye clinic with a 6-month history of photophobia and decreased vision in the right eye. His past ocular history is significant for a right chemical eye injury, which was treated elsewhere. His presenting vision is 6/36. Examination shows 3 clock-hours of peripheral conjunctivalization of the cornea, extending to the visual axis, which is also associated with stippled fluorescein staining. Which of the following is the best initial treatment option for this patient?
   A. Amniotic membrane transplant
   B. Anterior lamellar keratoplasty
   C. Autologous limbal stem cell transplant
   D. Sequential sector conjunctival epitheliectomy

8. Which of the following findings regarding corneal impression cytology is suggestive of limbal stem cell deficiency?
   A. Absence of goblet cell
   B. Presence of cytokeratin (CK)-3
   C. Presence of CK-12
   D. Presence of CK-13

9. Which of the following corneal dystrophies has a different gene mutation from the others?
   A. Epithelial basement membrane dystrophy (or map-dot-fingerprint dystrophy)
   B. Granular dystrophy
   C. Meesmann dystrophy
   D. Thiel–Behnke dystrophy

10. A 25-year-old patient with keratoconus underwent an uncomplicated penetrating keratoplasty for visual rehabilitation. On the next day, the patient complains of a fixed dilated pupil with some headache. Examination of the eye shows a fixed and dilated pupil with a deep and quiet anterior chamber. The dilated pupil is not responsive to topical pilocarpine 2% drops. Otherwise there is no sign of ptosis. What should be the next step in your management?
    A. Check the patient's ocular motility
    B. Check the patient's IOP
    C. Organize a computed tomography angiogram of the head
    D. Organize an MRI head with contrast

11. A 75-year-old patient presents with vesicular rashes affecting the right side of the forehead and scalp and the base of the nose, respecting the midline of the face. On examination there are pseudodendritic changes on the cornea with mild intraocular inflammation. Which of the following statements concerning this scenario is true?
    A. This patient has a high risk of developing corneal denervation
    B. Oral aciclovir is not useful if it is started 72 hours after the onset of rashes
    C. Topical aciclovir should be used in this case
    D. Oral antibiotic should be started if there is evidence of bilateral periorbital swelling

12. A 53-year-old man, with a background of right penetrating keratoplasty performed 1 year ago, presents with a 3-day history of right eye photophobia and mildly reduced vision. He has recently recovered from a viral illness. Slit-lamp examination reveals a minimally red eye with mild papillary conjunctival changes and multiple subepithelial opacities within the corneal graft. Otherwise there is no sign of epithelial defect, stromal oedema, keratic precipitates, or anterior chamber activity. Which of the following options is the most appropriate management for this patient?
    A. Start on regular topical lubricants and reassure the patient
    B. Start on topical chloramphenicol 0.5% four times a day for 1 week and review the patient in a few weeks' time
    C. Start on topical prednisolone 0.5% twice a day and review in a few weeks' time
    D. Start on topical dexamethasone 0.1% four to six times a day and review the patient in a few days' time

13. Which of the following options regarding corneal arcus is correct?
    A. It may be associated with peripheral corneal thinning
    B. The lipid deposition is restricted to the stromal level
    C. It usually starts at 3 and 9 o'clock
    D. Ipsilateral corneal arcus may be associated with ipsilateral carotid artery disease

14. **Which layer of the cornea is affected by the copper deposition in Wilson's disease?**
    A. Epithelium
    B. Bowman's layer
    C. Stroma
    D. Descemet's membrane

15. **Which of the following conditions is associated with 'curly fibres' in Bowman's layer on histopathologic examination?**
    A. Meesmann epithelial dystrophy
    B. Reis–Buckler dystrophy
    C. Schnyder central crystalline dystrophy
    D. Thiel–Behnke dystrophy

16. **Which of the following options regarding keratoconus is NOT correct?**
    A. Breaks in the Bowman's layer is a diagnostic feature of keratoconus
    B. Posterior keratoconus is usually congenital and unilateral
    C. Posterior corneal curvature is usually not affected in keratoconus
    D. Belin Ambrosio Enhanced Ectasia Display is useful in detecting early keratoconus

17. **Which of the following statements regarding Peter's anomaly is correct?**
    A. It may be associated with systemic abnormalities such as cardiac and central nervous system malformations
    B. It is caused by a mutation of the *TIMP3* gene
    C. Approximately 20% of the patients develop glaucoma
    D. It is caused by developmental abnormalities of the corneal stroma

18. **A 14-year-old patient presents to the eye clinic with her mum, concerning about a recent increase in size of a 'lesion' on the white part of the eye. On examination, there is a minimally elevated, pigmented lesion on the conjunctiva near the limbus area with cystic changes and without vascularization or epithelial defect. She mentions that the pigmented lesion has been present for many years. What is the most likely diagnosis?**
    A. Conjunctival melanoma
    B. Conjunctival melanosis
    C. Conjunctival naevus
    D. Conjunctival papilloma

CLINICAL OPHTHALMOLOGY 1 | QUESTIONS

19. **Based on the evidence up to 2018, which of the following statements regarding the role of topical steroids in bacterial keratitis is true?**
    A. Patients with worse visual acuity at initial presentation benefit more with additional topical steroids than those with better presenting visual acuity
    B. Topical steroids hasten the healing time of bacterial keratitis
    C. Topical steroids increase the risk of corneal perforation compared to those without topical steroids
    D. Patients with *Nocardia* keratitis have a better visual outcome when additional topical steroids are given along with topical antibiotics

20. **Which of the following statements regarding Mooren's ulcer is correct?**
    A. It is a type of peripheral ulcerative keratitis associated with scleritis
    B. It may be associated with hepatitis C infection
    C. The ulcer is usually painless, which is a distinguishing feature from other types of peripheral ulcerative keratitis
    D. Bilateral disease usually has a less painful presentation, with better responsiveness to therapy compared to the unilateral disease

21. **A 30-year-old patient presents to the eye clinic with reduced vision in the right eye. Slit-lamp examination shows a beaten bronze appearance of the corneal endothelium with iris atrophy and peripheral anterior synechiae on gonioscopy. Examination of the left eye is entirely normal. Which of the following statements concerning this condition is correct?**
    A. This condition normally has an autosomal dominant inheritance
    B. It is more commonly found in men than in women
    C. Around 20% of the patients are affected by glaucoma
    D. PCR testing of the affected corneal endothelium may reveal HSV DNA

22. **Which of the following statements regarding primary acquired melanosis (PAM) is true?**
    A. Most conjunctival melanomas arise from PAM
    B. It is more commonly found in patients with darker skin
    C. Limbal conjunctiva is the most commonly affected area
    D. PAM with any degree of atypia is associated with an increased risk of developing melanoma

23. **Which of the following statements regarding pellucid marginal degeneration (PMD) is correct?**
    A. It affects both males and females equally
    B. The steepest area of cornea corresponds with the thinnest area of the cornea
    C. It is associated with against-the-rule astigmatism
    D. 'Crab-claw' pattern on corneal topography is a pathognomonic finding of PMD

24. **Which of the following statements regarding amniotic membrane is correct?**
    A. The use of amniotic membrane is contraindicated in patients with active herpes simplex viral keratitis
    B. Cryopreserved amniotic membrane has been shown to improve signs and symptoms of dry eye disease
    C. It has anti-inflammatory, antifibrotic, and wound healing properties but no antimicrobial properties
    D. Cryopreservation is currently the only technique to preserve amniotic membrane for clinical use

25. **A 70-year-old woman presents to the eye clinic with a 4-day history of right-sided conjunctival redness, jaw swelling, and fever. He has no previous medical or ocular history. She has two pet rabbits at home and denied any history of cat scratch or exposure. Examination reveals severe right conjunctival hyperaemia and multiple conjunctival nodules and ulceration. There is also associated pre-auricular and submandibular lymphadenopathy. Which of the following organisms is the most likely culprit in this scenario?**
    A. *Bartonella henselae*
    B. *Francisella tularensis*
    C. *Sporotrichum schenckii*
    D. *Treponema pallidum*

26. **A 25-year-old patient with advanced keratoconus underwent a deep anterior lamellar keratoplasty for visual rehabilitation. During the operation, there was an inadvertent perforation of the Descemet's membrane, necessitating a conversion of deep anterior lamellar keratoplasty (DALK) to penetrating keratoplasty (PKP). Which of the following statements is correct?**
    A. There is no significant difference in the graft rejection rate between PKP and DALK for keratoconus
    B. There is a significant increased risk of keratometric astigmatism after PKP compared to DALK
    C. The patient is likely to have a worse uncorrected visual acuity at 6 months with PKP compared to DALK
    D. The patient is likely to have a better corrected visual acuity at 6 months with PKP compared to DALK

27. **Which of the following statements regarding herpes zoster or shingles vaccination in the United Kingdom is true?**
    A. Shingles vaccination consists of inactivated/killed varicella-zoster virus
    B. It is available for all people of more than 70 years old
    C. Shingles vaccination could result in reactivation of herpes zoster keratitis
    D. People who had shingles previously do not benefit from shingles vaccination

28. According to the Collaborative Corneal Transplant Studies (CCTS), which of the following statements is correct?
   A. Human leukocyte antigen-A (HLA-A) antigen matching significantly reduces the risk of corneal graft rejection
   B. HLA-DR antigen matching significantly reduces the risk of corneal graft rejection
   C. ABO blood group matching may reduce the risk of corneal graft rejection
   D. Positive donor-recipient cross-match significant increases the risk of corneal graft rejection

29. A 3-year-old boy was brought in by his mum to the eye clinic with 2 weeks' history of itchy and painful eyes. He was treated by his general physician with topical chloramphenicol during the preceding week with no improvement. The boy was very uncooperative during the examination and you could only obtain a quick glance from slit-lamp examination, which revealed inflamed eyes with moderate papillary conjunctivitis. There was also a moderate size corneal plaque with epithelial defect at the superior paracentral cornea in the right eye. Measurement of IOP was not possible. The boy was started on topical olopatadine and topical prednisolone 0.5% four times a day. On examination during the following week, the corneal changes remained the same. Which of the following is the most appropriate next step for this child?
   A. Change topical prednisolone 0.5% to topical dexamethasone 0.1% six times a day
   B. Change topical chloramphenicol four times a day to topical levofloxacin six times a day
   C. Start the child on topical ciclosporin 0.1% once at night
   D. Arrange for the child to have removal of corneal plaque under general anaesthesia soon

30. Which of the following statements regarding the mechanism of action of Lifitegrast (recently approved for treatment of dry eye disease) is correct?
   A. Inhibits CD-20 antibody
   B. Inhibits cytotoxic T cells (CD8)
   C. Inhibits lymphocyte function-associated antigen 1
   D. Inhibits calcineurin/nuclear factor of activated T cells

31. Which of the following types of anterior segment dysgenesis is strongly associated with corneal leukoma, craniofacial, and central nervous system abnormalities?
   A. Aniridia
   B. Axenfeld-Rieger syndrome
   C. Peter's anomaly
   D. Trabeculodysgenesis

32. A 59-year-old hypermetropic female patient with a best corrected visual acuity of 6/5 in both eyes (OU) attends your clinic due to elevated IOP at her optician. She has gonioscopically occludable iridocorneal angles, IOP of 27 mmHg OD, and 32 mmHg OS. She has a notch in the neuroretinal rim in both optic discs, and evidence of early arcuate defects on perimetry. Which intervention is superior in terms of efficacy and cost-effectiveness?
    A. Clear lens extraction
    B. Peripheral iridoplasty
    C. Peripheral iridotomy
    D. Selective laser trabeculoplasty

33. Which of the following statements regarding the landmark glaucoma studies is correct?
    A. Advanced Glaucoma Intervention Study (AGIS) found that Caucasian patients had better IOP control if they had primary ALT
    B. Collaborative Normal Tension Glaucoma Study (CNTGS) found that over the study period almost two-thirds of patients did not progress even without treatment
    C. Early Manifest Glaucoma Study (EMGS) found that age, race, and optic disc haemorrhages were risk factors for progression
    D. Ocular Hypertension Study (OHTS) found that age, race, and optic disc haemorrhages were risk factors for progression

34. A patient attends clinic one day after a trabeculectomy operation on his right eye. His Snellen best corrected visual acuity is 6/36 OD and 6/9 OS. Which of the following is most likely to be TRUE?
    A. His IOP is 4 mmHg. His anterior chamber is shallow. You suspect overdrainage and a conjunctival leak and so check with topical fluorescein 2%
    B. His IOP is 4 mmHg. His anterior chamber is shallow. You suspect a partial/complete blockage of the sclerostomy may be the cause
    C. His IOP is 35 mmHg. His anterior chamber is shallow. You suspect retained viscoelastic may be the cause
    D. His IOP is 35 mmHg. His anterior chamber is shallow. You suspect aqueous misdirection may be the cause and start him on topical pilocarpine 2% immediately pending further management

35. A patient who has had a trabeculectomy within the last 4 weeks has the clinical appearance of a conjunctival wound leak. All of the following is most likely to be correct, **EXCEPT**:
    A. This can be associated with a risk of blebitis and endophthalmitis
    B. Any wound leak requires further surgery to ensure adequate closure to reduce the risk of postoperative infection
    C. Slow flow wound leak can be managed conservatively, including contact lens
    D. Is more likely in patients who have been on long-term ocular antihypertensive medication

36. **Which of the following statements about the side effects of acetazolamide is correct?**
    A. May increase the level of potassium in the blood
    B. Is safe to be used in patients with liver impairment
    C. Is associated with an elevation in blood pressure
    D. Is associated with Stevens–Johnson syndrome

37. **A general practitioner (GP) contacted you about a 55-year-old male patient who has presented to his practice with symptoms consistent with impotence. He has primary open angle glaucoma and the GP wondered about the possible side effect from his glaucoma medication. Which medication is MOST likely to be responsible?**
    A. Apraclonidine
    B. Bimatoprost
    C. Dorzolamide
    D. Levobunolol

38. **A 38-year-old female patient is referred into the clinic following a high IOP reading. On examination she has an IOP of 17 mmHg OD and 35 mmHg OS. The left iris appears paler and she has stellate keratic precipitates across the whole corneal endothelium. She has some circulating cells in the anterior chamber. Which of the following statements about this condition is TRUE?**
    A. Anterior chamber activity always requires aggressive treatment with topical steroids
    B. There are normally no associated posterior segment findings
    C. Trabeculectomy is known to be ineffective
    D. Cataract surgery in this condition is associated with an increased risk of intraoperative bleeding

39. **A 45-year-old, type 1 diabetic, male patient attends a follow-up appointment 1 month following a fresh vitreous haemorrhage in his right eye. He has had a previous vitrectomy due to the same condition in the same eye. On examination he has developed diffuse corneal oedema, anterior chamber activity, and an elevated IOP of 45 mmHg OD (15 mmHg OS). No hyphema is noted. The view is limited but the vitreous haemorrhage does not seem to have altered. Which of the following is MOST LIKELY to describe his problem?**
    A. Ghost cell glaucoma
    B. Posner–Schlossman syndrome
    C. Red cell glaucoma
    D. Schwartz–Matsuo syndrome

40. A 54-year-old female is referred to your clinic with suspected narrow angles. Her refraction is +4.75 D OD and +4.25 D OS. She is asymptomatic. Her IOP is 28 mmHg OD and 30 mmHg OS. On gonioscopic examination, you are able to visualize the trabecular meshwork for approximately 90° in each eye. Optic disc assessment, visual field testing, and optical coherence tomography of the optic disc and macula are all normal. Which of the following correctly summarizes your findings?
    A. Occludable angles
    B. Primary angle closure
    C. Primary angle closure glaucoma
    D. Primary angle closure suspect

41. Which category of IOP lowering medication suppresses aqueous production and increases uveoscleral outflow?
    A. α-2-adrenergic agonists
    B. β-blockers
    C. Carbonic anhydrase inhibitors
    D. Prostaglandin analogues

42. You see a 67-year-old male patient with ocular hypertension who takes topical latanoprost at night in both eyes. His IOP is 20 mmHg. After completing all your investigations, you are satisfied there is no evidence of conversion to open angle glaucoma. Which of the following best describes the timing of the next review appointment?
    A. 4–6 months
    B. 6–9 months
    C. 9–12 months
    D. 12–18 months

43. In patients with high hypermetropia and/or very short axial length, which of the following procedures is known to cause aqueous misdirection (also known as malignant glaucoma)?
    A. Cataract surgery
    B. Peripheral iridotomy
    C. Trabeculectomy
    D. All of the above

44. When is it most appropriate to perform laser trabeculoplasty on a patient with glaucoma?
    A. Patient with chronic open angle glaucoma taking ≥1 medication and inadequate IOP control
    B. First-line therapy in a patient with ocular hypertension or chronic open angle glaucoma
    C. Following laser peripheral iridotomy in primary angle closure glaucoma
    D. First-line therapy in a patient with primary or secondary angle closure glaucoma

45. A 75-year-old patient presents to the clinic with a 1-week history of right eye pain. Examination revealed a hypermature cataract with raised IOP and deep anterior chamber with cells and flare. What is the likely diagnosis of this case?
    A. Lens particle glaucoma
    B. Phacoanaphylatic glaucoma
    C. Phacolytic glaucoma
    D. Phacomorphic glaucoma

46. During routine cataract surgery you become aware that there is a posterior capsule rupture. A quadrant of the lens nucleus drops into the anterior vitreous. Which of the following statements is most likely to be correct?
    A. Stop phacoemulsification immediately. Introduce a dispersive viscoelastic. If the lens fragment is within reach proceed with the phaco probe with caution to remove from the anterior vitreous
    B. Proceed with caution to remove the remainder of the lens fragments from the anterior segment. You can then decide how to proceed
    C. Stop phacoemulsification immediately. Introduce a dispersive viscoelastic. Do not attempt to remove the lens fragment with the phaco probe. Safely close the operative site and arrange discussion with vitreo-retinal (VR) service to arrange for completion of surgery +/− intraocular lens (IOL) as a secondary procedure
    D. Stop phacoemulsification immediately. Take appropriate steps, and remove lens fragment with vitrector

47. The following statements about post-phacoemulsification cystoid macular oedema (CMO, or Irvine–Gass syndrome) are true, **EXCEPT**:
    A. If investigated with optical coherence tomography (OCT), many more patients will have CMO than observed clinically
    B. There is strong evidence to suggest that prostaglandin analogues should be stopped in those patients with pre-existing glaucoma of any subtype
    C. Diabetes mellitus is a risk factor
    D. Uveitis is a risk factor

48. During phacoemulsification you rupture the posterior capsule. Following successful anterior vitrectomy and removal of all lens matter, you decide a sulcus IOL will be needed. The initial lens selected was +18.00 D three-piece IOL. Which of the following lenses would most closely match this refractive plan, assuming no optic capture is possible?
    A. +16.00 D
    B. +17.00 D
    C. +18.00 D
    D. +19.00 D

49. **Which of the following statements is correct with regard to an outbreak of acute postoperative endophthalmitis?**
    A. Cease all bilateral cataract cases and consider cessation of all surgery
    B. The responsible organisms are mostly contaminants
    C. It is defined as an outbreak if more than two cases are traced back to one operating list
    D. Only cases that comprised a proven outbreak need to be reported as clinical incidents

50. **Which of the following is a potential cause for myopic refractive surprise?**
    A. Previous laser refractive surgery for hypermetropia
    B. Lower A constant
    C. Undiagnosed staphyloma
    D. All of the above

51. **You see a patient in clinic with bilateral inferonasal lens subluxation. There is no history of trauma. The patient is tall with thin limbs and extremities ('marfanoid'). Which of the following statements is correct?**
    A. The gene defect is most likely to be fibrillin
    B. Cataract surgery should be performed under general anaesthesia due to increased risk of intraoperative complications
    C. The metabolic abnormality results in increased bone density
    D. A blood or urine test could confirm the diagnosis of this autosomal recessive condition

52. **Which of the following statements should be read aloud as part of the 'Sign in' procedure according to the World Health Organization (WHO) surgical safety checklist for cataract?**
    A. Have all team members introduced themselves by name and role?
    B. What lens model and power is to be used?
    C. Is there any anticipated difficulty with patient positioning?
    D. Is the correct lens implant present?

53. **Which of the following statements regarding pseudoexfoliation syndrome (PXF) is true?**
    A. These patients have deeper iridocorneal angles
    B. The degree of PXF material correlates with the severity of zonular dehiscence
    C. Lenticular instability can always be managed with a capsular tension ring intraoperatively
    D. Is associated with Eastern European and Scandinavian population

54. **As a cataract surgeon, you may encounter a variety of problems during surgery. Which of the following statements is true?**
    A. Reverse pupil block is more common in myopes
    B. Bimanual irrigation/aspiration has been proven to be safer and more efficient than coaxial
    C. Shorter eyes are less likely to be associated with intraoperative aqueous misdirection
    D. Intraoperative floppy iris syndrome can be avoided if you ask patients to stop their α-blocker 2 weeks prior to surgery

55. **A patient calls the eye department 3 days following cataract surgery. They feel that the vision is reduced and the eye is red and light sensitive. Please select the most appropriate answer from the following:**
    A. Advise the patient to increase the topical steroid drops but have a low threshold for attending the eye casualty
    B. The most common causative organisms include *Staphylococcus aureus*, *Staphylococcus epidermis*, and *Streptococcus* spp.
    C. Consider early vitrectomy if the vision is better than perception of light
    D. In addition to intravitreal antibiotics, topical or intravitreal corticosteroids should also always be administered

56. **Which of the following does NOT reduce the risk of posterior capsular opacification?**
    A. Square edge design of the IOL optic
    B. Haptics with flexible arms and posterior flexion
    C. Complete overlapping of anterior capsulorrhexis and anterior surface of IOL optic
    D. Polishing of the posterior capsular after cleaning of lens cortex

57. **What effect does intravitreal silicone oil have in a pseudophakic eye?**
    A. It makes the refraction less hypermetropic
    B. It makes the refraction more hypermetropic
    C. No effect on refraction
    D. Variable effect on refraction

58. **Which of the following statements on toxic anterior segment syndrome is correct?**
    A. Examination usually reveals diffuse corneal oedema with presence of hypopyon
    B. It usually acts as a precursor of infective endophthalmitis
    C. It is caused by inadvertent introduction of infectious substances into the anterior segment
    D. It can be distinguished from postoperative inflammation based on its unresponsiveness to topical steroids

59. Which of the following diseases is most commonly associated with posterior subcapsular cataract?
   A. Alport syndrome
   B. Fabry's disease
   C. Lowe's syndrome
   D. Waardenburg syndrome

60. Compared to the standard phacoemulsification cataract surgery, which of the following is true regarding femtosecond laser-assisted cataract surgery (FLACS)?
   A. FLACS is associated with a lower risk of postoperative CMO
   B. FLACS is associated with a lower risk of posterior capsular rupture
   C. The risk of anterior capsular tear is similar between FLACS and standard phacoemulsification
   D. FLACS is more cost-effective

chapter 1

CLINICAL OPHTHALMOLOGY 1

ANSWERS

1. Answer: A

Management of herpetic simplex keratitis (HSK) is a popular exam topic. This question tests the knowledge on the landmark study—Herpetic Eye Disease Study (HEDS), which consists of six arms (three therapeutic arms, two prophylactic arms, and one observational arm). For epithelial HSK the treatment is purely with topical antiviral (commonly aciclovir/ganciclovir in the United Kingdom); the use of oral aciclovir is only indicated if patient could not tolerate topical antiviral. There is no evidence of reducing recurrence of HSK with the use of oral antiviral in patients with strictly epithelial disease. Mechanical debridement may provide additional benefit in epithelial HSK, according to a Cochrane review.

The Herpetic Eye Disease Study Group. A controlled trial of oral acyclovir for the prevention of stromal keratitis or iritis in patients with herpes simplex virus epithelial keratitis. The Epithelial Keratitis Trial. *Arch Ophthalmol* 1997;115(6):703–12.

Wilhelmus KR. Antiviral treatment and other therapeutic interventions for herpes simplex virus epithelial keratitis. *Cochrane Database Syst Rev* 2015;1:CD002898.

2. Answer: C

OCP is an uncommon cicatricial conjunctival disease that is diagnosed on clinical ground +/− immunohistopathologic evidence. A positive DIF test is diagnostic of OCP but a negative result does not exclude the diagnosis. Severely inflamed conjunctiva can result in extensive scarring, which may reduce the diagnostic yield of the conjunctival biopsy; therefore, biopsy should be obtained from tissue adjacent to an inflamed site. Identification of linear deposition of IgG, IgA (not IgE), and C3 complement factors at the epithelial basement membrane zone using DIF test is diagnostic of OCP. Conjunctival biopsy sample should be transported in Michel medium for immunohistochemical analysis, whereas formalin solution is used for histopathologic analysis for any evidence of neoplastic changes.

Ahmed M, et al. Ocular cicatricial pemphigoid: pathogenesis, diagnosis and treatment. *Prog Retin Eye Res* 2004;23(6):579–92.

3. Answer: B

Avellino corneal dystrophy is a rare corneal dystrophy that consists of lattice dystrophy and granular dystrophy. Therefore, Congo red stain is useful in detecting the amyloid deposits in Avellino corneal dystrophy. The corneal stains can be remembered by the following mnemonic:

> **M**arilyn **M**onroe **A**lways **G**ets **H**er **M**an in **LA** **C**ity, **S**he **L**ikes **O**bese man.
>
> **M**acular dystrophy – **M**ucopolysaccharide – **A**lcian blue stain;
>
> **G**ranular dystrophy – **H**yaline – **M**asson trichrome stain;

Lattice dystrophy – <u>A</u>myloid – <u>C</u>ongo red stain;

<u>S</u>chnyder dystrophy – <u>L</u>ipid – <u>O</u>il-red-O stain.

Kanski J, Bowling B. *Clinical Ophthalmology: A Systematic Approach*, 7th edition. Chapter 6: Cornea, pp. 216–21. Edinburgh/New York: Elsevier/Saunders, 2011.

4. Answer: D

In 2001 Dua et al. published a new classification on chemical eye injury and provided additional prognostic factors to predict the outcome of the injury. The main differences between Dua's classification and Roper-Hall classification are that the former includes limbal involvement (instead of limbal ischaemia) and conjunctival involvement due to its ability to re-epithelialize the cornea if there is limbal stem cell deficiency. The reasons for modifications are that limbal involvement (fluorescein staining of the limbus) is more objective and consistent than limbal ischaemia, which can vary considerably among clinicians, and conjunctival involvement predicts the extent of conjunctival stem cell loss, which plays a vital role when there is significant limbal stem cell deficiency. There is a saying—'*corneal epithelium is better than conjunctival epithelium; conjunctival epithelium is better than no epithelium*' (see also Table 1.1).

Table 1.1 Classification system for chemical eye injury

Grading	Limbal involvement (clock-hour)	Conjunctival involvement (%)	Prognosis
1	0	0	Very good
2	≤3	≤30	Good
3	>3–6	>30–50	Good
4	>6–9	>50–75	Good—guarded
5	>9–12	>75–<100	Guarded—poor
6	12 (total)	100 (total)	Very poor

Reproduced from *British Journal of Ophthalmology*, Dua, H. et al. A new classification of ocular surface burns. 85(11): 1379–83. http://dx.doi.org/10.1136/bjo.85.11.1379. Copyright © 2001, British Medical Journal. With permission from BMJ Publishing Group Ltd.

5. Answer: A

OSSN is the most common non-pigmented malignancy of the ocular surface. It encompasses a spectrum of diseases, ranging from conjunctival intraepithelial neoplasia (also known as Bowen's disease), which basement membrane is not affected, to squamous cell carcinoma. It usually presents as a unilateral vascularized limbal mass located at the interpalpebral fissure due to ultraviolet (UV) light exposure.

The incidence rate ranged between 0.03 and 1.9 per 100 000/year in the Caucasian population to around 3 per 100 000/year in the African population. The main risk factors for OSSN include immunosuppression (e.g. AIDS, post-organ transplantation, lymphoma, xeroderma pigmentosa), ultraviolet B radiation, smoking, and infectious diseases such as HIV-1 and -2, human papillomavirus (HPV), hepatitis B and C virus. More importantly, OSSN may manifest as the first sign of HIV in some cases; therefore, all patients presenting with OSSN should be checked for HIV/AIDS and other infectious diseases. Moreover, OSSN in HIV-positive patients are usually associated with larger and thicker tumour and a higher incidence of corneal, scleral, and orbital involvement.

Management of OSSN includes surgical resection and medical treatment, including topical mitomycin C, 5-fluorouracil, interferon α-2b, and cidofovir. The risk of recurrence following surgical treatment or topical medical treatment alone may be as high as 43%, highlighting the need of long-term post-treatment surveillance.

Cicinelli MV, et al. Clinical management of ocular surface squamous neoplasia: a review of the current evidence. *Ophthalmol Ther* 2018;7(2):247–62.

Kamal S, et al. Ocular surface squamous neoplasia in 200 patients: a case-control study of immunosuppression resulting from human immunodeficiency virus versus immunocompetency. *Ophthalmology* 2015;122(1688):94.

6. Answer: A

Several organisms have the ability to penetrate intact corneal epithelium and this group of organisms can be remembered using the following mnemonic '**CHANeLS**'.

C—Corynebacterium

H—Haemophilus influenza

A—Acanthamoeba

Ne—Neisseria gonorrhoea/meningitidis

L—Listeria

S—Shigella

Microbial keratitis caused by this group of organisms need to be treated aggressively to prevent permanent visual loss.

ASCRS. *Special Report: Acanthamoeba Keratitis.* July 2007. Available at: http://www.ascrs.org/sites/default/files/resources/Acanthamoeba%20Keratitis.pdf

Tjia KF, et al. The interaction between *Neisseria gonorrhoeae* and the human cornea in organ culture. An electron microscopic study. *Graefes Arch Clin Exp Ophthalmol* 1988;226:341–5.

7. Answer: D

The clinical scenario describes a patient with partial limbal stem cell deficiency (LSCD) following chemical eye injury. Signs of LSCD include epithelial opacity (due to a mixture of metaplastic corneal and conjunctival epithelial cells), stippled/delayed fluorescein staining, loss of palisades of Vogt, vortex/columnar keratopathy, superficial vascularization, and recurrent/persistent corneal epithelial defect.

The management of LSCD depends on the patient's symptoms, laterality of the affected eyes (e.g. unilateral vs. bilateral), the severity of the disease (e.g. partial vs. total), and the state of the ocular surface. In this case, this patient suffers from a partial LSCD and therefore sequential sector conjunctiva epitheliectomy should be attempted first before undergoing autologous limbal stem cell transplant. Anterior lamellar keratoplasty is much more invasive and does not address the underlying LSCD problem. Amniotic membrane transplant will not work in this case because it is mainly used to promote healing of corneal epithelial defect, which is absent in this case.

Dua HS, et al. Contemporary limbal stem cell transplantation—a review. *Clin Exp Ophthalmol* 2010;38:104–17.

Le Q, et al. The diagnosis of limbal stem cell deficiency. *Ocul Surf* 2018;16:58–69.

8. Answer: D

Impression cytology serves as a useful clinical tool for investigating LSCD. It is performed by applying a cellulose acetate filter paper to the ocular surface to remove the very superficial layers of ocular surface epithelium. The presence of goblet cells on the cornea indicates the invasion of conjunctival cells, which is a hallmark of LSCD. However, the absence of goblet cells on cornea does not exclude the diagnosis of LSCD. CK-13 and CK-19 are important conjunctival surface markers and the presence of these factors are suggestive of LSCD whereas CK 3 and CK 12 are corneal surface markers.

Le Q, et al. The diagnosis of limbal stem cell deficiency. *Ocul Surf* 2018;16:58–69.

Ramirez-Miranda A, et al. Keratin 13 is a more specific marker of conjunctival epithelium than keratin 19. *Mol Vis* 2011;17:1652–61.

9. Answer: C

Meesman's dystrophy is a rare epithelial corneal dystrophy with an autosomal dominant inheritance. It is caused by gene mutations at CK-3 and CK-12, which are both important cytokeratins for corneal epithelium. The rest of the corneal dystrophies listed in the answer options are all caused by mutations in the *BIGH3* gene, or known as transforming growth factor β-induced (TGFBI), on chromosome 5q31. The list of corneal dystrophies caused by TGFBI/**BIG**H3 mutation can be memorized as '**LARGE**' (BIG = LARGE).

L—Lattice dystrophy (Type 1 and Type 3A)

A—Avellino dystrophy (combination of granular and lattice dystrophy)

R—Reis–Buckler dystrophy/Theil-Behnke dystrophy (milder form of Reis–Buckler)

G—Granular dystrophy

E—Epithelial basement membrane dystrophy (in some cases)

Boutboul S, et al. A subset of patients with epithelial basement membrane corneal dystrophy have mutations in TGFBI/BIGH3. *Hum Mutat* 2006;27:553–7.

Han KE, et al. Pathogenesis and treatments of TGFBI corneal dystrophies. *Prog Retin Eye Res* 2016;50:67–88.

10. Answer: B

This scenario describes a patient who has developed a condition called Urrets-Zavalia syndrome (UZS), which is characterized by a fixed and dilated pupil usually following penetrating keratoplasty or other types of intraocular surgeries such as DALK, Descemet stripping endothelial keratoplasty, and cataract surgery, among others. The incidence of UZS following penetrating keratoplasty is estimated at 0–17.7%. The main risk factors for UZS are intraoperative iris injury, intraoperative or postoperative raised IOP (usually within 24 hours postoperative), leading to iris ischaemia. Therefore, checking the IOP should be the next step of the management plan in this patient. It is unlikely that the patient has suddenly developed a dilated pupil secondary to third nerve palsy, especially without any sign of ptosis. Therefore neuroimaging is not required at this stage. Checking the ocular motility is reasonable but should come after the measurement of IOP.

Isac MMS, Ting DSJ, et al. Spontaneous pupillary recovery in a patient with Urrets-Zavalia syndrome following Descemet's membrane endothelial keratoplasty. *Med Hypothesis Discov Innov Ophthalmol* 2019;8:7–10.

Spierer O, Lazar M. Urrets-Zavalia syndrome (fixed and dilated pupil following penetrating keratoplasty for keratoconus) and its variants. *Surv Ophthalmol* 2014;59:304–10.

11. Answer: A

This is a typical scenario of a patient presenting with herpes zoster ophthalmicus (HZO) with ocular involvement. The standard treatment of HZO is systemic antiviral treatment; for instance, oral aciclovir 800 mg five times a day for 7–10 days, which is the common first-line treatment in the United Kingdom. Topical aciclovir is commonly and inappropriately used by many clinicians when there are corneal changes; however, studies did not show any beneficial effect of topical aciclovir in early HZO. Starting oral aciclovir within 72 hours of the onset of rash significantly reduces the risk of post-herpetic neuralgia and ocular complications; however, it should still be considered in patients who present after 72 hours of the onset of rash, especially when there are still new lesions forming. Involvement of the base, side, or tip of the nose (Hutchinson's sign) increases the risk of ocular inflammation and corneal denervation by 3–4 times. Bilateral periorbital swelling is caused by gravitational oedema instead of spreading of infection; therefore, antibiotic is not warranted.

Neoh C, et al. Comparison of topical and oral acyclovir in early herpes zoster ophthalmicus. *Eye (Lond)* 1994;8:688–91.

Ting DSJ, et al. Herpes zoster ophthalmicus. *BMJ* 2019;364:k5234.

12. Answer: D

This case scenario describes an uncommon presentation of subepithelial/stromal corneal graft rejection, which is characterized by numerous subepithelial opacities resembling adenoviral keratitis (Krachmer's spots). The incidence of this type of stromal rejection ranges between 2% and 15%. Although this entity represents a low-grade rejection process, it may be associated with or heralds the onset of other types of graft rejection; therefore, frequent topical steroids with close monitoring are advisable. The absence of follicular conjunctivitis and presence of subepithelial opacities within the corneal graft only go against the diagnosis of adenoviral keratitis. Erring on the cautious side, the patient should be treated for possible stromal rejection in this case. Corneal graft rejection can take place in various layer of cornea (Table 1.2).

Table 1.2 Types of corneal graft rejection

Types of rejection	Clinical features
Epithelial	Epithelial rejection line
Stromal (low grade)	Subepithelial opacities (Krachmer's spots)
Stromal (high grade)	Stromal haze, oedema, and vascularization
Endothelial	Most common and debilitating type; corneal oedema, endothelial line (Khodadoust line), keratic precipitates, anterior chamber activity

Krachmer JH, Alldredge OC. Subepithelial infiltrates: a probable sign of corneal transplant rejection. *Arch Ophthalmol* 1978;96:2234–7.

Panda A, et al. Corneal graft rejection. *Surv Ophthalmol* 2007;52:375–96.

13. Answer: A

Corneal arcus is a common degenerative corneal disease caused by lipid deposition in the peripheral stroma. The change normally starts at 12 and 6 o'clock and slowly spreads circumferentially to cover the entire peripheral stroma. In advanced cases, the Bowman's layer and Descemet's membrane may also be affected. Corneal arcus is frequently associated with hypercholesterolaemia and the presence of corneal arcus in young patients should prompt the investigation for familial hypercholesterolaemia and hyperbetalipoproteinaemia. The central edge is usually blurred with a distinct peripheral margin, which may be sometimes associated with peripheral thinning, named 'senile furrow degeneration'. Ipsilateral corneal arcus is rare and has been reported to be associated with ipsilateral ocular hypotony (due to increased blood flow to the anterior segment) and contralateral carotid artery disease (due to reduced blood flow).

Barchiesi BJ, et al. The cornea and disorders of lipid metabolism. *Surv Ophthalmol* 1991;36:1–22.

14. Answer: D

Wilson's disease (WD) is a rare autosomal recessive systemic condition characterized by abnormal accumulation of copper in various parts of the body, notably the basal ganglia, liver, and eye. It is caused by a mutation of the gene that regulates copper transport protein (ATP7B). This transporting protein supplies copper to a glycoprotein called caeruloplasmin, which transports copper to other parts of the body via the blood. Defective ATP7B results in increased accumulation of copper in the liver and apocaeruloplasmin (non-copper binding form of caeruloplasmin), which is rapidly degraded in the blood stream. The diagnosis of WD can be made by increased serum and urinary copper levels, reduced serum caeruloplasmin, MRI brain of the basal ganglia showing increased intensity on T2 scan ('face of giant panda'), and liver biopsy (gold standard). The ocular signs include Kayser-Fleischer (KF) ring (brownish ring at the peripheral cornea at the Descemet's membrane) and sunflower cataract. KF ring is present in 50–60% of patients with isolated hepatic WD and in more than 90% of patients with neurologic involvement. Interestingly KF ring may disappear on D-penicillamine, the systemic treatment for WD that promotes urinary excretion of copper.

Kelly C, Pericleous M. Wilson disease: more than meets the eye. *Postgrad Med J* 2018;94:335–47.

15. Answer: D

Meesmann dystrophy is a rare, autosomal dominant, epithelial corneal dystrophy that is characterized by irregular thickening of the epithelial basement membrane and intraepithelial cysts. Reis–Buckler dystrophy is an autosomal dominant, corneal dystrophy that affects the Bowman's layer. Histopathologic examination normally reveals replacement of Bowman's layer and epithelial basement membrane with fibrous tissues. Thiel–Behnke dystrophy has similar features to Reis–Buckler dystrophy but with additional features of 'curly fibres' in Bowman layer on electron microscopy. Schnyder central crystalline dystrophy is associated with abnormal metabolism of lipid and around 50% of the affected patients have hypercholesterolaemia. Histopathologic examination typically shows deposition of cholesterol and phospholipids.

Kanski J, Bowling B. *Clinical Ophthalmology: A Systematic Approach*, 7th edition. Chapter 6: Cornea, pp. 212–23. Edinburgh/New York: Elsevier/Saunders, 2011.

16. Answer: C

Keratoconus is the most common corneal ectatic disorder, with an estimated prevalence of 1:2000. It is associated with eye rubbing and connective tissue diseases, including Marfan's syndrome, Ehlers–Danlos syndrome, osteogenesis imperfecta, and others. Both anterior and posterior corneal surfaces are affected in keratoconus. In fact, posterior corneal changes are often the first clinically detectable structural changes because epithelial remodelling may mask the early anterior surface changes. Belin Ambrosio Enhance Ectasia Display is a useful analytic tool (embedded in Pentacam software) to detect early keratoconus. It displays the anterior and posterior elevation data relative to the best-fit-sphere, which is calculated with a fixed optical zone of 8 mm, omitting the 4 mm zone around the elevated cone. Breaks in Bowman's layer is a diagnostic feature of keratoconus on histopathologic examination. Sometimes they may be seen as subepithelial reticular opacities on clinical examination if the breaks are filled with scar tissue. Posterior keratoconus is a rare, typically non-progressive ectatic disorder characterized by an increased curvature of the posterior corneal surface. It is usually congenital, unilateral, and sporadic in nature.

Mas Tur V, et al. A review of keratoconus: diagnosis, pathophysiology and genetics. *Surv Ophthalmol* 2017;62:770–83.

Silas MR, et al. Posterior keratoconus. *Br J Ophthalmol* 2018;102:863–7.

17. Answer: A

Peter's anomaly is a rare type of anterior segment dysgenesis syndrome characterized by central opaque cornea (leukoma). The pathogenesis is unclear but it is postulated that there is failure of separation of cornea and lens during embryogenesis. The corneal endothelium and Descemet's membrane does not develop properly, with opacity overlying the defected area. Some cases may be associated with corneal-lenticular adhesion or cataract (type 2). Most cases are sporadic but autosomal recessive and dominant inheritance have been reported. It is associated with mutations of several genes, including *PAX6* (associated with aniridia), *PITX2*, and *FOXC1* (associated with anterior segment dysgenesis/Axenfeld-Rieger syndrome). *TIMP3* gene mutation is linked to Sorsby fundus dystrophy. Approximately 50–70% patients develop glaucoma. Peter's anomaly may be associated with other ocular abnormalities such as persistent hyperplastic primary vitreous and microphthalmia, and systemic abnormalities affecting the heart, ear, CNS, and genitourinary systems. Peters-plus syndrome refers to patients with Peter's anomaly associated with cleft lip and palate, abnormal ears, short stature, and mental retardation.

Shigeyasu C, et al. Clinical features of anterior segment dysgenesis associated with congenital corneal opacities. *Cornea* 2012;31:293–8.

18. Answer: C

This scenario describes a typical presentation of conjunctival naevus, which is a benign melanocytic tumour of the conjunctiva. It is the most common conjunctival pigmented tumours with no gender predilection. Features suggestive of conjunctival naevus include unilaterality, focality of the lesion, chronicity, and the presence of cysts (in around 60%). Interestingly, conjunctival naevus expresses progesterone receptors, which might explain the changes during hormonal alternations such as puberty or pregnancy. These changes often raise clinical concern of conjunctival melanoma, increasing the number of unnecessary surgical excision of the lesion. Features suggestive of conjunctival melanoma include elevation of the lesion, immobility, and vascularity. Conjunctival melanosis is caused by excessive melanin production and retention of pigment by epithelial melanocytes. In contrast to conjunctival naevus, it does not elevate the surface of conjunctiva and not associated with cystic changes. It may be associated with periocular skin changes called naevus of Ota (oculodermal melanocytosis). Conjunctival papilloma is a benign conjunctival epithelial tumour characterized by lobulated changes with a central vascular core. They tend to be larger and in multiple numbers in children and adolescents than in adults.

Kaliki S, et al. Conjunctival papilloma: features and outcomes based on age at initial examination. *JAMA Ophthalmol* 2013;131:585–93.

Oellers P, Karp CL. Management of pigmented conjunctival lesions. *Ocul Surf* 2012;10:251–63.

19. Answer: A

The use of topical steroids in bacterial keratitis has always been a controversial issue. According to a recent Cochrane review of four randomized controlled trials, there is currently inadequate evidence showing that topical steroids improve visual acuity, infiltrate, scar size, corneal perforation rate, and healing time on bacterial keratitis when compared to topical antibiotics alone. However, on subgroup analysis, patients with low vision (counting fingers or worse) at baseline had 1.7 lines better vision at 3 months in the topical steroids group compared with placebo group. Central ulcers that were treated with topical steroids also had a better 3-month corrected-distance-visual-acuity (around two lines better) at 3 months compared to placebo. In addition, non-Nocardia ulcers have one-line visual improvement with additional topical steroids, whereas Nocardia ulcers have worse outcome with additional topical steroids when compared to placebo.

Austin A, et al. Update on the management of infectious keratitis. *Ophthalmology* 2017;124:1678–89.

Herretes S, et al. Topical corticosteroids as adjunctive therapy for bacterial keratitis. *Cochrane Database Syst Rev* 2014;10:CD005430.

20. Answer: B

Mooren's ulcer is an idiopathic peripheral ulcerative keratitis with complete absence of systemic disorder that is responsible for the progressive destruction of the cornea. It is usually painful and progressive, typically starting from the peripheral cornea and progresses circumferentially and centrally. The ulcer is concentric to the limbus, with the leading edges being undermined, infiltrated, and de-epithelialized. This also creates an overhanging edge at its central border. It is not associated with scleritis. Hepatitis C infection and hookworm infestation have been reported to be associated with Mooren's ulcer. Wood and Kaufman classified Mooren's ulcer into two types; type 1 ulcer usually affects older patients and mild in symptoms with good response to therapy, whereas the type 2 ulcer usually affects younger patients with a more aggressive clinical course and poorer response to therapy. However further studies have shown that bilateral disease has a more aggressive presentation with poorer response to treatment compared to unilateral disease. The treatment includes intensive topical steroids, conjunctival resection, systemic immunosuppression, and other additional surgeries such as lamellar keratoplasty and keratoepithelioplasty.

Chen J, et al. Mooren's ulcer in China: a study of clinical characteristics and treatment. *Br J Ophthalmol* 2000;84:1244–9.

Garg P, Sangwan VS. Mooren's ulcer. In: Krachmer JH, Mannis MJ, Holland EJ (eds). *Cornea*, 3rd edition. New York, NY: Elsevier, 2011.

21. Answer: D

This is a clinical scenario of a patient presenting with iridocorneal corneal (ICE) syndrome. ICE syndrome is a unique unilateral ocular disease characterized by irregular corneal endothelium with varying degrees of corneal oedema, iris atrophy, and peripheral anterior synechiae. It occurs sporadically and does not have a specific inheritance pattern. It consists of three clinical variants, which can be easily remembered as 'ICE': (a) **I**ris naevus/Cogan-Reese syndrome; (b) **C**handler syndrome (most common subtype (50%), typically presents with most significant extent of corneal oedema, with less iris findings); and (c) **E**ssential iris atrophy (usually has greater extent of iris atrophy, as the name suggested, with polycoria, ectropion uveae, and corectopia). High peripheral anterior synechiae extending above the Schwalbe's line is considered a pathognomonic feature of ICE syndrome. It is more commonly found in women than in men, between the age of 20 and 50 years. Around 50% of the patients with ICE also develop glaucoma.

Silva L, et al. The iridocorneal endothelial syndrome. *Surv Ophthalmol* 2018;63:665–76.

22. Answer: A

PAM is a potentially serious melanocytic lesion that affects the conjunctival epithelium and may progress to conjunctival melanoma. It has been estimated that 75% of the conjunctival melanoma arise from PAM. Bulbar conjunctiva (91%) is the most commonly affected area, followed by limbal conjunctiva (55%), cornea (23%), and forniceal conjunctiva. According to one of the largest studies in the literature, it found that 96% of patients with PAM were Caucasian. The most significant risk factor for both recurrence and progression to melanoma is the extent of PAM in clock-hours. PAM without or with mild atypia shows 0% progression to melanoma, whereas PAM with severe atypia shows progression to melanoma in 13% at 10-year follow-up.

Shields JA, Primary acquired melanosis of the conjunctiva: risks for progression to melanoma in 311 eyes. The 2006 Lorenz E. Zimmerman lecture. *Ophthalmology* 2008;115:511–19.

23. Answer: C

PMD is a rare, idiopathic, corneal ectatic disorder that affects the peripheral cornea, usually the inferior quadrant in a crescentic fashion. It more commonly affects males and the onset is usually between the second and fifth decades. It is usually associated with against-the-rule astigmatism and has a 'crab-claw' or 'kissing-dove' appearance on the corneal topography. However, studies have shown that keratoconus may also have similar appearance on corneal topography, highlighting the importance of interpreting the sign along with the pachymetry maps. In keratoconus, the steepest area of cornea corresponds with the thinnest area of cornea whereas in PMD, the steepest area of cornea is usually superior to the thinned area.

Jinabhai A, et al. Pellucid corneal marginal degeneration: a review. *Cont Lens Anterior Eye* 2011;34:56–63.

24. Answer: B

The use of amniotic membrane is becoming increasingly common in ophthalmology. It promotes epithelialization and exhibits anti-inflammatory, antifibrotic, antiangiogenic, and antimicrobial properties. It can be used for treatment of persistent epithelial defects, non-healing corneal ulcers, chemical eye injury, corneal perforation, bullous keratopathy, LSCD, conjunctival reconstruction, and dry eyes. It can also be used as an adjuvant therapy for herpetic epithelial keratitis to improve corneal epithelialization and reduce ocular surface inflammation. Amniotic membrane can be preserved using cryopreservation, lyophilization (freeze-drying), and air-drying techniques.

Cheng AMS, Tseng SCG. Self-retained amniotic membrane combined with antiviral therapy for herpetic epithelial keratitis. *Cornea* 2017;36:1383–6.

Jirsova K, Jones GLA. Amniotic membrane in ophthalmology: properties, preparation, storage and indications for grafting—a review. *Cell Tissue Bank* 2017;18:193–204.

McDonald MB, et al. Treatment outcomes in the DRy Eye Amniotic Membrane (DREAM) study. *Clin Ophthalmol* 2018;12:677–81.

25. Answer: B

This is a clinical scenario of Parinaud's oculo-glandular syndrome (POGS). POGS was first described in 1889 by Henri Parinaud on two patients with unilateral nodular or ulcerative conjunctivitis associated with regional lymphadenopathy. All the organisms listed in the answer options have been implicated in POGS. *Bartonella henselae*—the causative organism of cat scratch disease—is the most common cause of POGS; however, the clinical history specifies that the patient has no contact with cat, rendering the diagnosis unlikely. Francisella tularensis causes tularemia and it is also one of the more frequent causes of POGS. Most patients with tularemia contract the infection through contact with rabbits, ticks, and squirrels. *Sporotrichum schenckii*—another common cause of POGS—is an organism that causes ocular sporotrichosis, which is usually caused by trauma from contaminated vegetable matter or dirt. *Treponema pallidum* is a motile spirochete responsible for syphilis. The patient's age makes this diagnosis extremely unlikely in this scenario.

Altuntas EE, et al. Tularemia and the oculoglandular syndrome of Parinaud. *Braz J Infect Dis* 2012;16:90–1.

26. Answer: D

This is not an uncommon surgical scenario and having a good knowledge helps to counsel the patient better preoperatively. According to systematic reviews, there is strong evidence to suggest that best corrected visual acuity and uncorrected visual acuity are better with penetrating keratoplasty (PK) than DALK at 6 months or more, that refractive astigmatism and graft rejection are less with DALK, and with no difference in spherical equivalent and keratometric astigmatism.

Henein C, Nanavaty MA. Systematic review comparing penetrating keratoplasty and deep anterior lamellar keratoplasty for management of keratoconus. *Cont Lens Anterior Eye* 2017;40:3–14.

27. Answer: C

Shingles vaccination is available in the United Kingdom for people who are older than 70 but not beyond 80 years of age. It is still beneficial for people who had previous shingles to receive the vaccination to boost the immunity against further attack. It has been shown to reduce the incidence rate of shingles (by around 2-fold) and post-herpetic neuralgia (by around 2–3-fold). As the vaccine contains live-attenuated varicella-zoster virus, it may rarely result in reactivation of herpes zoster infection such as keratitis and HZO.

Jastrzebski A, et al. Reactivation of herpes zoster keratitis with corneal perforation after zoster vaccination. *Cornea* 2017;36:740–2.

Matthews I, et al. Assessing the effectiveness of zoster vaccine live: a retrospective cohort study using primary care data in the United Kingdom. *Vaccine* 2018; pii: S0264-410X(18):31166–6.

NHS. *Shingles Vaccine Overview*. Available at: https://www.nhs.uk/conditions/vaccinations/shingles-vaccination/

28. Answer: C

CCTS represents one of the landmark studies that was designed to evaluate the effect of donor-recipient histocompatibility matching and cross-matching on the survival of corneal transplants in high-risk patients. It was found that neither HLA-A, -B, nor –DR significantly reduces the risk of graft failure or incidence of rejection. Positive donor-recipient cross-match does not substantially increase the risk of corneal graft rejection. However, ABO blood group matching may reduce the risk of corneal graft failure and rejection.

The Collaborative Corneal Transplantation Studies (CCTS). Effectiveness of histocompatibility matching in high-risk corneal transplantation. The Collaborative Corneal Transplantation Studies Research Group. *Arch Ophthalmol* 1992;110:1392–403.

Van Essen TH, et al. Matching for human leukocyte antigens (HLA) in corneal transplantation—to do or not to do. *Prog Retin Eye Res* 2015;46:84–110.

29. Answer: D

This is a clinical vignette of vernal keratoconjunctivitis (VKC) with persistent non-healing corneal ulcer/plaque (also known as shield ulcer). The only way to treat this persistent complication of VKC is to remove the plaque to allow for corneal re-epithelialization. Unfortunately, the child could not cooperate during slit-lamp examination, otherwise corneal scrapping of the plaque should be attempted in the clinic before doing it under general anaesthesia. Changing the topical antibiotic and topical steroids will not improve the shield ulcer.

Addis H, Jeng BH. Vernal keratoconjunctivitis. *Clin Ophthalmol* 2018;12:119–23.

30. Answer: C

Lifitegrast is a recently Food and Drug Administration (FDA)-approved treatment for dry eye disease. It is a novel small molecule integrin that inhibits T-cell-mediated inflammation by blocking the binding of two important cell surface proteins, namely the lymphocyte function-associated antigen 1 and intercellular adhesion molecule 1. Rituximab is a monoclonal antibody that inhibits CD-20 whereas ciclosporin inhibits calcineurin/nuclear factor of activated T cells.

Perez VL, et al. Lifitegrast, a novel integrin antagonist for treatment of dry eye disease. *Ocul Surf* 2016;14:207–15.

31. Answer: C

In aniridia, other than iris hypoplasia, the most common other ocular findings to be aware of are peripheral corneal opacity (due to LSCD but not leukoma), cataract, optic nerve hypoplasia, foveal hypoplasia, and nystagmus. Trabeculodysgenesis is another word for primary congenital glaucoma. Axenfeld-Rieger anomaly is associated with iris and angle dysgenesis, but not typically leukoma.

Gould DB, John SW. Anterior segment dysgenesis and the developmental glaucomas are complex traits. *Hum Mol Genet* 2002;11:1185–93.

32. Answer: A

The vignette describes primary angle closure glaucoma (i.e. not just gonioscopic findings, but elevated IOP and evidence of glaucomatous optic neuropathy). The 'Effectiveness of early lens extraction for the treatment of primary angle closure glaucoma (EAGLE)' study is a landmark study evaluating the role of early lens extraction for the treatment of primary angle closure with IOP of 30 mmHg or greater, or primary angle closure glaucoma in 419 patients. The EAGLE study found that clear lens extraction showed greater efficacy, in terms of lower mean IOP and higher mean health status score, and cost-effectiveness as compared to laser peripheral iridotomy.

Azuara-Blanco A, et al. Effectiveness of early lens extraction for the treatment of primary angle-closure glaucoma (EAGLE): a randomised controlled trial. *Lancet* 2016;388:1389–97.

33. Answer: B

This is a challenging question that requires knowledge of the key findings of these landmark glaucoma trials. This should be considered a minimum level for the exam. For studies of any subspecialty, it is worth noting the study design, patient cohort/control/comparator groups, and key findings.

> AGIS found that Caucasian patients had better IOP control with primary trabeculectomy, and black patients with primary ALT. EMGS found age, optic disc haemorrhages, intraocular pressure, pseudoexfoliation and bilateral findings were risk factors, but not race. OHTS found age, high IOP, high cup-to-disc ratio, high PSD, low CCT were risk factors, but not optic disc haemorrhages or race.

Collaborative Normal Tension Glaucoma Study Group. The effectiveness of intraocular pressure reduction in the treatment of normal tension glaucoma. *Am J Ophthalmol* 1998;126:498–505.

Heijl A, et al. Reduction of intraocular pressure and glaucoma progression: results from the Early Manifest Glaucoma Trial. *Arch Ophthalmol* 2002;120:1268–79.

Kass MA, et al. The Ocular Hypertension Treatment Study: a randomized trial determines that topical ocular hypotensive medication delays or prevents the onset of primary open-angle glaucoma. *Arch Ophthalmol* 2002;120:701–13.

The AGIS Investigators. The Advanced Glaucoma Intervention Study (AGIS): 7. The relationship between control of intraocular pressure and visual field deterioration. *Am J Ophthalmol* 2000;130:429–40.

34. Answer: A

Overdrainage and conjunctival leaks do not go hand in hand, but the purpose of this answer is that if you suspect a leak, you should check with fluorescein 2% (Seidel test). Option B is incorrect because a blocked sclerostomy would typically be associated with a high postoperative pressure. Option C is incorrect as retained viscoelastic in the anterior chamber would typically result in a deep anterior chamber. Option D is incorrect as topical pilocarpine can cause further anterior displacement of the lens-iris diaphragm, worsening aqueous misdirection syndrome.

Murdoch I. Post-operative management of trabeculectomy in the first three months. *Community Eye Health* 2012; 25:73–5.

35. Answer: B

Options A, C, and D are all true. Option B is false because a conjunctival wound leak does not always necessitate surgery. It depends on the individual clinical picture. Observation may be reasonable if the leak is not deemed excessive. Parameters that may require surgery include: (a) profuse, constant leak; (b) conjunctival retraction; or (c) the location of the leak is at limbal edge. With regard to Option D, this is thought to be secondary to the deleterious effect of long-term eye drops on the health of the conjunctiva, increasing the risk of conjunctival wound leak. Take time to read the phrasing of the question carefully as this is a negatively phrased question, which is a common multiple-choice question (MCQ) style in the Fellowship of the Royal College of Ophthalmologists (FRCOphth) part 2 written exam.

Henderson HW, et al. Early postoperative trabeculectomy leakage: the incidence, time course and severity and its impact on surgical outcome. *Br J Ophthalmol* 2004;88:626–9.

36. Answer: D

Acetazolamide can cause a range of side effects, which all ophthalmologists should be familiarized with. These include metabolic acidosis, renal stone, renal impairment, hepatic impairment, Steven–Johnson syndrome, dizziness, electrolyte imbalance (e.g. hypokalaemia) and rarely hypo- or hyperglycaemia. It is also important to note that its use is contraindicated in patients with sulfonamide hypersensitivity.

National Institute for Health and Care Excellence (NICE). *Acetazolamide*. Available at: https://bnf.nice.org.uk/drug/acetazolamide.html#indicationsAndDoses

37. Answer: D

Impotence is a rare, but underreported side effect of topical β-blocker medication. Other side effects of topical β-blocker include bronchospasm, bradycardia, fatigue, peripheral coldness, and sleep disturbance with nightmares. It may also affect carbohydrate metabolism, causing hypo- or hyperglycaemia, and interfere with metabolic and autonomic responses to hypoglycaemia, masking the symptoms such as tachycardia. A cardioselective β-blocker, which has more selectivity to $β_1$ receptors than $β_2$ (bronchial) receptors, is preferred in patients with diabetes and asthma/chronic obstructive pulmonary disease (if no other group of medication is suitable).

National Institute for Health and Care Excellence (NICE). *Beta-Adrenoceptor Blocking Drugs*. Available at: https://bnf.nice.org.uk/treatment-summary/beta-adrenoceptor-blocking-drugs.html

38. Answer: D

The vignette describes a Fuchs' heterochromic cyclitis (FHC). 'Twig-like' vessels often form across the angle that can bleed during lens extraction, which is known as Amsler's sign. Some level of anterior chamber activity can be seen long term, which does not require management. Involvement of the posterior segment such as vitritis is often seen. Trabeculectomy is usually the first-line surgical option for FHC.

Jones NP. Glaucoma in Fuchs' heterochromic uveitis: aetiology, management and outcome. *Eye* 1991;5:662–7.

La Hey E, et al. Treatment and prognosis of secondary glaucoma in Fuchs' heterochromic iridocyclitis. *Am J Ophthalmol* 1993;116:327–40.

39. Answer: A

This is a rare secondary open angle glaucoma caused by degenerated red blood cells (ghost cells) from a previous vitreous haemorrhage, blocking the trabecular meshwork. To access the anterior chamber (AC) there must be some communication between the anterior and posterior segments, either from previous vitrectomy, trauma, capsulotomy, or zonular damage from another aetiology. These tan-coloured cells may be visible circulating in the AC or as a layer overlying the iridocorneal angle on gonioscopy. Aqueous suppressants are generally the first-line therapy, but patients may require AC washout, vitrectomy, or even trabeculectomy.

Posner–Schlossman syndrome is characterized by unilateral painless, cyclical, acute rises in IOP (40–80 mmHg) that typically affect young males. It is associated with AC inflammation, but the eye remains white. Red cell glaucoma describes the IOP elevation caused by hyphema and blockage of the trabecular meshwork. Schwartz–Matsuo syndrome may occur if this uncommon secondary open angle glaucoma follows a similar mechanical blockage of the trabecular meshwork, but is caused by photoreceptor outer segments released following a rhegmatogenous retinal detachment.

Shields MB. *Shields' Textbook of Glaucoma*, 5th edition. Philadelphia, PA: Lippincott Williams & Wilkins, 2005.

40. Answer: B

It is important to be familiar with the correct terminologies of primary angle closure. The following table (Table 1.3) is useful to show the spectrum of the disorder.

Table 1.3 Classifications of the spectrum of primary angle closure

	≥2 quadrants of ITC	Elevated IOP +/− PAS	GON
PACS	Present	Absent	Absent
PAC	Present	Present	Absent
PACG	Present	Present	Present

PACS, primary angle closure suspect; PACG, primary angle closure glaucoma; ITC, iridotrabecular contact; PAS, peripheral anterior synechiae; GON, glaucomatous optic neuropathy.

Data from Panda A, et al. Corneal graft rejection. *Surv Ophthalmol* 2007;52:375–96; and Krachmer JH, Alldredge OC. Subepithelial infiltrates: a probable sign of corneal transplant rejection. *Arch Ophthalmol* 1978;96:2234–7.

41. Answer: A

This is a common FRCOphth question. The following table (Table 1.4) is a useful summary:

Table 1.4 The effect of certain medications on intraocular pressure

	Uveoscleral	Aqueous production	Conventional outflow
PGA	↑		*
β-blocker		↓	
CAI		↓	
α_2-agonist	↑	↓	
Miotic	(↓)		↑

PGA, prostaglandin analogues; CAI, carbonic anhydrase inhibitor.

*Note also that prostamides (such as bimatoprost) also increase conventional outflow but PGAs do not. Interestingly, bimatoprost and pilocarpine also actually increase aqueous production, but at a rate that is not significant.

Tataru CP, Purcarea VL. Antiglaucoma pharmacotherapy. *J Med Life* 2012;5(3):247–51.

42. Answer: D

Anecdotal evidence across clinics in the United Kingdom shows that the review time for treated and untreated ocular hypertension (OHT) is often shorter than is clinically indicated, and NICE has tried to tackle this in their latest guidelines. Note that the following table (Table 1.5) is identical for either OHT patients on treatment, or patients with suspected chronic open angle glaucoma (COAG).

Table 1.5 Recommended review times for treated and untreated ocular hypertension (OHT)

Conversion to COAG	Control of IOP	Time to next assessment
Not detected, or uncertain	No	Review management plan and review 1–4 months
Uncertain	Yes	6–12 months
No conversion	Yes	12–18 months
Conversion	No or Yes	See COAG recommendations

© NICE (2017) NG81 Glaucoma: diagnosis and management. Available from www.nice.org.uk/guidance/ng81 All rights reserved. Subject to Notice of rights NICE guidance is prepared for the National Health Service in England. All NICE guidance is subject to regular review and may be updated or withdrawn. NICE accepts no responsibility for the use of its content in this product/publication.

43. Answer: D

This question highlights just how prone patients with small eyes can be to this acute iatrogenic secondary angle closure glaucoma. It is caused by aqueous drainage into the vitreous cavity resulting in anterior displacement of the vitreous, ciliary body, and lens, with subsequent secondary angle closure. Other procedures known to have resulted in aqueous misdirection include insertion of an aqueous shunt, or even initiation of miotic therapy.

Clinical features include myopic shift, raised IOP (40–80 mmHg) and a shallow or flat AC in the absence of pupil block. Anterior segment imaging findings include anterior displacement of the iris-lens diaphragm (which includes the ciliary body). Management should avoid miotics; therefore, it is imperative to differentiate from the clinically similar acute angle closure. In fact, the use of topical atropine can encourage posterior rotation of the ciliary body. A variety of treatments, including YAG anterior hyaloidotomy through an existing peripheral iridotomy, surgical peripheral irido-zonulo-hyaloidectomy (with or without anterior/core vitrectomy), have been described.

Shahid H, Salmon JF. Malignant glaucoma: a review of the modern literature. *J Ophthalmol* 2012;2012:852659.

44. Answer: A

Due to the relative very low side effect or complication profile, selective laser trabeculoplasty (SLT) may be successful in a number of different scenarios. The only national guidance available is for use in COAG. Importantly, again despite varied local practices, the guidance does not include an indication for ocular hypertension (OHT).

As the evidence is not yet established, and the current national guidance does not cover OHT, Option B is incorrect. Primary SLT is practised in glaucoma clinics throughout the United Kingdom, and may be more effective than eye drops in patient who have been taking various topical therapies for many years. The Cochrane collaboration reported that there is no evidence to determine the effectiveness of laser trabeculoplasty compared to contemporary medication in open angle glaucoma or ocular hypertension, but the LiGHT trial is likely to guide us further in this (results not yet published). Option C is incorrect; however, if there is angle deepening following peripheral iridotomy or cataract surgery, this may be an option. It appears safe in this subgroup of patients, and as effective as a prostaglandin analogue in the short term in reducing IOP, however, there is little current evidence on its long-term effectiveness. Option D is incorrect as there is currently little evidence in this area and eyes with narrow/occludable iridocorneal angles may be difficult or impossible for this modality of laser. These patients should have laser iridotomy or lens extraction instead.

De Moura CR, et al. Laser trabeculoplasty for open angle glaucoma. *Cochrane Database Syst Rev* 2007;(4):CD003919.

Garg A, Gazzard G. Selective laser trabeculoplasty: past, present, and future. *Eye (Lond)* 2018;32:863–76.

Vickerstaff V, et al. Statistical analysis plan for the Laser-1st versus Drops-1st for Glaucoma and Ocular Hypertension Trial (LiGHT): a multi-centre randomised controlled trial. *Trials* 2015;16:517.

45. Answer: C

Following is the summary of types of lens-induced glaucoma:
   (a) Lens particle glaucoma—a type of secondary open angle glaucoma caused by inflammation of the lens particle, after a breach in the lens capsule, either from surgery or trauma.
   (b) Phacomorphic glaucoma—a type of secondary angle closure glaucoma caused by large cataractous lens with resultant narrowing and blockage of the AC angle.
   (c) Phacolytic glaucoma—a type of secondary open angle glaucoma caused by leakage of the soluble lens protein of hypermature cataract into the AC, causing trabecular obstruction. There is no history of trauma or surgery.
   (d) Phacoanaphylatic glaucoma—a type of secondary open angle glaucoma caused by granulomatous inflammatory reaction to the lens antigen, usually after trauma or postoperative lens retention.

American Academy of Ophthalmology. *Lens Induced Glaucomas*. Available at: http://eyewiki.aao.org/Lens_Induced_Glaucomas

46. Answer: C

Option A is incorrect as using the phaco probe in the vitreous will cause greater traction on the vitreous, pulling more vitreous to the probe or out of the vitreous cavity. This is associated with greater risk of retinal damage. The phaco probe has no ability to 'cut' tissue like a vitrector has. Option B is incorrect as if there is already vitreous present, the outcome can be similar to answer A. Option D is incorrect as the College generally want you to take the most conservative steps, working as a general ophthalmologist. Posterior vitrectomy is a subspecialist skill, and should be carried out by a specialist VR surgeon.

Hong AR, Sheybani A, Huang AJ. Intraoperative management of posterior capsular rupture. *Curr Opin Ophthalmol* 2015;26:16–21.

47. Answer: B

Post-cataract surgery macular oedema (PCMO) or Irvine–Gass syndrome is a common cause for reduced vision after cataract surgery. Diabetes, retinal vein occlusion, epiretinal membrane, macular hole, and uveitis are the most important risk factors for PCMO. A recent systematic review of 13 articles did not show any evidence of prostaglandin analogue increasing the risk of PCMO regardless of the time point; therefore, there is no evidence to support stopping prostaglandin analogue before or during the course of cataract surgery.

Hernstadt DJ, Husain R. Effect of prostaglandin analogue use on the development of cystoid macular edema after phacoemulsification using STROBE statement methodology. *J Cataract Refract Surg* 2017;43:564–9.

Wielders LHP, et al. Prevention of macular edema after cataract surgery. *Curr Opin Ophthalmol* 2018;29:48–53.

48. Answer: B

When deciding to place an IOL into the sulcus, you need to be aware of the altered effective lens position (i.e. it will be more anterior). If the refractive power is unchanged, this lens would focus the image slightly in front of the retina. This would result in a more myopic result than initially intended. You therefore need to reduce the power. Although somewhat arbitrary, removing 0.5–1.0 D (depending of the original lens power) is an effective way of doing this with some degree of accuracy. There is a useful website for calculation of the lens power difference between in-the-bag and sulcus implant.

If optic capture were possible (due to an intact anterior rhexis which had been sized appropriately for capturing the IOL optic), you would not need to change the IOL power as the relative IOL position would be the same (or very close to) the IOL position if it was inserted into the bag.

Doctor Hill. *Calculating Bag vs. Sulcus IOL Power*. Available at: http://www.doctor-hill.com/iol-main/bag-sulcus.htm

Millar ER, et al. Effect of anterior capsulorhexis optic capture of a sulcus-fixated intraocular lens on refractive outcomes. *J Cataract Refract Surg* 2013;39:841–4.

49. Answer: A

The majority (60–80%) of the postoperative endophthalmitis (POE) cases are caused by commensal organisms, mainly *Staphylococcus* and *Streptococcus* spp. More than two cases traced back to one operating list should certainly raise suspicion, as should a rate higher than 0.4%, or a number of cases within a few days/weeks. However, this does not define an outbreak, as clusters of cases can mimic an outbreak. The statistical method should be discussed with the local microbiology team. All cases of POE should be reported as clinical incidents.

Royal College of Ophthalmologists. *Ophthalmic Services Guidance: Managing an Outbreak of Postoperative Endophthalmitis*. July 2016. Available at: https://www.rcophth.ac.uk/wp-content/uploads/2016/07/Managing-an-outbreak-of-postoperative-endophthalmitis.pdf

50. Answer: A

Common causes of refractive surprises are summarized in Table 1.6:

Table 1.6 Potential causes for myopic refractive surprise

Myopic surprise	Hypermetropic surprise
Previous hyperopic laser	Previous myopic laser
Higher A constant	Lower A constant
Retained viscoelastic behind IOL	Undiagnosed staphyloma
Poor biometry, incorrect IOL calculation, poor surgical wound construction, incorrect IOL positioning	

In terms of management of refractive surprise, the most important factor is to take time to fully assess the patient:
(a) Was the biometry accurate with the correct formula chosen?
(b) Was the correct IOL put in?
(c) On clinical examination, is there any evidence of previously unrecognized or new pathology: keratoconus, oedema, poor wound construction, previous refractive surgery?
(d) Is the IOL positioned correctly?

It is worth repeating the biometry, keratometry, and corneal topography. It is only then you can begin to consider the most appropriate management plan, which may require use of contact lenses, laser treatments, or returning to theatre for IOL exchange.

Alio JL, et al. Management of residual refractive error after cataract surgery. *Curr Opin Ophthalmol* 2014;25:291–7.

51. Answer: D

The diagnosis is homocystinuria, which is an autosomal recessive metabolic disorder of methionine, leading to an abnormal accumulation of homocysteine and its metabolites in blood and urine. It is caused by deficiency of cystathionin β-synthase enzyme. Be aware that marfanoid is a description of their stature and not a diagnosis of Marfan's syndrome. Option B is incorrect as this suggests a diagnosis of Marfan's syndrome, which the typical ectopic position of the lens is superotemporally. General anaesthesia is associated with increased risk of thromboses in those with homocystinuria and should be avoided if possible. In addition, osteoporosis is common in these patients depending on their genotype.

Kumar T, et al. Homocystinuria: therapeutic approach. *Clin Chim Acta* 2016;458:55–62.

52. Answer: C

The WHO checklist provides a list of checks that needs to be performed before giving anaesthesia ('Sign in'), before start of cataract surgery ('Time out'), and upon completion of cataract surgery ('Sign out'). Checking for any difficulty in positioning should form part of the checks during 'Sign in' stage. All the other options should be checked during the 'Time out' stage. In most hospitals, special requirement for positioning would have been assessed as part of the preoperative assessment rather than at the time the patient is brought into the operating theatre. All other answers are correct.

NHS and National Patient Safety Agency. *Surgical Safety Checklist: For Cataract Surgery Only*, 2010. Available at: https://www.rcophth.ac.uk/wp-content/uploads/2014/12/2010_PROF_062_Cataract_Surgery_Checklist.pdf

53. Answer: D

In pseudoexfoliative (PXF) eyes, the angles are typically narrower. There is a limit to which a capsular tension ring will be effective, usually less than 3 clock-hour involvement. Also note that vitreous can come forward via the area of zonular dehiscence, even the posterior capsule is intact. Interestingly the degree of PXF material does not correlate with the severity of zonular dehiscence or the prevalence of PXF glaucoma.

PXF can cause problems intraoperatively during cataract surgery due to poor pupil dilation and zonular instability. Steps to help combat difficulties include:

- Extensive discussion with the patient preoperatively so they are aware of the potential problems
- Pupil manipulation (e.g. iris hooks, Malyugin ring)
- Adequate hydrodissection (minimizing torsional forces on the zonules during lens rotation)
- Minimal phaco energy
- Capsule tension ring if zonular dehiscence is observed. If phacodonesis is visualized at the slit lamp, it may be appropriate to refer to VR for cataract surgery
- Gentle, slow movement of instruments

Shingleton BJ, et al. Pseudoexfoliation and the cataract surgeon: preoperative, intraoperative, and postoperative issues related to intraocular pressure, cataract, and intraocular lenses. *J Cataract Refract Surg* 2009;35:1101–20.

54. Answer: A

Reverse pupil block is more common in myopes. It can cause acute rise in IOP and can be painful for the patient. The simplest way to resolve this is to use a second instrument to lift the iris anteriorly, relieving the pupil block. There is no evidence to prove that bimanual irrigation/aspiration is safer than coaxial method. Shorter eyes are more likely to be associated with intraoperative aqueous misdirection. This highest risk group is patients with nanophthalmia. Even relatively short-term use of α-antagonists can result in lifelong risk of intraoperative floppy iris syndrome (IFIS) and stopping the medication preoperatively does not reduce the risk. However, alfuzosin may have a lower risk of IFIS than tamsulosin. Intracameral phenylephrine and/or iris manipulation (e.g. iris hooks, Malyugin ring) may help.

Chang DF, et al. Prospective masked comparison of intraoperative floppy iris syndrome severity with tamsulosin versus alfuzosin. *Ophthalmology* 2014;121:829–34.

55. Answer: B

Although Option A sounds like a reasonable advice, the vignette should raise your concern about a possible diagnosis of postoperative endophthalmitis, so you are obliged to review the patient as soon as is possible. The Endophthalmitis Vitrectomy Study (EVS) showed a threefold improvement in attaining 6/12 for those with a vision of perception of light (N.B. patients with vision of non-perception of light were excluded from the study). Although topical or intravitreal corticosteroids are frequently administered as part of the treatment of postoperative endophthalmitis, there is little evidence to confirm the effect and therefore such practice cannot be enforced in all cases.

Endophthalmitis Vitrectomy Study Group. Results of the Endophthalmitis Vitrectomy Study. A randomized trial of immediate vitrectomy and of intravenous antibiotics for the treatment of postoperative bacterial endophthalmitis. *Arch Ophthalmol* 1995;113:1479–96.

56. Answer: D

Studies have shown that polishing the posterior capsule after lens cortex cleaning had no significant role in delaying or preventing posterior capsular opacification (PCO). Other factors listed in the options and acrylic hydrophobic lens have been shown to reduce the risk of PCO.

Khalifa MA. Polishing the posterior capsule after extracapsular extraction of senile cataract. *J Cataract Refract Surg* 1992;18:170–3.

Pandey SK, et al. Posterior capsule opacification: a review of the aetiopathogenesis, experimental and clinical studies and factors for prevention. *Indian J Ophthalmol* 2004;52:99–112.

57. Answer: B

Intravitreal silicone oil can result in significant refractive changes in phakic, pseudophakic, and aphakic eyes. In phakic and pseudophakic eyes, as the silicone oil fills up the vitreous cavity, the concavity of the anterior part of the silicone oil at the interface of the posterior lens renders the eye more hypermetropic. Effectively it acts like a concave lens. Conversely, the convexity of the anterior part of the silicone oil acts as a convex lens, rendering the eye less hypermetropic.

Hotta K, Sugitani A. Refractive changes in silicone oil-filled pseudophakic eyes. *Retina* 2005;25:167–70.

58. Answer: A

Toxic anterior segment syndrome (TASS) is a sterile postoperative inflammatory reaction caused by non-infectious substances that enter the anterior segment, resulting in inflammation and toxic damage to intraocular tissues. It typically starts within 24 hours of cataract surgery or other anterior segment surgeries compared to 3–7 days in postoperative endophthalmitis—the main differential diagnosis of TASS. The clinical characteristics of TASS include severe pain, eye redness, severe anterior segment inflammation with fibrins and hypopyon, diffuse limbal-to-limbal corneal oedema, negative Gram stain and culture results, and improvement with topical steroids.

Mamalis N, et al. Toxic anterior segment syndrome. *J Cataract Refract Surg* 2006;32:324–3.

59. Answer: B

Fabry's disease is a rare X-linked lysosomal storage disorder caused by deficiency in α-galactosidase A enzyme. Ocular abnormalities include vortex keratopathy, congenital cataract, and tortuous conjunctival and retinal vessels. The severity of vascular tortuosity may predict the level of impairment of cardiac and renal functions. Anterior lenticonus is most commonly associated with Alport's syndrome (characterized by nephritic haematuria and deafness), Lowe's syndrome, and Waardenburg's syndrome. The following article provides a good summary of all types of childhood cataract.

Amaya L, et al. The morphology and natural history of childhood cataracts. *Surv Ophthalmol* 2003;48:125–44.

Sodi A, et al. Ocular manifestations of Fabry's disease: data from the Fabry Outcome Survey. *Br J Ophthalmol* 2007;91:210–14.

60. Answer: C

Based on a Cochrane review of 16 randomized controlled trials, there is insufficient evidence to suggest that FLACS is more superior than standard cataract surgery, in terms of visual acuity, anterior and posterior capsular tears, postoperative CMO and elevated IOP, patient-reported outcomes, and cost-effectiveness.

Day AC, et al. Laser-assisted cataract surgery versus standard ultrasound phacoemulsification cataract surgery. *Cochrane Database Syst Rev* 2016;7:CD010735.

chapter 2

CLINICAL OPHTHALMOLOGY 2

QUESTIONS

1. A 23-year-old male presents with an acute inferior macular on retinal detachment following blunt trauma to the right eye. Slit-lamp examination shows a clear lens, and a retinal dialysis within the inferonasal quadrant with no posterior vitreous detachment. The subretinal fluid encroaches on the inferior arcades. Which would be the most likely primary surgical option used to repair the retinal detachment?
   A. Pneumatic retinopexy
   B. Scleral buckle and cryotherapy
   C. Suprachoroidal buckle
   D. Vitrectomy, endolaser, and gas endotamponade

2. A patient presents with a longstanding total retinal detachment. Retinal examination shows fixed retinal folds, with a preretinal membrane extending across 4 clock hours. The membrane is anterior to the equator. What grade of proliferative retinopathy (PVR) does the patient have?
   A. PVR A
   B. PVR B
   C. PVR CA-4
   D. PVR CP-4

3. Which of the following microorganisms are most commonly isolated in cases of postphacoemulsification bacterial endophthalmitis in Europe?
   A. β-haemolytic streptococci
   B. Coagulase-negative staphylococcus
   C. Gram-negative bacteria (including *Pseudomonas* species)
   D. *Staphylococcus aureus*

4. **According to the European Society of Cataract & Refractive Surgeons (ESCRS) study of prophylaxis of postoperative endophthalmitis after cataract surgery, which of the following risk factors was associated with an increased risk of postoperative endophthalmitis?**
   A. Immunosuppressed patient
   B. Not giving an intracameral injection of cefuroxime
   C. Reusable equipment
   D. Sutureless wound closure

5. **Which of the following statements describes a stage 2 full-thickness macular hole (Gass classification)?**
   A. A central round retinal defect <400 microns diameter, no Weiss's ring, rim of elevated retina
   B. A central yellow spot, loss of foveolar depression, no vitreofoveolar separation
   C. A central round retinal defect ≥400 microns diameter, no Weiss's ring, rim of elevated retina, with or without prefoveolar opacity
   D. A central round retinal defect, rim of elevated retina, Weiss's ring, with or without prefoveolar opacity

6. **Which of the following complications of diabetic retinopathy are an indication for three port pars plana vitrectomy?**
   A. Non-clearing vitreous haemorrhage
   B. Taut posterior hyaloid face
   C. Tractional retinal detachment involving the macula
   D. All of the above

7. **Which of the following conditions is ocriplasmin licensed and approved by NICE to treat?**
   A. Vitreomacular adhesion
   B. Full-thickness macular hole with a minimum linear diameter (MLD) of 450 microns
   C. Vitreomacular traction with epiretinal membrane
   D. Full-thickness macular hole (with an MLD of 250 microns) with vitreomacular traction present

8. **Which of the following about optic disc pit maculopathy is true?**
   A. It affects both sexes equally
   B. It commonly manifests during childhood
   C. The commonest presentation is with subretinal fluid
   D. It is usually associated with a choroidal coloboma

9. **Where is the mostly likely position of the retinal tear in Figure 2.1 (shaded area represents the area of detached retina)?**
    A. Inferonasal
    B. Inferotemporal
    C. Superonasal
    D. Superotemporal

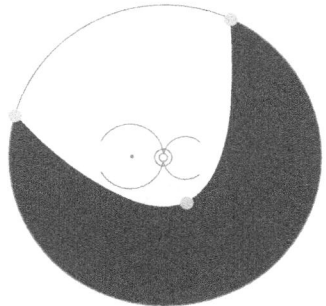

Figure 2.1

10. **Which of the following is NOT an associated risk factor for central retinal vein occlusion?**
    A. Diabetes mellitus
    B. High plasma viscosity due to blood dyscrasia
    C. Hypertension
    D. Longer axial length

11. **Which of the following conditions is associated with angioid streaks?**
    A. Diabetes insipidus
    B. Mercury toxicity
    C. Paget's disease
    D. Sarcoidosis

12. **A 34-year-old myopic (−9.00) female presents with worsening vision and distortion in her left eye. She has no past ocular history. Visual acuity is 82 and 49 EDTRS letters in the right eye (OD) and left eye (OS), respectively. An optical coherence tomography angiography (Figure 2.2) scan of the left eye shows the following appearance. Which treatment option would you recommend?**
    A. Focal argon laser
    B. Intravitreal aflibercept 40 mg/ml
    C. Observation
    D. Triamcinolone acetate

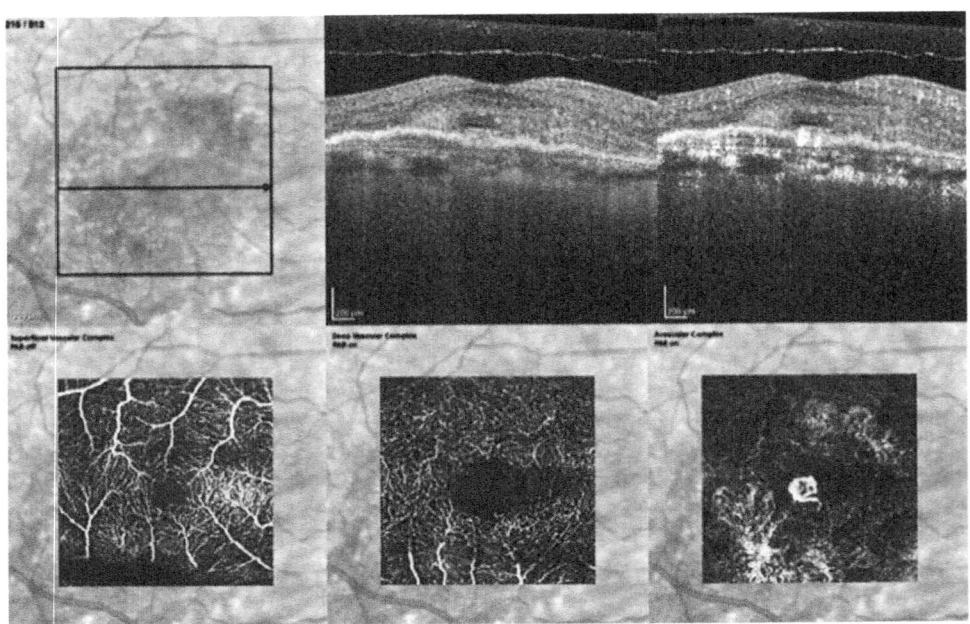

Figure 2.2

13. Which of the following conditions can cause an electronegative electroretinogram (ERG)—full field, bright flash in scotopic conditions?
    A. Acute macular neuroretinopathy
    B. Best's disease
    C. Retinitis pigmentosa
    D. X-linked retinoschisis

14. An asymptomatic 19-year-old female is referred to the eye clinic with an abnormal appearance to the optic nerve margins. An ocular B-scan confirms hyper-reflective deposits within the nerve head consistent with optic disc drusen. Which of the following conditions are associated with optic disc drusen?
    A. Alport's syndrome
    B. Gronblad–Strandberg syndrome
    C. Retinitis pigmentosa
    D. All of the above

15. A 7-year-old male presents with bilateral retinal detachments due to giant retinal tears. He is known to have hearing difficulties and his older brother and father have also previously undergone treatment for retinal detachments. Which of the following is the most likely underlying diagnosis?
    A. Familial exudative vitreoretinopathy
    B. Knobloch syndrome
    C. Stickler syndrome
    D. X-linked retinoschisis

16. Which of the following studies reported that intensive blood sugar control reduced the mean risk of developing diabetic retinopathy by 76% in type 1 diabetes?
    A. Diabetes Control and Complications Trial (DCCT)
    B. Diabetic Retinopathy Study (DRS)
    C. United Kingdom Prospective Diabetes Study (UKPDS)
    D. Wisconsin Epidemiological Study of Diabetic Retinopathy (WESDR)

17. The Early Treatment for Diabetic Retinopathy Study (ETDRS) is a landmark trial. It reported results on the timing of panretinal photocoagulation (PRP) in proliferative diabetic retinopathy (PDR) and the outcome of focal laser treatment in the management of diabetic maculopathy. All of the following statements were used to define clinically significant diabetic maculopathy (CSMO), **EXCEPT**:
    A. Retinal thickening at or within 500 μm of the fovea
    B. Any microaneurysm or haemorrhage within one-disc diameter of the centre of fovea with associated best corrected visual acuity of 6/12 or worse
    C. Hard exudates at or within 500 μm of the fovea if associated with adjacent retinal thickening
    D. An area or areas of retinal thickening one-disc area in size, at least part of which is within one-disc diameter of the fovea

18. The Diabetic Retinopathy Study (DRS) demonstrated a 60% reduction in severe visual loss (defined as vision less than 5/200 at two or more consecutive follow-up visits) in eyes treated with panretinal photocoagulation compared with controls. Which of the following examination findings indicated high-risk PDR?
    A. New vessels at the optic disc (NVD) >1/4 of disc diameter
    B. NVD without vitreous haemorrhage
    C. New vessels elsewhere (NVE) ≥1/2 of disc diameter with vitreous haemorrhage
    D. Tractional retinal detachment

19. Which of the following trial results provide evidence for the use of fluocinolone acetonide intravitreal implant in the management of chronic diabetic macular oedema?
    A. BEVORDEX
    B. FAME A and B
    C. Protocol S (Diabetic Retinopathy Clinical Research Network—DRCR net)
    D. VIVID and VISTA

20. A pseudophakic, type 2 diabetic patient presents with worsening vision due to a centre involving macular oedema, central macular thickness (CMT) 370 microns. He has no previous ocular treatment. Which of the following treatments is the most appropriate choice for management in this case?
    A. Aflibercept
    B. Dexamethasone intravitreal implant
    C. Focal argon laser
    D. Ranibizumab

21. A 63-year-old male is referred via his optometrist with worsening vision in both eyes. He reports a steady decline over a number of years with some metamorphopsia. Retinal examination was normal other than bilateral capillary abnormalities in the perifoveal region of each eye. Optical coherence tomography (Figure 2.3A) and blue reflectance (Figure 2.3B) showed the following characteristic appearances. What is the most likely diagnosis?
    A. Bilateral retinal vein occlusions
    B. Diabetic maculopathy
    C. Macular telangiectasia Type 1
    D. Macular telangiectasia Type 2

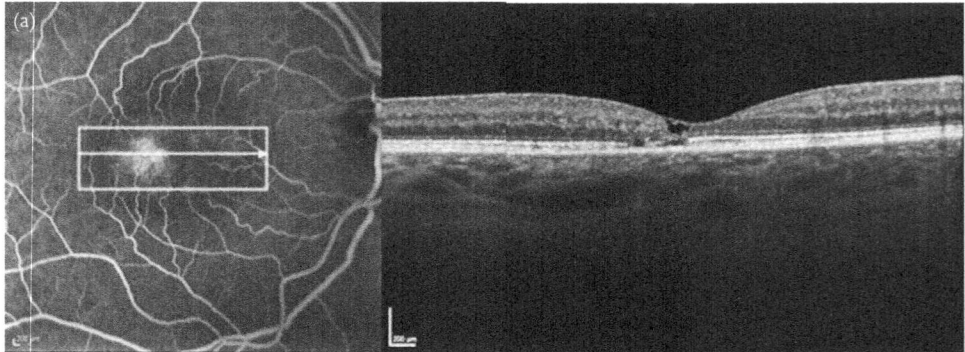

Figure 2.3

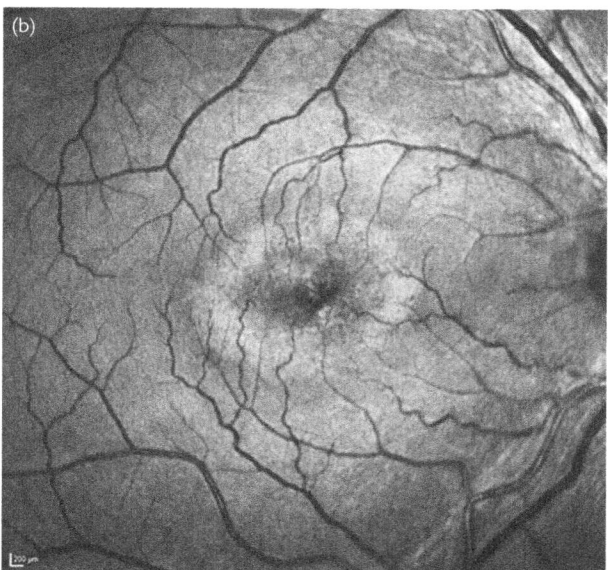

Figure 2.3 Continued

22. A 34-year-old female patient presents with worsening vision in her left eye. Fundal exam shows epiretinal membrane causing macular pucker, a pinkish mass with surrounding subretinal exudation is seen within the inferotemporal quadrant (Figure 2.4). Which of the following is the most likely diagnosis?
    A. Amelanotic choroidal melanoma
    B. Intermediate uveitis
    C. Retinal cavernous haemangioma
    D. Vasoproliferative tumour

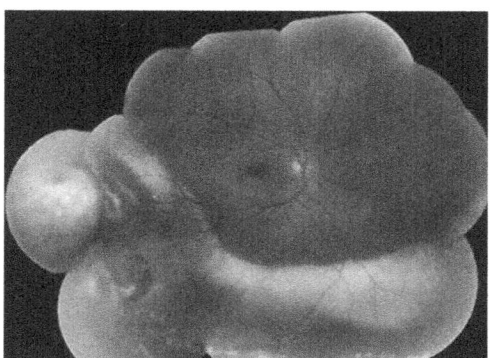

Figure 2.4

Reprinted by permission from Springer Nature: Nature, Eye, 24(3): 468–471, Retinal vasoproliferative tumours. Rennie, I. https://doi.org/10.1038/eye.2009.305. Copyright © 2010, Springer Nature.

23. **Which of the following medications could be best considered for the treatment of a non-resolving central serious chorioretinopathy (CSCR) with worsening vision?**
    A. Eplerenone
    B. Isoniazid
    C. Prednisolone
    D. Rifampicin

24. **Which of the following vitamins is associated with cystic changes at the macula?**
    A. Vitamin B_1
    B. Vitamin B_2
    C. Vitamin B_3
    D. Vitamin B_6

25. **Photodynamic therapy (using verteporfin) is a treatment option in all of the following, EXCEPT:**
    A. Central serous chorioretinopathy
    B. Choroidal haemangioma
    C. Macular telangiectasia type 2
    D. Polypoidal choroidal vasculopathy

26. **A 35-year-old female presents to the eye clinic with a 2-week history of right eye metamorphopsia. She is highly myopic (−8 D). Her corrected distance visual acuity is 6/18 OD and 6/6 OS. Slit-lamp examination revealed a small area of retinal pigment epithelial disturbance with subretinal fluid at the macula of the right eye. Which of the following treatment regimens is most appropriate for this patient?**
    A. A single intravitreal ranibizumab injection followed by monthly clinical observation with further top-up injections as required
    B. A loading dose of 3 monthly intravitreal ranibizumab injections followed by monthly observation with further top-up injection as required
    C. A loading dose of 3 monthly intravitreal aflibercept injections followed by monthly follow-up with further top-up injection as required
    D. A loading dose of 3 monthly intravitreal aflibercept injections followed by 2-monthly injections up to a 1-year time point

27. **Which of the following statements regarding intravitreal lampalizumab injection for dry age-related macular degeneration is correct?**
    A. Lampalizumab inhibits complement factor H
    B. Lampalizumab does not reduce the enlargement of geographic atrophy
    C. The benefit of lampalizumab is influenced by the complement factor I-profile biomarker
    D. It is associated with higher risk of postintravitreal injection endophthalmitis

28. **A 59-year-old female patient presents with gradual deterioration of the central vision. She had previously undergone mastectomy for breast cancer and has been taking tamoxifen medication for past 3 years. What is the most likely changes you will see on fundus examination?**
    A. White-yellow intraretinal crystals in the macular or paramacular area with or without oedema
    B. Ring-shaped yellow-orange crystals in the superficial retina
    C. Narrowing of the retinal arterioles with wrinkling of the retinal surface
    D. Retinal microangiopathy consisting of cotton wool spots and retinal haemorrhages

29. **Which of the following fits with the description of 'multiple intraretinal blood-filled saccules with bunch-of-grapes appearance'?**
    A. Capillary haemangioma
    B. Cavernous haemangioma
    C. Racemose haemangioma
    D. Vasoproliferative tumour

30. **Which of the following statements regarding cancer-associated retinopathy (CAR)/melanoma-associated retinopathy (MAR) is NOT correct?**
    A. optical coherence tomography (OCT) of the macula usually shows thinning of the inner retina
    B. The late stage of the disease may resemble the appearance of retinitis pigmentosa
    C. Antirecoverin antibody has been associated with CAR
    D. CAR usually affects rods more than cones

31. **A 45-year-old woman had recently undergone a thyroidectomy for a benign, large-sized multinodular goitre. She presents to the eye emergency department 1 week later with a right-sided mild droopy eyelid. The findings of the pupil examination are detailed in Table 2.1. What pharmacological tests can be performed that day to help confirm the diagnosis?**
    A. Topical tropicamide 1%
    B. Topical pilocarpine 10% followed by hydroxyamphetamine 1%
    C. Topical apraclonidine 1%
    D. Topical phenylephrine 10%

Table 2.1 Pupil examination findings

Right pupil	Findings	Left pupil
2 mm	Bright	2.5 mm
3 mm	Dim	4 mm
Brisk	Light reflex	Brisk
Normal	Near response	Normal

32. A 26-year-old female presents with one pupil larger than the other which she noticed in the mirror. There is no pain associated but she had fallen over last week with no head injury. On examination there was no ptosis, no diplopia. In bright condition, pupils measured 3.5 mm (right) and 6.5 mm (left); in dim condition, the pupils measured 6.5 mm (right) and 7 mm (left). There was no relative afferent pupillary defect (RAPD). What would be the most likely slit-lamp findings?
    A. Heterochromia of the irides
    B. Iris transillumination
    C. Posterior synechiae
    D. Sectoral palsy of iris sphincter

33. Which of the following about the prognosis of non-arteritic anterior ischaemic optic neuropathy is correct?
    A. The involvement of the fellow eye is estimated at about 15–25% over 5 years
    B. About 50% of the affected patients have a final visual outcome of 6/60 or worse
    C. The recurrence rate in the affected eye is around 25%
    D. Around 5% of the affected eyes will recover at least 3 Snellen visual acuity over time

34. Which of the following statements about idiopathic intracranial hypertension (IIH) is correct?
    A. Long-term use of systemic corticosteroids is a recognized risk factor
    B. The gender predilection is not influenced by puberty
    C. Normal neuroimaging with normal cerebrospinal fluid (CSF) constituents is essential to make the diagnosis of IIH
    D. The recent IIH treatment trial (IIHTT) showed that acetazolamide was effective in improving the visual field defect in IIH patients with severe visual field loss (mean deviation worse than −12 dB)

35. An 87-year-old female presented to the eye emergency department with sudden loss of vision in her right eye. This had come on 2 hours before attending the hospital. She has been losing weight over the past 3 months and had a chronic headache. She had been surviving on soup and hot drinks as she found it painful to eat. On examination her visual acuity was perception of light OD and 6/9 OS. She complained of slight blurring of vision in her left eye while in the emergency department. The erythrocyte sedimentation rate (ESR) was 126 mm/h and C-reactive protein (CRP) was 42 mg/L. What would be the most likely finding on examination of her right eye?
    A. Normal optic nerve
    B. Optic atrophy
    C. Optic disc oedema with retinal cotton wool spots
    D. Telangiectasia of optic nerve head

36. **A 47-year-old man presents to eye casualty with sudden onset vertical diplopia. He had noticed the diplopia developing over a 2-week period changing from being intermittent to constant. He felt that the diplopia was not present when he woke in the morning but came on as soon as he got up and went downstairs. On examination he had normal visual acuity of 6/9 OD and 6/6 OS. See Table 2.2 for the ocular motility measurements. What additional test would you do next?**
    A. Bielchowsky head tilt test
    B. Measurement of pupils
    C. Magnetic resonance imaging (MRI) scan of head
    D. Thyroid function tests

Table 2.2 Ocular motility measurements

	1^R/L	
12^R/L	10^ R/L	4^R/L
	16^R/L	

Courtesy of the European Society of Cataract and Refractive Surgeons (ESCRS). Reprinted from ESCRS Guidelines for Prevention and Treatment of Endophthalmitis Following Cataract Surgery: Data, Dilemmas and Conclusions 2013. Peter Barry, Luis Cordoves, Susanne Gardner. https://education.escrs.org/wp-content/uploads/2018/08/ENGLISH_2018_updated.pdf

37. **In a patient with suspected tonic pupil, which of the following pharmacological tests is useful in establishing the diagnosis?**
    A. Topical apraclonidine 0.5%
    B. Topical cocaine 4%
    C. Topical pilocarpine 0.1%
    D. Topical pilocarpine 1%

38. **In a patient with suspected ocular myasthenia, which of the following tests would you perform next?**
    A. Chest X-ray
    B. Computed tomography (CT) scan of head
    C. Ice pack test
    D. Tensilon test

39. A 17-year-old male presented to the eye department with a 2-week history of painless reduction in vision in his right eye. He was fit and well and had just completed his basic army training. He had no history of injury and was on no medication. He had no peripheral neurological signs. His best corrected visual acuity was recorded as 6/18 OD and 6/6 OS. He had no **RAPD** but his colour perception on Ishihara plates was reduced to 3/15 OD and 14/15 OS. He had an **MRI** head and orbits which was normal. On examination of his fundus, he had a crowded small optic nerve head and apparent swelling of the nerve fibre layer around the optic nerve. Two weeks later, his vision had deteriorated to 6/60 OD and 6/18 OS. What would you expect to find on visual field testing?
    A. Bitemporal hemianopia
    B. Centrocaecal scotoma
    C. Homonymous hemianopia
    D. Peripheral visual field defect with tunnel vision

40. Which features of a third nerve palsy would indicate an ischaemic aetiology?
    A. Aberrant regeneration
    B. Improvement towards the end of the day
    C. Pupil-sparing with inferior rectus weakness
    D. Recovery after 3 months

41. A 58-year-old man presents with sudden change in vision in his right eye. He had started to notice that the TV was not so clear the evening before but thought it was tiredness. He has been treated for hypertension for past 6 years. He is otherwise well. His blood pressure on examination is 133/78. Visual acuity on examination is 6/7.5 OD and 6/6 OS. He felt his vision was blurred when he looked down. There is a **RAPD** in the right eye. What features would you expect to see on fundal examination?
    A. Inferior retinal detachment
    B. Large cup-to-disc ratio
    C. Macular haemorrhage
    D. Optic nerve oedema

42. A 60-year-old patient, type 2 diabetic, presented to the eye emergency department with a sudden drooping of the right upper eyelid with diagonal diplopia. On examination there was a 3 mm ptosis with restriction of eye movement on adduction of the right eye. Both pupils were equal and reactive to light. He underwent an urgent CT brain scan which is normal. The patient presents to you a week later in the clinic. He complains of ongoing symptoms and examination findings remains the same. What is the most appropriate next step?
    A. CT angiography of the circle of Willis
    B. Daily pupil check
    C. Follow-up in 2 months' time and advise the patient to return if there is any sudden deterioration
    D. MRI head with no contrast

43. A 53-year-old male presented to the eye department with a 6-month history of reduction in visual acuity in both eyes. He was very thin in appearance and smelled strongly of cigarette smoke and looked unkempt. Visual function when he attended was 6/24 OD and 6/36 OS. He had reduced colour vision in both eyes, 2/15 OD and 1/15 OS. Both optic nerves appeared pale on fundal examination. What other features would you want to explore in his history?
    A. Any current treatment for tuberculosis
    B. Any recent visit to optometrist
    C. Any recent bariatric surgery
    D. Any recent eye injury

44. A 35-year-old healthy man presents to the eye clinic with intermittent visual disturbance, described as 'vision jumping up and down' in the right eye for 2 weeks. He mentions that he has been undergoing quite a lot of stress recently. Slit-lamp examination revealed a low amplitude, high-frequency torsional nystagmoid movement in the right eye only. Examination of the left eye is otherwise unremarkable. Which of the following topical medication has been tried for this clinical condition with reported success?
    A. Apraclonidine
    B. Dexamethasone
    C. Dorzolamide
    D. Timolol

45. Which of the following risk factors is associated with a higher risk of multiple sclerosis in patients with optic neuritis?
    A. Pain on eye movement
    B. Severe optic disc swelling
    C. Non-perceptive of light (NPL) vision
    D. Male sex

46. Which of the following features is associated with right-sided, non-dominant, parietal lobe infarction?
    A. Dysgraphia
    B. Left-right disorientation
    C. 'Pie in the sky' visual field defect
    D. Visual neglect

47. See-saw nystagmus is most likely to be seen in which of the following conditions?
    A. Cerebellar arteriovenous malformation
    B. Craniopharyngioma
    C. Parietal lobe infarction
    D. Temporal lobe tumour

48. A 72-year-old patient, with a background of hypertension, presents to the eye clinic with a sudden onset of right droopy eyelid and double vision. He also appears to be losing balance towards the right side. Otherwise there is no associated tremor or weakness of the limbs. Ocular examination of the right eye revealed a 3 mm ptosis and weakness in adduction and elevation on abduction. What is the most likely diagnosis in this case?
    A. Benedikt syndrome
    B. Claude's syndrome
    C. Nothnagel syndrome
    D. Weber syndrome

49. A 73-year-old diabetic man presented to eye casualty with a 2-day history of double vison and a unilateral partial ptosis of his left upper eyelid. He felt that images were separated vertically and twisted. He could move his eye upwards a little. He had slight discomfort around his left eye. His vision was equal in both eyes at 6/6 Snellen and on examination he had no anisocoria, both pupils were equal in light and dark. What is the most likely diagnosis in a man of his age?
    A. Aneurysm
    B. Cavernous sinus meningioma
    C. Ischaemia
    D. Myasthenia gravis

50. Which of the following features is most likely seen in Parinaud dorsal midbrain syndrome?
    A. Convergence insufficiency
    B. Light-near dissociation
    C. Pursuit movement is affected earlier than saccadic movement
    D. Upward gaze palsy

51. A 52-year-old healthy male patient presents to the eye department with a 2-week history of intermittent visual disturbance, described as a persisting after-image lasting for 10–15 min after looking at certain objects. He was started on a medication a few weeks prior to the onset of this symptom. Which of the following drugs is most likely implicated in this clinical scenario?
    A. Carbamazepine
    B. Vigabatrin
    C. Quinine
    D. Topiramate

52. Which of the following genetic mutations carries the best prognosis for Leber's hereditary optic neuropathy?
    A. 1669
    B. 3460
    C. 11778
    D. 14484

53. Which of the following features is suggestive of bilateral superior oblique palsies?
    A. Chin-up head posture
    B. Excyclotorsion >10°
    C. Prominent A pattern
    D. Bilateral failure of abduction in depression

54. A 34-year-old female presented to A&E with sudden loss of vision in her left eye. Visual acuity was recorded as 6/12 OD and no perception of light OS. She described an ache across her forehead. There was no history of trauma and her general health was good. On examination she had normal eye movements, her eyes were white and quiet, and she had normal pupil reactions. What is the most likely diagnosis?
    A. Central retinal artery occlusion (CRAO)
    B. Leber's hereditary optic neuropathy (LHON)
    C. Optic neuritis
    D. Unexplained visual loss

55. A lung-transplant patient on immunosuppression presents with a large focus of retinitis in one eye associated with patchy haemorrhages and vascular occlusion. Aqueous sampling is positive for cytomegalovirus (CMV) and negative for herpes simplex types 1 and 2 and varicella zoster virus. Peripheral blood is positive for CMV with high viral load. What is the most appropriate therapeutic strategy for this patient?
    A. Intravitreal foscarnet injection alone
    B. Intravitreal foscarnet plus oral valaciclovir
    C. Intravitreal foscarnet plus oral valganciclovir
    D. Intravitreal foscarnet plus intravenous aciclovir

56. A patient with a history of type 2 diabetes (diet controlled) and hypertension is attending for an assessment of diabetic retinopathy. A recent HbA1C is 54 mmol/mol. What is the correct interpretation of this value?
    A. The HbA1C value demonstrates excellent control
    B. A target HbA1c is <48 mmol/mol
    C. A HbA1C <58 mmol/mol indicates excellent control
    D. The HbA1C value is satisfactory control

57. A dual energy X-ray absorptiometry (DEXA) bone scan for a 65-year-old patient on long-term oral steroid (prednisolone 10 mg/day) is reported as T score −2.6. The patient is on long-term calcium D3 supplementation. What is the interpretation and correct action?
    A. The T score indicates normal bone density and no further therapy is necessary
    B. The T score indicates osteopaenia, but no further bone protection therapy is necessary
    C. The T score indicates osteopaenia and further protection therapy is necessary
    D. The T score indicates osteoporosis and further protection therapy is necessary

58. Erythema chronicum migrans is associated with which following organism?
    A. *Borrelia burgdorferi*
    B. *Bartonella henselae*
    C. *Treponema pallidum*
    D. *Leptospira interrogans*

59. A 28-year-old male with known Budd–Chiari syndrome and an inflammatory arthritis presents with acute onset headaches and horizontal diplopia. Thrombophilia screen is negative but inflammatory markers are raised. Examination reveals bilateral VI nerve pareses and papilloedema. What is the most likely cause for his papilloedema?
   A. Cerebellopontine angle tumour causing cerebrospinal fluid obstruction
   B. CSF outflow obstruction at the level of foramen magnum
   C. Dural venous sinus thrombosis
   D. Pituitary apoplexy

60. A 34-year-old female is referred to the eye emergency department by her optician for assessment of suspected disc swelling. The patient is 37/40 pregnant and overweight. She reports minor visual blur but her visual acuity is 6/9 in both eyes. Examination reveals bilateral mild disc swelling with sparse flame haemorrhages and cotton wool spots at the posterior poles and peripheral retina in both eyes with macular subretinal fluid. Her blood pressure is 153/93. MRI of the brain is otherwise normal. What is the most likely diagnosis?
   A. Diabetic retinopathy
   B. Hypertensive retinopathy
   C. Posterior reversible encephalopathy syndrome
   D. Purtscher-like retinopathy

61. Which of the following about hemifacial spasm is correct?
   A. It is caused by anomalous vascular compression of the facial nerve
   B. It is more common in males
   C. The peak onset is usually 20–30 years of age
   D. It has an autosomal recessive inheritance pattern

62. During a fluorescein angiography procedure, a 52-year-old female becomes acutely unwell. On arrival you find her reclined, pale, tachypnoeic, and clammy with a capillary refill time in excess of 5 seconds. An urticarial skin rash is present. Her blood pressure is 74/35, pulse rate 120 bpm. She appears frightened and confused. The emergency response team has been called. The acute management of this patient should include:
   A. Intravenous hydrocortisone 100 mg and chlorphenamine 10 mg
   B. Intravenous hydrocortisone 200 mg and chlorphenamine 10 mg
   C. Intramuscular adrenaline (1:1000) 500 μg
   D. 500–1000 ml bolus 0.9% saline fluid challenge

63. **Which of the following is associated with saddle nose deformity?**
    A. Polyarteritis nodosa
    B. Relapsing polychondritis
    C. Takayasu arteritis
    D. Tuberculosis

64. **Which of the following combination regarding the medical condition and deficiency of the enzyme is correct?**
    A. Albinism—tyrosinase enzyme
    B. Fabry's disease—phytanic acid alpha-hydrolase
    C. Galactosaemia—galactokinase enzyme
    D. Refsum disease—hexosaminidase A

65. **Which of the following treatment options is best for a functioning pituitary tumour producing prolactin?**
    A. Dopamine agonist therapy
    B. Dopamine antagonist therapy
    C. Radiation therapy
    D. Trans-sphenoidal surgery

66. **Which of the following statements regarding congenital Zika syndrome (CZS) is correct?**
    A. Around 20% of the patients will have some ocular findings
    B. There is currently a licensed vaccine for Zika viral infection
    C. Anterior segment abnormalities are most commonly reported in CKZ
    D. It is transmitted to human via mosquito from the *Aedes* genus

67. **A 30-year-old man presents to the accident and emergency department with shortness of breath over the past 2 weeks. He also mentions that he tends to bleed easily and examination shows signs suggestive of oculocutaneous albinism. What is the most likely diagnosis?**
    A. Chédiak–Higashi syndrome
    B. Griscelli syndrome
    C. Hermansky–Pudlak syndrome
    D. Waardenburg syndrome

68. **Which of the following visual phenomenon/syndromes describes patients with cortical blindness who can see moving targets but not stationary targets?**
    A. Anton syndrome
    B. Blue field entoptic phenomenon
    C. Charles Bonnet syndrome
    D. Riddoch phenomenon

69. Which of the following about migraine is true?
   A. Patients with migraine with aura are at increased risk of ischaemic stroke
   B. Need to have at least three typical attacks to meet the criteria of migraine with aura
   C. The headache usually precedes the visual aura
   D. It is more common in men

chapter 2

CLINICAL OPHTHALMOLOGY 2

ANSWERS

1. Answer: B

The most likely surgical option among UK-based surgeons is a scleral buckle and cryotherapy. Vitrectomy with endotamponade could be performed, but due to the absence of a posterior vitreous detachment and inferior location of the retinal break, it is less likely in the primary setting. Pneumatic retinopexy is unlikely to be used, as the retinal break is inferiorly placed. Suprachoroidal buckling (viscoelastic injected into the suprachoroidal space) is an option, but currently has not gained widespread popularity.

Heimann H, et al. Scleral buckling versus primary vitrectomy in rhegmatogenous retinal detachment: a prospective randomized multicenter clinical study. *Ophthalmology* 2007;114:2142–54.

Shanmugam PM, et al. Novel techniques in scleral buckling. *Indian J Ophthalmol* 2018;66:909–15.

2. Answer: C

The term and classification of proliferative vitreoretinopathy (PVR) was first introduced in 1983 by the Retina Society Terminology to describe a unique clinical entity that is characterized by massive vitreous traction and preretinal proliferation. This was subsequently updated to its current classification in 1991 and it is divided into three categories:

Grade A—vitreous haze, pigment clumps, and pigment clusters on inferior retina

Grade B—wrinkling of inner retinal surface, retinal stiffness, vessel tortuosity, rolled edge of retinal break

Grade CP—full-thickness retinal folds or subretinal strands posterior to equator. This can be further divided into focal, diffuse, and subretinal subtypes.

Grade CA—full-thickness retinal folds or subretinal strands anterior to equator. This can be further divided into anterior and circumferential subtypes.

Reprinted from *American Journal of Ophthalmology*, 112(2), Machemer, R. et al. An update classification of retinal detachment with proliferative vitreoretinopathy. pp. 159–65. https://doi.org/10.1016/S0002-9394(14)76695-4. Copyright © 1991, with permission from Elsevier Inc. All rights reserved.

For full details of the classification, please refer to the following references.

Di Lauro S, et al. Classification for proliferative vitreoretinopathy (PVR): an analysis of their use in publication over the last 15 years. *J Ophthalmol* 2016;2016:7807596.

Machemer R, et al. An update classification of retinal detachment with proliferative vitreoretinopathy. *Am J Ophthalmol* 1991;112(2):159–65.

3. Answer: B

Coagulase-negative staphylococcus are the most commonly isolated microorganisms in bacterial endophthalmitis post cataract surgery in Europe. The ESCRS Guidelines for Prevention and Treatment of Endophthalmitis Following Cataract Surgery gives detailed information on the management of endophthalmitis.

Table 2.3 offers a summary of common microorganisms in postoperative endophthalmitis.

Table 2.3 Common microorganisms in postoperative endophthalmitis

Prevalence	Microorganisms
33–77%	Coagulase-negative staphylococci (e.g. *S. epidermidis*)
10–21%	*Staphylococcus aureus*
9–19%	α- and β-haemolytic streptococci, and *S. pneumonia*
6–22%	Gram-negative bacteria including *Pseudomonas aeruginosa*
Up to 8%	Fungi (*Candida* sp., *Aspergillus* sp., *Fusarium* sp.)

Courtesy of the European Society of Cataract and Refractive Surgeons (ESCRS). Reprinted from ESCRS Guidelines for Prevention and Treatment of Endophthalmitis Following Cataract Surgery: Data, Dilemmas and Conclusions 2013. Peter Barry, Luis Cordoves, Susanne Gardner. https://education.escrs.org/wp-content/uploads/2018/08/ENGLISH_2018_updated.pdf

Barry P, et al. *ESCRS Guidelines for Prevention and Treatment of Endophthalmitis Following Cataract Surgery: Data, Dilemmas and Conclusions*, 2013. Available at: https://education.escrs.org/wp-content/uploads/2018/08/ENGLISH_2018_updated.pdf

4. Answer: B

The ESCRS Guidelines for Prevention and Treatment of Endophthalmitis Following Cataract Surgery identified a number of risk factors; see following link.

Barry P, et al. *ESCRS Guidelines for Prevention and Treatment of Endophthalmitis Following Cataract Surgery: Data, Dilemmas and Conclusions*, 2013. Available at: https://education.escrs.org/wp-content/uploads/2018/08/ENGLISH_2018_updated.pdf

5. Answer: A

This biomicroscopic classification is still widely used within vitreoretinal clinics. Optical coherence tomography has also been used to classify full-thickness macular holes and provide prognostic indicators for the risk of non-closure following surgery (Table 2.4).

Table 2.4 Gass classification

Grading	Clinical features
Stage 1	1A—Foveolar detachment with a loss of foveal contour and lipofuscin-coloured spot 1B—Foveolar detachment with lipofuscin-coloured ring
Stage 2	Full-thickness hole of <400 μm in diameter size + no complete PVD
Stage 3	Full-thickness hole of >400 μm in diameter size + no complete PVD
Stage 4	Full-thickness hole of >400 μm in diameter size + complete PVD

Adapted from *American Journal of Ophthalmology*, 119(6), Gass, J. Reappraisal of biomicroscopic classification of stages of development of a macular hole. pp. 752–759. https://doi.org/10.1016/S0002-9394(14)72781-3. Copyright © 1995, with permission from Elsevier Inc. All rights reserved.

Duker JS, et al. The International Vitreomacular Traction Study Group classification of vitreomacular adhesion, traction, and macular hole. *Ophthalmology* 2013;120:2611–9.

Gass JD. Reappraisal of biomicroscopic classification of stages of development of a macular hole. *Am J Ophthalmol* 1995;119:752–9.

6. Answer: D

All of the aforementioned complications of diabetic retinopathy are indications for vitrectomy. The Diabetic Retinopathy Vitrectomy Study (DRVS) was conducted to establish the benefit of early

vitrectomy in patients with severe vitreous haemorrhage from PDR. The main results reported are as follows:
- Six-hundred-and-sixteen eyes with recent severe diabetic vitreous haemorrhage reducing visual acuity to 5/200 (equivalent to 2/60) or less for at least 1 month were randomly assigned to either **early vitrectomy** or **deferral of vitrectomy** for 1 year.
- At 2 years' follow-up, vision of 10/20 (or 6/12) = 25% (early vitrectomy group) vs. 15% (deferral group).
- In patients with type 1 diabetes, who were on the average younger and had more-severe proliferative retinopathy, there was a clear-cut advantage for early vitrectomy, as reflected in the percentage of eyes recovering visual acuity of 10/20 or better (36% vs. 12% in the deferral group, p = 0.0001). No such advantage was found in the type 2 diabetes group (16% in the early group vs. 18% in the deferral group), but evidence that this advantage differed by diabetes type was of borderline significance.

[No authors]. Early vitrectomy for severe vitreous hemorrhage in diabetic retinopathy. Two-year results of a randomized trial. Diabetic Retinopathy Vitrectomy Study Report 2. The Diabetic Retinopathy Vitrectomy Study Research Group. *Arch Ophthalmol* 1985;103:1644–52.

7. Answer: D

Ocriplasmin is a small fragment of plasmin enzyme designed for enzymatic vitreolysis. The use of ocriplasmin is supported by the evidence of two large phase 3 clinical trials:

(a) Microplasmin for Intravitreal Injection-Traction Release without Surgical Treatment (MIVI-TRUST)—6 months follow-up
(b) Ocriplasmin for Treatment for Symptomatic Vitreomacular Adhesion Including Macular Hole (OASIS)—24 months follow-up

A summary of the results can be seen in Table 2.5:

Table 2.5 Results of two large phase 3 clinical trials for use of ocriplasmin

Studies	Ocriplasmin (O)	Control (C)	VMT release	p value	FTMH closure	p value
MIVI-TRUST	464	188	26.5% (O) vs. 10.1% (C)	<0.001	40.6% (O) vs. 10.6% (C)	<0.001
OASIS	146	74	41.7% (O) vs. 6.2% (C)	<0.001	30.0% (O) vs. 15.4% (C)	0.163

MIVI-TRUST, Microplasmin for Intravitreal Injection-Traction Release without Surgical Treatment; OASIS, Ocriplasmin for Treatment for Symptomatic Vitreomacular Adhesion Including Macular Hole.

Ocriplasmin is recommended as an option for treating vitreomacular traction in adults, but only if:
- An epiretinal membrane is not present **AND**
- They have a stage II full-thickness macular hole with a diameter of 400 micrometres or less **AND/OR**
- They have severe symptoms.

Khan MA, Haller JA. Ocriplasmin for treatment of vitreomacular traction: an update. *Ophthalmol Ther* 2016;5:147–59.

National Institute for Health and Care Excellence (NICE). *Ocriplasmin for Treating Vitreomacular Traction. Technology Appraisal Guidance [TA297].* Available at: https://www.nice.org.uk/guidance/ta297/chapter/1-Guidance

8. Answer: A

Optic disc pit maculopathy is a rare condition affecting ~50% of all people with a congenital optic disc pit at some point in their life. The prevalence of congenital pits is thought to be approximately 1:5000 and the incidence of pit maculopathy ~1 in 2 million per annum in the United Kingdom. There is no sex predilection, and the median age of presentation is ~35 years old. The commonest fluid pattern at presentation is subretinal fluid with multilayered intraretinal fluid. Subretinal fluid alone is rare. Congenital pits are only rarely associated with a coexisting choroidal coloboma. There is an approximately 75% chance of anatomical success with surgery. Surgery can take a variety of forms, mostly vitrectomy based. Resolution of sub- and intraretinal fluid is often slow and a prolonged follow-up period is advised, before considering revision surgery.

Steel DHW, et al. Optic disc pit maculopathy: a two-year nationwide prospective population-based study. *Ophthalmology* 2018;pii: S0161–6420(18):30774–7.

9. Answer: C

The development of subretinal fluid within rhegmatogenous retinal detachments follows certain patterns. Retinal breaks can be located by looking at the distribution of the subretinal fluid and applying certain principles. These principles or rules were first described by Harvey Lincoff in 1971 and still hold true for retinal examination today (Lincoff's rule).

Lincoff H, Gieser R. Finding the retinal hole. *Arch Ophthalmol* 1971;65:565–9.

10. Answer: D

Identifying any underlying systemic or ocular causes is an important part of the investigation and management of retinal vein occlusion. A comprehensive list of all reported associations and management can be found within the RCOphth retinal vein occlusion guidelines. The RCOphth recommendation on investigations for retinal vein occlusions (RVO) in the eye clinic has changed significantly from 2010 to 2015. Current recommendation includes:

(a) Medical history
(b) BP measurement
(c) Serum glucose estimation
(d) FBC and ESR

Further medical tests are probably best performed by the patient's physician. In the aforementioned question, all the choices have been reported other than longer axial length. A number of studies have reported on associations with central vein occlusion.

[No authors]. Risk factors for central retinal vein occlusion. The Eye Disorders Case-Control Study Group. *Arch Ophthalmol* 1996;114:545–54.

Elman MJ, et al. The risk for systemic vascular diseases and mortality in patients with central retinal vein occlusion. *Ophthalmology* 1990;97:1543–8.

Royal College of Ophthalmologists. *Clinical Guidelines: Retinal Vein Occlusions (RVO),* 2015. Available at: https://www.rcophth.ac.uk/wp-content/uploads/2015/07/Retinal-Vein-Occlusion-RVO-Guidelines-July-2015.pdf

11. Answer: C

Angioid streak refers to linear, cracked-line dehiscence of the Bruch's membrane, with secondary changes in the choriocapillaris and retinal pigment epithelium. It can be an ocular manifestation of systemic disease and candidates should be familiar with the most common associated systemic conditions. It is also a recognized cause for choroidal neovascular membrane. A useful acronym for remembering them is **'PAPER-CLIP'**.

P—Pseudoxanthoma elasticum (or Gronblad–Strandberg syndrome)

A—Acromegaly

P—Paget's disease of bone

E—Ehler–Danlos syndrome

R—Red cell abnormality (e.g. sickle cell disease, haemolytic anaemia, hereditary spherocytosis)

C—Calcification (e.g. hypercalcinosis, hyperphosphataemia)

L—Lead poisoning

I—Idiopathic

P—Phakomatoses (e.g. neurofibromatosis, Sturge–Weber syndrome, tuberous sclerosis)

Gurwood AS, Mastrangelo DL. Understanding angioid streaks. *J Am Optom Assoc* 1997;68:309–24.

12. Answer: B

Figure 2.2 demonstrates a choroidal neovascular membrane—flow within a vascular network within the 'avascular' zone of the retina. Optical coherence tomography angiography has become increasingly widespread and candidates should be familiar with the basic concepts of the imaging. Candidates should also be familiar with the NICE guidance for the management of choroidal neovascular membranes, which is a common VIVA question. Focal argon laser would not be appropriate in this case due to the risk of scarring and recurrence. Triamcinolone could be considered as a treatment option; however, aflibercept and ranibizumab are licensed alternates. Aflibercept is licensed by NICE for the treatment of myopic choroidal neovascular membranes—a link to the guidance is provide in the further reading.

National Institute for Health and Care Excellence (NICE). *Age-related Macular Degeneration. NICE Guideline [NG82]*. Available at: https://www.nice.org.uk/guidance/NG82

13. Answer: D

Electrodiagnostic tests are an essential part of the investigation into retinal disorders and are frequently tested within the FRCOphth Part 2 examination. An (electro) negative full field ERG usually describes an International Society for Clinical Electrophysiology of Vision (ISCEV) standard maximal response in which the b-wave is smaller than a normal or minimally reduced a-wave and indicates dysfunction that is postphototransduction. The commonest causes are:

- X-linked retinoschisis
- Congenital stationary night blindness (CSNB)
- Central retinal artery occlusion
- Central retinal vein occlusion (ischaemic)
- Melanoma-associated retinopathy
- Birdshot chorioretinopathy
- Batten disease

Best disease causes abnormal electro-oculogram (EOG) result with a reduced Arden (light peak: dark trough) of ≤ 1.5 (normal is ≥1.8).

Robson AG, et al. Unilateral electronegative ERG of non-vascular aetiology. *Br J Ophthalmol* 2005;89:1620–6.

14. Answer: D

Optic disc drusen consists of acellular intracellular and extracellular deposits that often become calcified over time. They are typically buried early in life and generally become superficial, and therefore visible, later in childhood, at the average age of 12 years. Most commonly they occur in isolation, however, there are many associated ocular and systemic conditions, including retinitis pigmentosa, pseudoxanthoma elasticum, and angioid streaks, Alagille syndrome, among others. It is important to keep these in mind. A comprehensive overview is given in the following article:

Chang MY, Pineles SL. Optic disk drusen in children. *Surv Ophthalmol* 2016;61:745–58.

15. Answer: C

The most likely answer is Stickler syndrome, though all of the listed conditions can cause retinal detachment. Stickler syndrome is a type of hereditary connective tissue disorder of fibrillar collagen associated with retinal detachment, congenital megalophthalmos, deafness, cleft palate, Pierre Robin sequence, joint hypermobility, and premature arthritis. It is the commonest cause of rhegmatogenous retinal detachment in childhood. Human vitreous is primarily composed of types 2, 9, and 11 collagens and mutations affecting the genes encoding all these three collagens can cause Stickler syndrome.

The risk of retinal detachment depends on the underlying genetic abnormality. The majority of the cases seen by ophthalmologists are type 1 Stickler syndrome, with an inheritance pattern of autosomal dominant. Candidates should be familiar with the most common form of inherited vitreoretinopathy.

Table 2.6 offers a summary of the types and characteristics of Sticker syndrome.

Table 2.6 Types and characteristics of Sticker syndrome

Type	Gene	Features
Type 1	COL2A1	Membranous vitreous anomaly, megalophthalmos, deafness, arthropathy, cleft palate
Type 2	COL11A1	Beaded vitreous anomaly, megalophthalmos, deafness, arthropathy, cleft palate
Type 3	COL11A2	Normal vitreous and ocular phenotype, deafness, arthropathy, cleft palate
Type 4	COL9A1, COL9A2	Recessive inheritance, deafness, myopia, vitreoretinopathy, epiphyseal dysplasia
Ocular-only	COL2A1	Membranous vitreous anomaly, megalophthalmos. No systemic features
Other	Unknown	Hypoplastic vitreous, deafness, arthropathy, cleft palate

Reprinted by permission from Springer Nature: Nature, *Eye*, 25: 1389–400. Stickler syndrome, ocular-only variant and a key diagnostic role for ophthalmologists. Snead, M. et al. https://doi.org/10.1038/eye.2011.201. Copyright © 2011, Springer Nature.

Snead MP, et al. Stickler syndrome, ocular-only variant and a key diagnostic role for ophthalmologists. *Eye (Lond)* 2011;25:1389–400.

16. Answer: A

The DCCT reported the aforementioned finding. Modifiable risk factors within the management of diabetic retinopathy include glycaemic control, blood pressure, and lipid levels.

The RCOphth guidelines (Section 6) gives an excellent summary of the findings in trials that have looked each of the aforementioned risk factors, candidates for the FRCOphth should be similar with these findings.

Royal College of Ophthalmologists. *Diabetic Retinopathy Guidelines,* December 2012. Available at: https://www.rcophth.ac.uk/wp-content/uploads/2014/12/2013-SCI-301-FINAL-DR-GUIDELINES-DEC-2012-updated-July-2013.pdf

17. Answer: B

All the options are criteria of CSMO, except for Option B, which is one of the criteria used by national screening committee for referring patients with diabetic maculopathy (M1 grade) to hospital eye service. M0 refers to no maculopathy.

The following excerpt is taken from the RCOphth Diabetic retinopathy guidelines and provides a summary of the results of focal laser for CSMO. In patients with CSMO and normal visual acuity, the ETDRS data indicated a trend towards benefit in laser treated patients, i.e. a 10% to 5% reduction in incidence of visual loss of two lines of Snellen acuity equivalent (Level 1 evidence). It is important to note that benefit in the ETDRS was taken as a delay in progression of visual loss (i.e. that even when photocoagulation treatment was applied there was still an increasing incidence of visual loss, albeit at a slower rate). It is also worth noting that 'treatable lesions' (i.e. leaking microaneurysms or diffuse macular leakage) were identified by fluorescein angiography. In the absence of clinically detectable retinal thickening (CSMO) fluorescein angiographic evidence of leakage is not normally regarded as an indication for treatment in routine clinical practice. The advent of OCT has altered the situation somewhat, in that very early intraretinal fluid that may not be seen on fundal examination may be visualized on OCT, and the data from the ETDRS cannot necessarily be extrapolated to that group of patients. In other words, focal laser reduces the risk of moderate visual loss (2 Snellen-line vision) by 50% in eyes with CSMO.

Reproduced from RCOphth Diabetic retinopathy guidelines https://www.rcophth.ac.uk/wp-content/uploads/2014/12/2013-SCI-301-FINAL-DR-GUIDELINES-DEC-2012-updated-July-2013.pdf

Department of Health (NHS England). *Public Health Functions to be Exercised by NHS England,* 2013. Available at: https://assets.publishing.service.gov.uk/government/uploads/system/uploads/attachment_data/file/256492/22_nhs_diabetic_eye.pdf

Royal College of Ophthalmologists. *Diabetic Retinopathy Guidelines,* December 2012. Available at: https://www.rcophth.ac.uk/wp-content/uploads/2014/12/2013-SCI-301-FINAL-DR-GUIDELINES-DEC-2012-updated-July-2013.pdf

18. Answer: C

The DRS and ETDRS are landmark trails whose results were adopted worldwide. Both trials used 'high-risk' examination findings to help determine which patients should undergo PRP and when. High-risk findings were defined as:

1. NVD ≥1/3 disc area
2. Any NVD with vitreous haemorrhage
3. NVE ≥ ½ disc area with vitreous haemorrhage

High-risk PDR was also defined as **three or more** of the following high-risk characteristics (HRCs):

1. Presence of vitreous haemorrhage or preretinal haemorrhage

2. Presence of any active neovascularization
3. Location of neovascularization on or within one-disc diameter of the optic disc
4. NVD > 1/3 disc area or NVE > ½ disc area

Section 10 of the RCOphth Diabetic retinopathy guidelines provides a summary of the findings of these trials and recommendations for management of all grades of diabetic retinopathy.

Royal College of Ophthalmologists. *Diabetic Retinopathy Guidelines*, December 2012. Available at: https://www.rcophth.ac.uk/wp-content/uploads/2014/12/2013-SCI-301-FINAL-DR-GUIDELINES-DEC-2012-updated-July-2013.pdf

19. Answer: B

Fluocinolone acetonide (FA) intravitreal implant is a NICE approved treatment for the management of chronic diabetic macular oedema. FAME A and B were identical randomized trials that evaluate the efficacy of fluocinolone acetonide.

The primary outcome reported in the FAME trials was the proportion of people with an improvement of best corrected visual acuity (BCVA) by ≥15 letters at 2 years. Following are the main results:

- Improvement of BCVA at 2 years: 28% (0.2 µg/day) vs. 16% (sham)
- Cataract extraction: 41% vs. 51% vs. 7%
- VA at 3 years:
    - Overall: 29% vs. 28% vs. 19%
    - With chronic diabetic macular oedema (DMO) >3 years: 34% (FA 0.2 µg/day) vs. 13% (sham)
    - With chronic DMO <3 years: 22% (FA 0.2 µg/day) vs. 28% (sham)

Interestingly the benefit was only significant in patients who have had chronic DMO for longer than 3 years. A summary of the findings can be found in the following NICE Technology appraisal guidance.

Protocol S reported visual outcomes in patients receiving panretinal photocoagulation versus intravitreal ranibizumab for PDR over a 2-year period (non-inferiority randomized trial). The BEVORDEX study was the first head-to-head randomized clinical trial of bevacizumab versus a slow-release intravitreal dexamethasone implant (DEX-implant; Ozurdex; Allergan Inc., Irvine, CA) for diabetic macular oedema. The VIVID and VISTA trials compared the efficacy and safety of intravitreal aflibercept injection with macular laser photocoagulation for diabetic macular oedema over 3 years.

National Institute for Health and Care Excellence (NICE). *Fluocinolone Acetonide Intravitreal Implant for Treating Chronic Diabetic Macular Oedema After an Inadequate Response to Prior Therapy. Technology Appraisal Guidance [TA301]*, 2013. Available at: https://www.nice.org.uk/guidance/ta301/chapter/3-The-manufacturers-submission

20. Answer: B

Dexamethasone intravitreal implant (700 µg) is approved by NICE for the management of a centre involving diabetic macular oedema, in pseudophakic patients with a CMT of less than 400 µm. Anti-VEGF therapy is also approved by NICE, however, the CMT must be greater than 400 µm. Focal argon laser could be considered if fluorescein angiography shows areas of leakage that are affecting the fovea. These areas may be close to the foveal avascular zone and are therefore unsuitable for focal laser.

National Institute for Health and Care Excellence (NICE). *Aflibercept for Treating Diabetic Macular Oedema*, 2015. Available at: https://www.nice.org.uk/guidance/ta346/resources/aflibercept-for-treating-diabetic-macular-oedema-pdf-82602611201221

National Institute for Health and Care Excellence (NICE). *Dexamethasone Intravitreal Implant for Treating Diabetic Macular Oedema*, 2015.
Available at: https://www.nice.org.uk/guidance/ta349/resources/dexamethasone-intravitreal-implant-for-treating-diabetic-macular-oedema-pdf-82602616240069

National Institute for Health and Care Excellence (NICE). *Ranibizumab for Treating Diabetic Macular Oedema*, 2013. Available at: https://www.nice.org.uk/guidance/ta274/resources/ranibizumab-for-treating-diabetic-macular-oedema-pdf-82600612458181

21. Answer: D

The most likely answer is macular telangiectasia (Mac Tel) type 2. Diabetic maculopathy and bilateral RVO would be in the differential diagnoses; however, the OCT and confocal blue reflectance are indicative of Mac Tel type 2. Figure 2.3A shows 'internal limiting membrane (ILM) drape'. This is a later imaging feature of Mac Tel type 2 and occurs secondarily to loss of the outer nuclear layer and ellipsoid zone, which can progress into larger cysts (often called 'cavitation') eventually encompassing all retinal layers. Confocal blue reflectance (Figure 2.3B)—increased reflectance of blue light (488 nm)—is seen in Mac Tel type 2 and is thought to occur due to loss of macular pigments and structural alterations.

Macular telangiectasia types:

Type 1—congenital and unilateral. Possibly a variant of Coats disease. Uncommon.

Type 2—acquired and bilateral. The most common form of the three types. Usually found in middle-aged or older patients.

Type 3—poorly understood primarily occlusive phenomena which is quite rare.

American Academy of Ophthalmology. *Macular Telangiectasia*, 2015. Available at:http://eyewiki.aao.org/Macular_telangiectasia

Charbel Issa P, et al. Macular telangiectasia type 2. *Prog Retin Eye Res* 2013;34:49–77.

22. Answer: D

Vasoproliferative tumours are uncommon retinal lesions that may occur in isolation (primary) or in association with another ocular condition (secondary). They may be unilateral or bilateral and have a predilection for the peripheral inferior temporal quadrant of the retina. Vasoproliferative tumours can be associated with abnormalities of the macular, including epiretinal membrane formation and cystoid macular oedema.

Rennie IG. Retinal vasoproliferative tumours. *Eye (Lond)* 2010;24:468–71.

23. Answer: D

A range of medical treatment has been investigated for the treatment of CSCR with no clearly accepted preferred management. Endogenous and exogenous corticosteroids can have a role in the pathogenesis of CSCR. Spironolactone and eplerenone are both aldosterone antagonist agents with possible evidence of efficacy, though a recent randomized controlled trial, VICI, showed no effect (awaiting publication). Rifampicin, but not isoniazid, is an antituberculous medication which is thought to facilitate catabolism of endogenous steroids. It causes a proliferation of the smooth endoplasmic reticulum and an increase in the cytochrome P- 450 content in the liver, thus affecting the metabolism and bioavailability of endogenous corticosteroids, consequently possibly aiding in resolution of CSCR.

Nicholson B, et al. Central serous chorioretinopathy: update on pathophysiology and treatment. *Surv Ophthalmol* 2013;58:103–26.

Willcox A, et al. Clinical efficacy of eplerenone versus placebo for central serous chorioretinopathy: study protocol for the VICI randomised controlled trial. *Eye* (Lond) 2019;33:295–303.

24. Answer: C

Vitamin B_3 (or niacin/nicotinic acid) has been associated with cystic changes at the macula. However, there is no leakage on the fundus fluorescein angiography (FFA) despite the cystic changes. It has been postulated that the drug causes direct toxic effect on Muller cell, resulting in intracellular oedema. Similar clinical finding of non-leaking macular oedema may be seen in other conditions such as juvenile X-linked retinoschisis, retinitis pigmentosa, and Goldmann-Favre syndrome (a severe form of enhanced S-cone syndrome).

Domanico D, et al. Ocular effects of niacin: a review of the literature. *Med Hypothesis Discov Inno Ophthalmol* 2015;4:64–71.

25. Answer: C

Photodynamic therapy (PDT) can be used to treat vascular abnormalities that arise within the retinal and choroidal circulation. Photodynamic therapy with verteporfin causes release of free radicals when the verteporfin is activated by the laser energy. The reaction that ensues between the free radicals and blood vessel endothelial cell membranes cause locally increased histamines, thromboxane, and TNF-α, all immune modulation factors. The anti-inflammatory response can lead to series of events including vasoconstriction, thrombosis, increased vascular permeability, blood stasis, and hypoxia. Many ocular conditions can be treated with PDT—the following article summarizes the evidence for PDT in each of the conditions listed earlier. Macular telangiectasia type 2 has no proven treatment unless it is complicated by choroidal neovascularization, which can be treated by anti-VEGF.

American Academy of Ophthalmology. *Photodynamic Therapy (PDT)*, 2017. Available at: http://eyewiki.aao.org/Photodynamic_Therapy_(PDT)

26. Answer: A

This is a clinical vignette of myopic choroidal neovascularization (CNV). Myopic CNV is typically seen as a small, flat, greyish membrane that may have a hyperpigmented border if chronic or recurrent. There appears to be three main stages of myopic CNV: the first phase results in direct damage to photoreceptors; the second phase is the regression of CNV, resulting in the formation of a fibrous pigmented scar (also known as the Förster-Fuchs' spot); and the third phase is the formation of atrophy around the regressed CNV.

Evidence has suggested that myopic choroidal neovascular membrane (CNVM) behaves differently from age-related CNVM whereby the myopic CNVM usually requires less intravitreal anti-VEGF injections. The phase 2 (REPAIR) and phase 3 (RADIANCE) trials showed that patients who received *pro re nata* (PRN) regimens of ranibizumab were able to achieve significantly greater gains in best corrected visual acuity than verteporfin photodynamic therapy (vPDT). The median of required injections was 2–4 injections.

Wong TY, et al. Myopic choroidal neovascularisation: current concepts and update on clinical management. *Br J Ophthalmol* 2015;99:289–96.

27. Answer: B

Lampalizumab is a selective complement factor D inhibitor. Two identically designed phase 3 randomized controlled trials, Chroma and Spectri, examined its efficacy and safety for treating geographic atrophy secondary to age-related macular degeneration. Unfortunately, the treatment did not reduce the enlargement of geographic atrophy compared to sham injection at 48 weeks. The risk of endophthalmitis was similar to other intravitreal anti-VEGF treatment studies.

Holz FG, et al. Efficacy and safety of lampalizumab for geographic atrophy due to age-related macular degeneration: Chroma and Spectri phase 3 randomized clinical trials. *JAMA Ophthalmol* 2018;136:666–77.

28. Answer: A

Tamoxifen is an antioestrogen drug frequently used for breast cancer. The incidence of tamoxifen retinopathy is extremely low and usually presents after 3 years of treatment or after a total cumulative dose of more than 100 g. Option B refers to the changes observed in patients who are taking canthaxanthin, which is a naturally occurring carotenoid used for skin pigmentation in vitiligo. Option C refers to the changes observed in patients who are taking vigabatrin, an antiepileptic medication. Option D refers to the changes in patients taking interferon alpha, which is used in treatment of Kaposi's sarcoma, chronic hepatitis C, leukaemia, and lymphoma, among others.

Nencini C, et al. Retinopathy induced by drugs and herbal medicines. *Eur Rev Med Pharmacol Sci* 2008;12:293–8.

Tang RJ, et al. Retinal changes associated with tamoxifen treatment for breast cancer. *Eye (Lond)* 1997;11:295–7.

29. Answer: B

The main types of retinal vascular tumours are listed in the options. Capillary haemangioma is an uncommon benign hamartoma of the retina, consisting of capillary-like vessels. It is characterized by red nodular lesions with dilatation and tortuosity of the feeding artery and draining vein. Cavernous haemangioma is a benign hamartoma of retinal vessels, usually large-calibre and thin-walled, characterized by a 'bunch-of-grapes' appearance of the lesion with blood-filled saccules. Racemose haemangioma is a rare retinal arteriovenous malformation, which may be associated with Wyburn-Mason syndrome. Vasoproliferative tumour is usually a dome-shaped appearance retinal lesion, commonly located at the inferior temporal peripheral retina with telangiectatic vessels on the surface of the lesion.

Wang W, Chen L. Cavernous hemangioma of the retina: a comprehensive review of the literature (1934–2015). *Retina* 2017;37:611–21.

30. Answer: D

CAR is the most common intraocular paraneoplastic retinopathy. The most common primary tumours are small-cell lung carcinoma followed by gynaecologic and breast malignancies. The average age of symptom onset is 65 years. The symptoms are mainly caused by the dysfunction of rod and cone photoreceptors. Patients typically present with photosensitivity, photopsia, glare, reduced central vision, and colour vision. **CAR** normally affects **C**ones > **R**ods and MAR affects rods more than cones. The fundus usually appears normal at the initial stage but may have optic nerve pallor, attenuated retinal arterioles, and retinal pigment epithelial thinning and mottling at later stage, mimicking retinitis pigmentosa. Electroretinogram in CAR typically shows global retinal dysfunction with severely reduced photopic a- and b-waves. OCT may show severe macular atrophy with thinning of the outer retina (not inner retina) and loss of photoreceptors and inner segment/outer segment (IS/OS) junction.

Rahimy E, Sarraf D. Paraneoplastic and non-paraneoplastic retinopathy and optic neuropathy: evaluation and management. *Surv Ophthalmol* 2013;58:430–58.

31. Answer: C

This is a clinical vignette of right Horner's syndrome occurring after thyroidectomy due to inadvertent damage to the oculosympathetic pathway. It is important to establish the diagnosis of Horner's as this enables the correct investigations to be performed so that any treatable cause is identified. After clinical examination, confirmation is usually done using pharmacological tests. The classic test is using cocaine 4% or 10%. This will dilate a normal pupil but not a Horner's pupil. If cocaine is not available, then apraclonidine 0.5% or 1% can be used. Cocaine blocks the reuptake of norepinephrine at the neuromuscular junction so the normal pupil dilates as there are more norepinephrine available; however, the pupil affected by a Horner's has little or no norepinephrine to be blocked so the pupil will dilate poorly.

Apraclonidine 1% is an alpha2-agonist and in normal patients causes pupil constriction; however, the drug also has weak alpha1-agonist property which promotes pupil dilatation. Therefore, in a pupil that has been sympathetically denervated, the pupil dilator muscle develops super sensitivity to the alpha1-agonist property of apraclonidine so the Horner's pupil will dilate. Hydroxyamphetamine test is useful as it will dilate a normal or preganglionic Horner's but not a postganglionic Horner's pupil. In addition, adrenaline 1:1000 and phenylephrine 1%, which are weak alpha1-agonists, have also been used to localize a Horner's pupil. They dilate a Horner's pupil that is caused by postganglionic lesion (due to denervation hypersensitivity) but not by central or preganglionic lesion.

Cambron M, et al. Apraclonidine and my pupil. *Clin Auton Res* 2011;21:347–51.

Gao Z, Crompton JL. Horner syndrome: a practical approach to investigation and management. *Asia Pac J Ophthalmol (Phila)* 2012;1:175–9.

Giannaccare G, et al. Horner syndrome following thyroid surgery: the clinical and pharmacological presentations. *J Ophthalmic Vis Res* 2016;11:442–4.

32. Answer: D

This is a clinical vignette of left Adie's tonic pupil. Many patients with a tonic pupil present with anisocoria. Often this has been noticed by family members and there is usually no clear history of the time of onset. A tonic pupil is found in approximately two people per 1000 in the general population. The usual features are a dilated pupil with a sluggish response to light and poor response to near. There are usually vermiform movements of the iris tissue. The condition is caused by ciliary ganglion or short ciliary nerve damage. The responses in the pupil function are related to the ciliary ganglion fibres. Most of the ciliary ganglion fibres are used for accommodation (about 95%) and so the accommodation response of the ciliary muscles is more likely to be spared than the iris sphincter muscles.

There is no specific cause, but a tonic pupil has been associated with herpes zoster, Lyme disease, sarcoidosis, and inflammatory conditions such as giant cell arteritis and rheumatoid arthritis that may cause a ciliary ganglionitis. Other local causes include orbital trauma (blunt or penetrating) and orbital tumours. Females are affected more often that males at approximately 3:1. Systemic neurological conditions that have been associated with tonic pupils include dysautonomias such as Shy–Drager syndrome. It is vital to examine the eye thoroughly as paralysis of the third cranial nerve can cause a dilated pupil, but there are usually other associated features.

Wilhelm H. Disorders of the pupil. *Handb Clin Neurol* 2011;102:427–66.

33. Answer: A

The vision can deteriorate over 2 weeks after the initial presentation and usually stabilizes by 2 months. The prognosis of the affected eye is usually good; about 50% will have a final vision of

6/9 or better and 25% will have a final vision of 6/60 or worse. Around 15–40% eyes will recover 3 Snellen vision over time. There is a 10–20% chance of deterioration of vision of the affected eye at 2 years compared to the initial presentation. The risk of recurrence of the disease in the same eye was reported at 3–8%. The risk of fellow eye involvement is estimated at 15–25% over 5 years. The Eyewiki website provides a very good summary on this topic.

American Academy of Ophthalmology. *Non-Arteritic Anterior Ischemic Optic Neuropathy (NAION)*, 2019. Available at: http://eyewiki.aao.org/Non-Arteritic_Anterior_Ischemic_Optic_Neuropathy_(NAION)

34. Answer: C

IIH is a neurological disorder characterized by increased intracranial pressure of unknown origin. It typically affects overweight women of childbearing age. Before puberty, it affects boys and girls equally whereas after puberty, women are nine times more likely to be affected than men. The Friedman or modified Dandy diagnostic criteria for IIH include: (1) normal neurological evaluation with exception of cranial nerve abnormalities; (2) normal neuroimaging showing normal brain parenchyma without hydrocephalus or mass; (3) normal CSF constituents; (4) presence of papilloedema; and (5) elevated CSF opening pressure during lumbar puncture (more than 25 cm of water in adults and more than 28 cm of water in children). The recent IIHTT showed that acetazolamide is a well-tolerated first-line therapy in IIH patients with mild visual field loss (perimetric mean deviation between −2 dB and −7 dB) but not in severe visual field loss. Drugs that may be associated with intracranial pressure can be remembered as '**STAIN-LONG**':

S—Steroid withdrawal (after long-term use)

T—Tetracycline and derivatives

A—Vitamin A and retinoids

I—Indomethacin

N—Nitrofurantoin

L—Lithium

O—Oral contraceptive pills

N—Nalidixic acid

G—Growth hormone

Madriz Peralta G, Cestari DM. An update of idiopathic intracranial hypertension. *Curr Opin Ophthalmol* 2018;29:495–502.

35. Answer: C

This clinical scenario is highly suggestive of giant cell arteritis (GCA), which is a systemic vasculitis which tends to affect persons >50 years old. The incidence rate of GCA tends to increase with increasing age. It is much more common in the Western world. GCA rarely occurs in patients aged between 30 and 50 years but there are isolated case reports. GCA affects males and females equally and the mean age of onset is 70 years of age. It most commonly affects cranial branches of arteries from the arch of the aorta, and loss of vision in one or both eyes occurs in up to 50% of patients.

Classically patients present with a temporal headache and jaw claudication which can lead to weight loss as the patient finds eating difficult. Visual symptoms may be the presenting feature of the disease. A normal/borderline ESR/CRP is possible and in a patient with a high clinical suspicion of GCA it is still prudent to treat this. The gold standard for diagnosis is still a temporal artery biopsy. A positive temporal artery biopsy will reveal intimal thickening of the blood vessels and there will be necrosis of parts of the arterial wall and there is formation of granulomas containing multinucleated giant cells. Other investigations performed in some hospitals include ultrasound scanning demonstrating a 'halo sign' which may be due to thickening of the artery wall.

Vodopivec I, Rizzo JF 3rd. Ophthalmic manifestations of giant cell arteritis. *Rheumatology (Oxford)* 2018;57:ii63–72.

36. Answer: B

The table demonstrates an ocular motility problem suggestive of right inferior rectus weakness—large R/L at right gaze and down gaze. Isolated inferior rectus weakness may manifest as the presenting sign of myasthenia gravis. This patient may have myasthenia gravis but no comment has yet been made on the pupil responses. It is important to endure that there is no evidence of pupil involvement as this would indicate development of a third nerve palsy, which would require different investigations. Myasthenia gravis will not have any involvement of the pupillary muscles.

Spoor TC, Shippman S. Myasthenia gravis presenting as an isolated inferior rectus paresis. *Ophthalmology* 1979;86:158–60.

37. Answer: C

The iris sphincter is highly sensitive to substances similar to acetylcholine and therefore when a substance similar to acetylcholine is instilled then the pupil response is highly active, so the abnormal pupil constricts even in response to weak stimulation. With time aberrant regeneration may develop of the fibres supplying the ciliary muscle increasing nerve supply to the iris sphincter muscles. Adie syndrome or Homes-Adie syndrome is characterized by pupillary changes with reduced or lost deep tendon reflexes.

Wilhelm H. Disorders of the pupil. *Handb Clin Neurol* 2011;102:427–66.

38. Answer: C

The ice pack test has been used now for some time and has gained more interest as it is a simple bedside test that can be performed with little discomfort to the patient and little risk (unlike the Tensilon test which can lead to cardiovascular collapse). The ice is applied to the dropped eye lid for 2–5 min and pre- and post-ice measurements of lid position are taken. A positive result is if the eye lid opens by 2 mm or more. The ice causes improvement in the signs of ptosis by cooling the skeletal muscle tissue and therefore cooling the activity of the acetyl cholinesterase enzyme. The Tensilon test used to be readily available but it is now difficult to source edrophonium so other tests are required. After confirming the diagnosis of myasthenia gravis (MG), chest X-ray can be utilized to diagnose thymoma in patients with MG but the sensitivity ranges between 45% and 80%; CT chest is a more definite way to image thymoma. Treatment involves the use of pyridostigmine and an immunosuppressant such as prednisolone and/or azathioprine.

Natarajan B, et al. Accuracy of the ice test in the diagnosis of myasthenic ptosis. *Neurol India* 2016;64:1169–72.

39. Answer: B

This clinical vignette is suggestive of LHON. It tends to affect males more than females, with males having a higher risk of visual loss (up to 80%) than females (up to 35%). The visual loss is painless and tends to affect both eyes eventually, often within the space of a few weeks to months. The visual loss is often severe usually in the range of 6/60 to hand movements with central or centrocaecal scotomas. There is often a family history of visual loss and it is important to take a thorough family history in any cases presenting with this type of optic neuropathy. Prognosis is poor for most patients with LHON and the main treatment involves low vision assessments.

The differential diagnoses for bilateral sequential optic neuropathy include anterior ischaemic optic neuropathy (which tends to affect patients >40 years old who often have associated risk factors such as diabetes, atherosclerosis, or collagen vascular disorders such as systemic lupus erythematosus), and demyelination, which is a possibility in this man. It is always important to exclude neuromyelitis optica (NMO) in bilateral optic nerve disease but this man has no other neurological symptoms. It would be important to take a blood test for Aquaporin-4 antibody and consider a lumbar puncture.

Kim US, et al. Leber hereditary optic neuropathy-light at the end of the tunnel? *Asia Pac J Ophthalmol (Phila)* 2018;7:242–5.

40. Answer: D

Most ischaemic third nerve palsies show signs of recovery within 3 months. If there are any signs of aberrant regeneration in a third nerve palsy such as upper lid retraction and pupil constriction on eye movement, then an alternative diagnosis must be sought as this is often a sign of compression from a slow growing tumour such as meningioma in the cavernous sinus or aneurysm. Pupil-sparing with single muscle weakness is indicative of partial third nerve palsy, which may be a sign of compressive lesion. Third nerve palsy will not have any diurnal variation, unlike cases of ocular myasthenia.

Kung NH, Van Stavern GP. Isolated ocular motor nerve palsies. *Semin Neurol* 2015;35:539–48.

41. Answer: D

This man is describing blurring of vision in his inferior field of vision and therefore an inferior retinal detachment would give a superior field defect. He would usually also describe floaters and flashing lights. A macular haemorrhage would be more likely to give a central scotoma and more significant reduction in visual acuity. The most likely diagnosis in this case is non-arteritic anterior ischaemic optic neuropathy (NA-AION) and this is often associated with the 'disc-at-risk' where the cup-to-disc ratio is small and the disc often appears crowded and hyperaemic. Optic nerves affected by GCA can also be crowded, so other features need to be taken into account but a large cup-to-disc ratio would be uncommon with NA-AION.

Hayreh SS. Ischemic optic neuropathy. *Prog Retin Eye Res* 2009;28:34–62.

42. Answer: A

All patients with a partial third nerve palsy (e.g. partial ptosis, preservation of some eye movements supplied by the third nerve) that is pupil-sparing should undergo imaging with angiography of some type either CT angiogram or MR angiogram, particularly looking at the area of posterior communicating artery. This is because even if the patient is high risk for an ischaemic third nerve palsy (e.g. diabetes in this case), there is still a risk that the pupil may eventually dilate after compression from an aneurysm.

Saito R, et al. Pupil-sparing oculomotor nerve paresis as an early symptom of unruptured internal carotid-posterior communicating artery aneurysms: three case reports. *Neurol Med Chir (Tokyo)* 2008;48:304–6.

43. Answer: A

This clinical scenario describes a patient who is thin with possibly malnutrition. However, there is no option for questioning on the nutrition intake. The patient may have been suffering from a chronic illness such as tuberculosis. Therefore, before performing any further investigations, it is important to know if the patient had been taking any prescribed antituberculosis drugs as ethambutol can cause optic neuropathy which can present several months after commencing the drug.

Optic neuropathy may occur in 1% of patients taking ethambutol at the World Health Organization (WHO) recommended dose. Patients who develop symptoms or signs of ethambutol optic neuropathy should be referred to the ethambutol-prescribing physician immediately for discontinuation or dose reduction of the drug. Several studies have examined the potential value of optical coherence tomography in screening for ethambutol optic neuropathy (EON). There was reduction of retinal nerve fibre layer thickness in patients with clinically significant EON; however, its ability to detect such changes in patients taking ethambutol without visual symptoms has yet to be confirmed.

Chamberlain PD, et al. Ethambutol optic neuropathy. *Curr Opin Ophthalmol* 2017;28:545–51.

44. Answer: D

This is a clinical vignette of superior oblique myokymia (SOM), which is characterized by unilateral (often the right eye), low amplitude (less than 4°), high frequency (more than 50 Hz), torsional, nystagmoid movement of superior oblique muscle. It normally occurs in otherwise healthy individuals and is frequently triggered by fatigue, stress, or excessive caffeine intake. There is no definitive treatment for SOM but various medications, including topical/systemic β-blockers, carbamazepine, phenytoin, baclofen, gabapentin, memantine, botulinum toxin injections, have been tried with success. In some cases SOM may be linked with neurovascular compression of the trochlear nerve; therefore neuroimaging is recommended in recurrent or longstanding cases.

Zhang M, et al. Superior oblique myokymia. *Surv Ophthalmol* 2018;63:507–17.

45. Answer: A

Various factors have been reported in determining the risk of multiple sclerosis in patients with optic neuritis. Factors associated with lower risk of MS include:

1. Male sex
2. Optic disc swelling
3. Atypical optic neuritis features such as absent pain, vision is NPL, and severe disc swelling with haemorrhage

Essentially, patients presenting with typical symptoms of demyelinating optic neuritis have a higher risk of developing MS. In addition, the length of optic nerve being involved and involvement of intracanalicular segment are poor visual prognostic factors.

Optic Neuritis Study Group. Multiple sclerosis risk after optic neuritis final optic neuritis treatment trial follow-up. *Arch Neurol* 2008;65:727–32.

46. Answer: D

Right-sided, non-dominant, parietal lobe infarction may result in left-sided visual neglect and pie-on-the-floor visual field defect (inferior quadrantanopia) as opposed to pie in the sky visual field defect that is observed in temporal lobe infarction. Left-sided, dominant, parietal lobe infarction may result in Gerstmann's syndrome, which is characterized by left-right disorientation, finger agnosia (inability to name or recognize fingers), dysgraphia (inability to write), and dyscalculia (inability to calculate).

Ting DS, et al. Visual neglect following stroke: current concepts and future focus. *Surv Ophthalmol* 2011;56:114–34.

47. Answer: B

See-saw nystagmus is a rare ophthalmic manifestation with less than 50 cases reported in the literature. It is a type of disconjugate, torsional nystagmus in which one eye rises and intorts while the other eye falls and extorts in one cycle, and reverse in the next cycle. The most common cause is parasellar masses (including pituitary tumour, craniopharyngioma), mesodiencephalic disease, brainstem stroke, trauma, multiple sclerosis, and congenital disease.

Drachman DA. See-saw nystagmus. *J Neurol Neurosurg Psychiat* 1966;29:356–61.

48. Answer: C

Various fascicular third nerve syndromes have been described in the literature. Table 2.7 shows a summary of the four syndromes listed in the option.

Table 2.7 Various fascicular third nerve syndromes

Syndromes	Third nerve palsy + other features	Lesion site
Benedikt	Contralateral intention tremor	Red nucleus/paramedian midbrain
Claude	Contralateral ataxia	Midbrain
Nothnagel	Ipsilateral ataxia	Superior cerebellar peduncle
Weber	Contralateral hemiparesis	Cerebral peduncle

American Academy of Ophthalmology. *Acquired Oculomotor Nerve Palsy*, 2019. Available at: http://eyewiki.aao.org/Acquired_Oculomotor_Nerve_Palsy

49. Answer: C

Ischaemia is the most common cause of all acquired third cranial nerve palsies (around 40%) but in all cases of acquired third nerve palsy, an underlying aneurysm must be excluded as there is always this risk in all cases of third nerve palsy. A pupil-sparing third nerve palsy may well be ischaemic but partial third nerve palsy which is pupil-sparing may still be caused by an aneurysm. Both ischaemic and aneurysmal third nerve palsies may be painful. Patients with a third nerve palsy should all undergo imaging to exclude an aneurysm at the time of presentation.

Fang C, et al. Incidence and etiologies of acquired third nerve palsy using a population-based method. *JAMA Ophthalmol* 2017;135:23–8.

50. Answer: B

Parinaud dorsal midbrain syndrome is a neurological disorder caused by damage of the vertical gaze centre located at the rostral interstitial nucleus of medial longitudinal fasciculus. This results in a constellation of symptoms and signs, which can be remembered by the mnemonic '**DULL-PC**'. Saccadic movement is usually affected first followed by smooth pursuit and vestibulo-ocular reflex.

D—Downward gaze in primary position (sun-setting sign)
U—Upward gaze palsy
L—Light-near dissociation
L—Lid retraction (Collier's sign)
P—Papilloedema (commonly present)
C—Convergence retraction nystagmus

It is noteworthy to mention that the doll's head manoeuvre could elevate the eyes as this is a supranuclear palsy. The presence of light-near dissociation is due to the pretectal involvement of the lesion, resulting in more damage to the afferent light pathway with relatively preserved accommodative pathway; therefore, patients will have impaired pupillary light reflex but preserved near response. Convergence retraction nystagmus is best elicited on upgaze saccades, which can be brought on by asking the patient to track a downwardly rotating optokinetic drum. The co-contraction of all horizontal extraocular muscles results in inward pulling of the globe. As medial rectus is a stronger muscle than lateral rectus, a convergence movement is shown. The most common cause is dependent on the age group: pinealoma (children), multiple sclerosis (20s–30s), and upper brainstem stroke (elderly).

Feroze KB, Patel BC. Parinaud syndrome. In: *StatPearls* [Internet]. Treasure Island (FL): StatPearls Publishing 2018. Available at: https://www.ncbi.nlm.nih.gov/books/NBK441892/

51. Answer: D

This is a clinical vignette describing a patient with palinopsia, which is a visual phenomenon characterized by persistence or recurrence of visual images after the removal of initial stimulus. It may be caused by disease affecting the parieto-occipital pathway or some medications, including topiramate (an antiepileptic drug), trazadone, risperidone, mirtazapine, and acetazolamide. It was proposed that the increased serotonergic activity secondary to 5-HT_2 receptors of these medications predispose to the manifestation of palinopsia. Carbamazepine has been shown to effective in treating palinopsia.

Yun SH, et al. Topiramate-induced palinopsia: a case series and review of the literature. *J Neuroophthalmol* 2015;35:148–51.

52. Answer: D

LHON is a disease caused by point mutations in the mitochondrial DNA. The most important prognostic factor for visual recovery in patients with LHON is the gene mutation status. There are three main types of mutation:

(a) 14484 mutation: 37—71% chance of some degree of visual improvement
(b) 11778 mutation: 4% chance of improvement
(c) 3460 mutation: similar to 11778 but numbers are too small for comparison

Other positive prognostic factors include age of onset of <20 years, and especially <10 years of age.

Newman NJ. Treatment of Leber hereditary optic neuropathy. *Brain* 2011;134:2447–50.

53. Answer: B

Superior oblique (SO) palsy is a common cause of vertical strabismus. Bilateral SO palsy is most commonly due to trauma. There are five features that are suggestive of bilateral SO palsy. A useful mnemonic is '**CRAVE**':

C—Chin-down head posture
R—Reversing hyperdeviation on left gaze (R/L) and right gaze (L/R)
A—Adduction failure in depression
V—Prominent V pattern
E—Excyclotorsion >10°

Note that patients with bilateral SO palsy usually do not have a head tilt. Congenital SO palsy will have a large vertical prism fusion range and high concomitance as compared to new onset acquired lesion.

Kushner BJ. The diagnosis and treatment of bilateral masked superior oblique palsy. *Am J Ophthalmol* 1988;105:186–94.

54. Answer: D

At this presentation it is not possible to be certain of the definite diagnosis, so a tentative diagnosis of unexplained visual loss is the best diagnosis. Until further examination and investigations have been performed, you will not be able to offer a diagnosis. The patient could have any of the suggested diagnoses, so it is best to wait until further tests are available. Often at the onset of optic neuritis there is a more gradual visual loss rather than immediately presenting with NPL but there are cases described with this presentation. LHON rarely presents with sudden loss of vision but often there is not a RAPD at presentation so this diagnosis should still be considered. In addition, there may be optic nerve head crowding/oedema with telangiectatic vessels visible on fundus examination. Most patients with CRAO usually have a RAPD at presentation, especially if the vision is NPL.

Griffiths PG, Ali N. Medically unexplained visual loss in adult patients. *Curr Opin Neurol* 2009;22:41–5.

55. Answer: C

CMV causes significant morbidity and mortality in immunocompromised individuals. Systemic antiviral therapy with adjunctive intravitreal therapy is the standard approach. Intraocular treatment alone (Option A) is only appropriate if systemic therapy is strongly contraindicated such as severe myelosuppression or nephrotoxicity. Systemic treatment protects the other eye. Systemic antiviral therapies for CMV are ganciclovir, valganciclovir, foscarnet, cidofovir, and leflunomide. Valganciclovir is an oral pro-drug and avoids intravenous administration needed for ganciclovir. Foscarnet is the standard intravitreal medication used in the United Kingdom (ganciclovir is an alternative agent). Intravenous acyclovir or high-dose valaciclovir (the oral pro-drug) are used to treat herpes simples and varicella zoster acute retinal necrosis (ARN). In ARN there is evidence that combined systemic and intravitreal therapy may yield greater therapeutic efficacy than systemic treatment alone. All systemic antiviral drugs have significant toxicity profiles and require monitoring: valganciclovir is myelotoxic and nephrotoxic and foscarnet and cidofovir are nephrotoxic.

Port AD, et al. Cytomegalovirus retinitis: a review. *J Ocul Pharmacol Ther* 2017;33:224–34.

Schoenberger SD, et al. Diagnosis and treatment of acute retinal necrosis: a report by the American Academy of Ophthalmology. *Ophthalmology* 2017;124:382–92.

56. Answer: B

UK NICE guidelines for diabetic control are available. Candidates are not expected to recall these guidelines in detail but should have an understanding for the FRCOphth of HbA1C interpretation to counsel patients appropriately. In type 2 diabetes, for patients on diet/lifestyle management +/– single oral drug therapy the target HbA1C is <48 mol/mol. The level here is therefore suboptimal and diet and lifestyle advice are appropriate, and drug modification by the patient's physician may be necessary. In those with drug hypoglycaemia, the target is relaxed to a target level of 53 mmol/mol. Levels <48 mmol/mol represent good control. In patients on a single drug with HbA1C >58 mmol/mol intervention with diet lifestyle/drug intervention is recommended to a target of 53 mmol/mol.

National Institute of Health and Care Excellence (NICE). *Type 2 Diabetes in Adults: NICE Guideline [NG28]*, 2015. Available at: https://www.nice.org.uk/guidance/ng28/chapter/recommendations#dietary-advice-2

57. Answer: D

DEXA bone T score compares the bone density against a normal, healthy young female adult. A T score of –2.6 SD indicates osteoporosis. Glucocorticosteroids increase the risk of fracture of the hip and spine and loss of bone mineral density. In the United Kingdom, the femoral neck T score is used to calculate fracture risk, using an online tool called FRAX® (available online). Important clinical risk factors considered in the FRAX assessment are low body mass index (BMI), lack of weight-bearing exercise, smoking, and alcohol (>3 u/day), secondary causes of osteoporosis, history of fragility fractures, and family history of hip fracture and osteoporosis. In general, DEXA bone scan is recommended for those exposed/anticipated to continuous oral corticosteroid (any dose) for >3 months.

The National Osteoporosis Guideline Group (NOG, March 2017; see Table 2.8) recommends with regard to glucocorticoid-induced osteoporosis:

- Women and men age >70 years with a previous fragility fracture, or taking high doses of glucocorticoids (>7.5 mg/day prednisolone), should be considered for bone protective therapy.
- In other individuals fracture probability should be estimated using FRAX with adjustment for glucocorticoid dose.
- Bone protective treatment should be started at the onset of glucocorticoid therapy in individuals at high risk of fracture.
- Alendronate and risedronate are first-line treatment options.

Table 2.8 Bone densitometry scores

T score	Condition
0 to −1 SD	Normal
−1 SD to −2.5 SD	Osteopenia
Below −2.5 SD	Osteoporosis

NOGG 2017: Clinical guideline for the prevention and treatment of osteoporosis. Available online at https://www.sheffield.ac.uk/NOGG/NOGG%20Guideline%202017.pdf

FRAX Fracture Risk Assessment Tool. Available at: https://www.sheffield.ac.uk/FRAX/

58. Answer: A

Lyme borreliosis is a tick-borne bacterial infection. *B. burgdorferi* is inoculated via a tick bite. After a period of days to 3 weeks, the typical primary lesion, erythema migrans, commences. The lesion has a target appearance with erythema and induration at the centre (the tick bite) and at the spreading margin. The appearance is unique and can be used to diagnose Lyme disease, supplemented by serological testing. *B. henselae* is responsible for cat-scratch disease; the associated ocular diseases are oculoglandular syndrome, keratitis, neuroretinitis, and uveitis, and a pustular reaction may be seen at the entry site (caused by cat-scratch). *L. interrogans* is associated with a macular skin rash and *T. pallidum*, which causes syphilis, is associated with a painful chancre at the primary stage and in the secondary stages, maculopapular rash (usually on the trunk), maculopapular eruptions on the soles and palms, and condylomata.

Bush LM, Vazquez-Pertejo MT. Tick borne illness-Lyme disease. *Dis Mon* 2018;64:195–212.

59. Answer: C

The key here is avoiding confusion between the Budd–Chiari and Arnold–Chiari syndromes. The latter involves anatomical anomaly at the foramen magnum predisposing to cerebellar tonsillar descent and potential brain stem compression. Budd–Chiari syndrome refers to thrombosis of the hepatic portal vein. In a young male with arthritis and a major vessel thrombosis, Behçet's disease, which is a well-recognized cause of dural sinus thrombosis, should be near the top of the differential.

Yazici H, et al. Behcet syndrome: a contemporary view. *Nat Rev Rheumatol* 2018;14:107–19.

60. Answer: B

The concern here is pre-eclamptic toxaemia a condition that affects 3–5% of pregnancies and is characterized by development of new onset hypertension in the second half of pregnancy and proteinuria. Blood pressure tends to run lower in pregnancy with readings above 140/90 sufficient to diagnose hypertension. Widespread endothelial dysfunction relating to arterioles causes damage to vascular beds. Posterior reversible encephalopathy syndrome caused by pre-eclamptic cortical oedema (which will be highlighted on MRI brain) is a well-recognized cause of visual loss in this condition, however, a more marked drop in acuity would be expected in cortical blindness. Diabetes either arising *de novo* in pregnancy (gestational diabetes) or gestational acceleration of established diabetes would be more likely to produce blot haemorrhages, microaneurysms, and exudates rather than the features described which are typical of hypertensive retinopathy. Purtscher (traumatic cause) or Purtscher-like (non-traumatic cause) retinopathy is a type of microvascular occlusive retinal disease characterized by cotton wool spots, Purtscher flecken (pathognomonic sign), and retinal haemorrhages. The findings are usually centred around peripapillary area.

Tadin I, et al. Hypertensive retinopathy and pre-eclampsia. *Coll Antropol* 2001;25Suppl:77–81.

61. Answer: A

Hemifacial spasm (HFS) is a sporadic, rarely autosomal dominant, condition characterized by involuntary synchronous tonic and/or clonic contraction of facial muscles. It is caused by dysfunctional facial nerve usually as a result of anomalous vascular compression of the facial nerve, which can be visualized on high resolution MRI. The anterior inferior cerebellar artery and posterior inferior cerebellar artery are the most common compressing single vessels. It has a female predominance with a peak onset of 40–60 years of age.

Green KE, et al. Treatment of blepharospasm/hemifacial spasm. *Curr Treat Options Neurol* 2017;19:41.

62. Answer: C

This patient is in anaphylactic shock. The cause here is anaphylaxis on the basis of recent exposure to an allergen (fluorescein dye), the presence of an urticarial skin rash with acute cardiovascular compromise, and an urticarial skin rash. The correct answer is dependent on familiarity with the management of acute anaphylaxis. While less severe reactions (for adults) may be treated with intravenous (IV) 200 mg hydrocortisone and intravenous 10 mg chlorphenamine, this patient is in anaphylactic shock. The UK Resuscitation Council Guidelines emphasize the early use of intramuscular (IM) adrenaline in anaphylaxis, usually the dose is 0.5 mg (0.5 ml of adrenaline 1:1000). IV adrenaline should only be used by personnel with specialist training. Once IM adrenaline has been given, an IV fluid bolus of crystalloid fluid is recommended. Colloids should ideally be avoided in the context of allergy as they may contain potential allergens.

UK Resuscitation Council Guidelines. *Anaphylaxis*, 2008. Available at: https://www.resus.org.uk/anaphylaxis/emergency-treatment-of-anaphylactic-reactions/

63. Answer: B

Saddle nose deformity results from a depression caused by a decrease in the structural support of the cartilaginous or bony framework deep to the nasal soft tissue envelope. It can be caused by various conditions, including trauma, surgery, inflammatory diseases (e.g. granulomatosis with polyangiitis, relapsing polychondritis, sarcoidosis, and Crohn's disease), and infection (e.g. syphilis, leprosy, and septal abscesses).

Pribitkin EA, Ezzat WH. Classification and treatment of the saddle nose deformity. *Otolaryngol Clin North Am* 2009;42:437–61.

64. Answer: A

Tyrosinase is responsible for melanin synthesis and absence or reduced tyrosinase will lead to albinism. Fabry's disease is caused by deficiency in alpha-galactosidase A. Galactosaemia is caused by deficiency in galactose-1-phosphate uridyltransferase, whereas Refsum disease is caused by deficiency in phytanic acid alpha-hydrolase.

Poll-The BT, et al. The eye in metabolic diseases: clues to diagnosis. *Eur J Paediatr Neurol* 2011;15:197–204.

65. Answer: A

Pituitary adenoma represents 12–15% of symptomatic intracranial tumour. They usually occur in adults, rarely in childhood, and are mostly isolated but 3% are associated with multiple endocrine neoplasia type 1. They can be divided into macroadenoma (10 mm or more) vs. microadenoma (<10 mm), or functioning vs. non-functioning tumours. Functioning tumours are associated with hormonal secretion; therefore, they are detected earlier and smaller (microadenoma). The most common type is prolactinoma followed by growth hormone-secreting adenoma. Prolactinoma can result in gynaecomastia, amenorrhoea, and galactorrhoea (known as 'Forbes-Albright syndrome') and infertility in women and gynaecomastia, hypogonadism, and impotence in men. The treatment for prolactinoma is bromocriptine—a dopamine agonist—which inhibits the release of prolactin.

On the other hand, non-functioning tumours do not produce excess hormone and may cause hypopituitarism due to mass effect. The most common type is gonadotrophic adenoma. Most ophthalmologic symptoms and signs are secondary to mass effects caused by macroadenoma.

Patients with pituitary adenoma need to be referred to Endocrinology immediately as many patients develop pan-hypopituitarism and need a full review of all the hormone levels. Many patients have a functioning pituitary adenoma which responds to medical treatment and early intervention ensures less comorbidity such as hypertension and cardiovascular disease. If the pituitary tumour is non-functioning, then the patient would be referred for surgery.

Oki Y. Medical management of functioning pituitary adenoma: an update. *Neurol Med Chir (Tokyo)* 2014;54:958–65.

66. Answer: D

Zika virus is an arbovirus primarily transmitted to humans via the *Aedes* genus mosquito. It can lead to Guillain–Barré syndrome and congenital birth abnormalities, including neurologic, ophthalmic, audiologic, and skeletal abnormalities (now called CZS). Around 70% of the patients will some form of ocular abnormalities. Posterior segment abnormalities such as loss of retinal pigment epithelium, perivascular choroidal inflammatory infiltrates, chorioretinal atrophy, and retinal haemorrhages, are the most common ophthalmic findings in CZS. Other ophthalmic abnormalities include iris coloboma, glaucoma, cataract, and lens subluxation findings. Currently there is no licensed vaccine or treatment for Zika viral infection.

de Oliveira Dias JR, et al. Zika and the eye: pieces of a puzzle. *Prog Retin Eye Res* 2018;66:85–106.

67. Answer: C

All the options listed are syndromic forms of albinism. Chédiak–Higashi syndrome (CHS) is a rare autosomal recessive disorder characterized by recurrent severe pyogenic infections, progressive neurologic abnormality, and mucosal disease. The many 'i's in the name of the syndrome can help candidates to link the disease to **I**nfection. Griscelli syndrome is characterized by neurologic deficit, with or without immunologic impairment. It is distinguished from CHS by the lack of giant intracellular granules seen in CHS. Hermansky–**P**udlak syndrome is **p**latelet deficiency (resulting in bleeding), **p**ulmonary disease, and granulomatous colitis. Waardenburg syndrome is characterized by iris heterochromia, broad nasal root, and white forelock.

American Academy of Ophthalmology. *Albinism*, 2014. Available at: http://eyewiki.aao.org/Albinism

68. Answer: D

These are several interesting visual phenomenon/syndromes that the candidates should be familiar with. Anton syndrome refers to patients with cortical blindness who deny their blindness. This is due to bilateral retrochiasmal visual pathway diseases such as bilateral occipital lobe infarction. Blue field entoptic phenomenon describes the phenomenon of multiple tiny dots moving rapidly along wavy lines in the visual field, which is caused by the moving white blood cells within the superficial retinal capillaries. Charles Bonnet syndrome refers to formed and unformed visual hallucination in patients with bilateral poor vision. They usually have good insights when they are experiencing hallucination. Pulfrich phenomenon refers to patients seeing targets moving towards them when the targets are moving perpendicular to the line of sight (i.e. laterally). It usually occurs in optic nerve diseases. Riddoch phenomenon refers to the preserved awareness of moving but not stationary stimuli.

Arcaro MJ, et al. Psychophysical and neuroimaging responses to moving stimuli in a patient with the Riddoch phenomenon due to bilateral visual cortex lesions. *Neuropsychologia* 2018; pii: S0028-3932(18):30204-5.

69. Answer: A

Migraine is a debilitating chronic neurologic disorder with a global prevalence of 12%. It is more common in female than male, with an estimated ratio of 3:1. Migraine is typically unilateral, pulsating, moderate-severe pain, lasting 4–72 hours, and associated with nausea and/or vomiting or photophobia/phonophobia. The criteria for migraine with aura are defined by at least two typical attacks of migraine with some form of aura symptoms (e.g. visual, sensory, motor, etc.). A recent meta-analysis found an increased risk of ischaemic stroke and myocardial infarction in patients with migraine with aura.

Meir RW, Dhadwal S. Primary headaches. *Dent Clin North Am* 2018;62:611–28.

Vgontzas A, Burch R. Episodic migraine with and without aura: key differences and implications for pathophysiology, management and assessing risks. *Curr Pain Headache Rep* 2018;22:78.

chapter 3

CLINICAL OPHTHALMOLOGY 3

QUESTIONS

1. **Which of the following statements about childhood sight impairment in the United Kingdom is true?**
    A. The prevalence of childhood amblyopia with an acuity worse than LogMAR 0.3 is 5%
    B. The mortality rate among children in the year following diagnosis of severe visual impairment is 1%
    C. Annual age group specific incidence childhood visual impairment was reported to be highest in the first year of life
    D. Congenital cataract remains an important cause of severe sight impairment

2. **Which of the following statement regarding Sturge–Weber syndrome (SWS) is correct?**
    A. Ocular changes are seen in over 75% of patients on the ipsilateral side to the port wine stain
    B. The incidence of SWS without port wine stain is 10%
    C. 90% of the glaucoma cases seen in SWS patients are of congenital or early onset
    D. Choroidal haemangioma is seen in up to 25%

3. **Which of the following eyes with retinopathy of prematurity can be followed conservatively?**
    A. Zone 1, Stage 3 with Plus disease
    B. Zone 1, Stage 3 without Plus disease
    C. Zone 2, Stage 3 without Plus disease
    D. Zone 2, Stage 2, with Plus disease

4. **The minimum required diagnostic criteria to diagnose congenital (infantile) esotropia is:**
    A. The range of the angle of strabismus is 40–50 prism dioptres
    B. Some children neurological status is abnormal
    C. The refractive error correction eliminates strabismus in some children
    D. Asymmetric optokinetic nystagmus characterized by robust temporal to nasal response and erratic nasal to temporal response

5. **These are the features of Sticklers syndrome, EXCEPT:**
   A. Stickler syndrome is usually autosomal dominant and caused by type 2 collagen abnormality
   B. Stickler syndrome type III is commonly associated with ocular problems
   C. Up to 10% may develop glaucoma
   D. Stickler syndrome is the leading cause of retinal detachment in children, and retinal tears or detachments occur in up to 50% of sufferers

6. **Congenital cataract features include:**
   A. Persistent fetal vasculature can be associated with a posterior plaque outside or involving the posterior capsule of a clear lens
   B. Posterior polar cataract is genetically determined with autosomal recessive the common mode of inheritance
   C. Posterior subcapsular opacities involve the cortex and posterior capsule
   D. Spontaneous rupture of the posterior lenticonus is common and results in total hydrated cataract

7. **Which of the following type of strabismus is usually associated with stable angle of deviation?**
   A. Convergence excess esotropia
   B. Microtropia
   C. Nystagmus blockage syndrome
   D. Uncorrected anisometropia

8. **The standard management option for type II Duane syndrome includes:**
   A. Surgery of the extraocular muscle can eliminate innervation abnormality in some cases
   B. Abnormal head posture can be corrected by surgery in over 80% of the cases
   C. Surgery is commonly performed to improve fusion
   D. Prisms commonly used to treat anomalous head posture

9. **The characteristics features of juvenile X-linked retinoschisis include:**
   A. DNA sequencing detects RS1 mutation in 50% of cases
   B. Electronegative electroretinogram (ERG) is seen in both focal and macular ERG and full-field ERG
   C. In X-linked juvenile retinoschisis, optical coherence tomography (OCT) reveals cystic spaces primarily in the outer nuclear and inner plexiform layers of the retina
   D. Fluorescein angiography may reveal leakage at the macula cystic area

10. Which of the following statements concerning primary congenital glaucoma is true?

A. Primary congenital glaucoma occurs sporadically and is familial in less than 5% of cases
B. Epiphora is present on first presentation in under 5% of children with primary congenital glaucoma
C. Neuroretinal rim thinning preferentially occurs superiorly and inferiorly resulting in vertical cupping of the disc
D. Ketamine has little effect on the intraocular pressure measurement during examination under anaesthesia

11. A seven-year girl presents to the eye emergency department with sudden onset of convergent squint. Her management options include:

A. Base-in prisms on the contralateral side
B. Bimedial recession as an urgent procedure
C. Botox on the ipsilateral lateral rectus muscle
D. Cycloplegic refraction and prescribe glasses

12. Which of the following features of congenital monocular elevation deficiency (MED) is correct?

A. The affected eye is commonly the fixating eye
B. Hypotropia of the affected eye on the affected side present as orthophoria in primary gaze
C. It is usually due to inferior oblique weakness
D. Chin-down as compensatory head position

13. Which of the following features of strabismus is usually observed in thyroid eye disease?

A. Inferior rectus is the most commonly affected extraocular muscle with hypertropia as the presenting feature
B. Pain with eye movement is seen in at least 30% of affected patient
C. During superior rectus recession, connection points between the superior rectus and upper eyelid elevators improve upper eyelid retraction
D. The order of surgery is orbital decompression followed by corrective eyelid procedures then strabismus surgery

14. A nine-year-old child presents with intermittent right divergent squint and she measures 45 prism dioptres base-in for distance and 20 dioptres base-in for near. Her ocular movements are full. Factors taken into consideration during management plan include:

A. Tenacious proximal fusion in addition to AC/A ratio play important roles in distance/near discrepancy
B. Both distance and near stereopsis is normal during the manifest phase
C. Magnitude of deviation is the single factor that gives information about the 'quality' of control
D. Evidence of fusion in the presence of a manifest deviation is indicative of normal correspondence

15. An 18-month-old child has been referred with sudden onset of strabismus and abnormal red reflex. On examination a solid unilateral retinal lesion is identified and a provisional diagnosis of retinoblastoma is made. Which of the following statements regarding management of retinoblastoma is correct?
    A. The primary objective in the management is to preserve vision
    B. Unilateral tumour stage III, IV, and V are generally managed with enucleation
    C. Bilateral tumours are treated with chemoreduction for at least one of their two involved eyes
    D. Plaque radiotherapy is generally reserved for small tumours less than 3 mm in size

16. Which of the following statements about rhabdomyosarcoma is correct?
    A. The most common extracranial solid childhood tumour
    B. Embryonal and alveolar subtypes have distinct genetic alterations that may play in the pathogenesis of the tumours
    C. Orbital tumours are more likely to have alveolar histologic subtype
    D. Orbital tumours commonly present with ophthalmoplegia

17. Kearns–Sayre syndrome features include:
    A. Onset before 8 years of age
    B. Cerebellar syndrome
    C. Cerebrospinal fluid protein level greater than 10 mg/dL
    D. Cardiomyopathy

18. A 26-year-old female presents to an eye department with vertical diplopia and defective elevation of the eye. The feature that is suggestive of acquired Brown syndrome include:
    A. Diplopia when the patient looks up and to the ipsilateral side
    B. Lack of significant hypotropia observed in the primary position
    C. Compensatory head posture with chin down and ipsilateral face turn
    D. Audible or palpable click on ocular rotations up and contralateral side

19. Which of the following statements about neurofibromatosis type 1 is correct?
    A. More than 50% of patients with NF1 have learning difficulties
    B. Lab tests are useful in the diagnosis of NF1
    C. Lisch nodules is the most characteristic feature in children over six years of age
    D. Choroidal hamartomas are well-defined, elevated lesions found in the midperiphery of the retina

20. **Which of the following features describes the acute phase in Leber's hereditary optic neuropathy?**
    A. Bilateral simultaneous acute loss of vision
    B. Visual loss is severely reduced to 6/60 or less in two weeks
    C. Central scotoma is the characteristic field defect
    D. Pupillary reflexes are preserved

21. **Which of the following statements regarding the management of congenital fibrosis of extraocular muscles (CFEOM) is true?**
    A. Successful surgery at a young age may avoid the loss of vision in one or both eyes
    B. The order of management is to correct the lid position followed by strabismus surgery
    C. One of the goals of the surgery is to eliminate abnormal eye movements
    D. Forced duction test has very limited value in the management of CFEOM

22. **A two-and-a-half-year-old child presents to the eye department with a squint. On examination her near angle of deviation was 45 prism dioptres (PD) and her distant angle of deviation was 30 PD. Her refractive error was +2.25 D in each eye after cycloplegic refraction. Her ocular movements were full. What is the most likely working diagnosis?**
    A. Early onset esotropia
    B. Non-refractive accommodative esotropia
    C. Partial accommodative esotropia
    D. Refractive accommodative esotropia

23. **Which of the following features is most commonly seen in child with X-linked ocular albinism?**
    A. Compound myopic astigmatism
    B. Positive-angle Kappa
    C. Normal binocular function
    D. Progressive reduction in visual acuity

24. **A newborn is referred with tense, non-pulsatile swelling located below the medial canthus. The immediate management include:**
    A. Liaise with paediatrician and commence systemic antibiotics as prophylaxis as the risk of secondary infection is high
    B. Observe for 2 weeks, during which time most spontaneously improve
    C. Organize an urgent MRI scan to make an accurate diagnosis
    D. Surgical treatment is necessary to remove the swelling in most cases

25. In a 6-year-old child with an orbital floor fracture due to blunt trauma of the inferior orbital rim you would expect:
    A. Red inflamed eye
    B. Restricted upgaze
    C. No vomiting or fainting
    D. No long-term sequelae with conservative management

26. In acute severe traumatic optic neuropathy (TON) with associated with major head trauma, which of the following statements is most likely to be true?
    A. Computed tomography (CT) of the optic canal is commonly abnormal
    B. Fundoscopy is commonly abnormal
    C. High-dose steroids are indicated
    D. Intervention is unlikely to result in improvement

27. Which of the following signs would you expect to see in a patient presenting with a suspected direct carotico-cavernous fistula (CCF) after a deceleration injury but not in a spontaneous indirect CCF?
    A. Acute painful proptosis
    B. Cranial bruit
    C. Dilated episcleral vessels
    D. Raised intraocular pressure (IOP)

28. Which individual variable at presentation is the strongest predictor of visual outcome using the ocular trauma score (OTS)?
    A. Endophthalmitis
    B. Globe rupture
    C. Presence of relative afferent pupillary defect
    D. Visual acuity

29. Which of the following features is pathognomonic for abusive head trauma (or shaken baby syndrome)?
    A. Haemorrhagic retinoschisis
    B. Trilaminar retinal haemorrhages
    C. Perimacular folds
    D. No pathognomonic sign has been identified

30. A patient is shot in the face with a shot gun. The eye is hypotonous with a total hyphaema so there is no fundal view. On CT scan the globe appears disrupted with metallic foreign bodies in the retro-orbital space but no intraocular foreign body. Which of the following best classifies her ocular injury according to the Birmingham Eye Trauma Terminology system (BETT)?
    A. Lamellar laceration
    B. Penetrating laceration
    C. Perforating laceration
    D. Ruptured globe

31. A 4-year-old child presents as an emergency with a 2-day history of unilateral periocular swelling, redness, and proptosis. Which of the following is **NOT** an essential emergency investigation?
    A. Full blood count
    B. Temperature
    C. Plain film X-ray face
    D. Weight

32. Which of the following is most commonly found in ptosis secondary to aponeurotic dehiscence?
    A. Low skin crease
    B. Normal levator function
    C. Reduced Bell's phenomenon
    D. Reduced marginal reflex distance (MRD)-2

33. Which of the following is the commonest cause of trichiasis worldwide?
    A. Entropion
    B. Ocular cicatricial pemphigoid (OCP)
    C. Steven–Johnson syndrome (SJS)
    D. Trachoma

34. A 53-year-old lady, with a background of asthma, presented with a 5-day history of periorbital inflammation, initially thought to be cellulitis but non-responsive to antibiotics. She rapidly developed proptosis and restricted eye movements. CT orbits showed inflammatory stranding throughout periorbital and intraconal fat, and oedema of the extraocular muscles. Orbital biopsy of the rectus muscles and orbital fat showed eosinophilic rich infiltration extending through the walls of medium-sized blood vessels with extravascular granulomas. Which of the following is the most likely diagnosis?
    A. Churg–Strauss syndrome
    B. Granulomatosis with polyangiitis (GPA)
    C. Idiopathic orbital inflammatory disease
    D. Sarcoidosis

35. Which of the following is associated with type 2 blepharophimosis syndrome?
    A. Epicanthus tarsalis
    B. Gene mutation in *FOXL2*
    C. Primary ovarian failure
    D. Increased interpupillary distance

36. Which of the following is the recommended management of dysthyroid optic neuropathy (DON)?
    A. Intravenous steroid
    B. Oral steroid
    C. Radiotherapy
    D. Selenium

37. Which of the following investigations must be performed prior to surgery for upper lid ptosis in an 8-year old child with neurofibromatosis type 1 (NF1)?
    A. Clotting assay
    B. CT orbits
    C. MRI orbits
    D. Visual field test (VFT)

38. In a patient treated for myasthenia with long-term oral steroids, which of the following would be the best regime for steroid cover for a patient undergoing ptosis correction?
    A. 100 mg intramuscular hydrocortisone just before the local anaesthetic
    B. 100 mg intravenous hydrocortisone just before the local anaesthetic
    C. Double oral dose for 24 hours postoperative
    D. 100 mg intramuscular hydrocortisone just before the local anaesthetic and double oral dose for 24 hours postoperative

39. A 48-year-old male presents with a 6-day history of unilateral 2 mm proptosis and painful eye movements with mild upper lid swelling and ptosis. For which of the following radiological appearances would it be appropriate to undertake a therapeutic trial of steroids without orbital biopsy?
   A. Single muscle enlargement on MRI
   B. Adjacent sinus mucosal thickening
   C. Diffuse contrast enhanced orbital signal on MRI with extension though the superior orbital fissure
   D. Enlarged lacrimal gland on CT

40. During a surgical decompression for acute compressive optic neuropathy which of the paranasal sinuses will **NOT** be entered?
   A. Ethmoid
   B. Frontal
   C. Maxillary
   D. Sphenoid

41. A 52-year-old Caucasian male patient, with a background of treated colonic cancer, is referred to the oculoplastic clinic for a growing eyelid lesion. He has a strong family history for colonic cancer. Ophthalmic examination reveals lid changes suggestive of sebaceous cell carcinoma. What is the most likely diagnosis?
   A. Bazex syndrome
   B. Gardner syndrome
   C. Gorlin–Golz syndrome
   D. Muir–Torre syndrome

42. Which of the following is the best indicator of activity in thyroid eye disease?
   A. Diplopia
   B. Upper lid oedema
   C. Pain
   D. Reduced colour vision

43. A 40-year-old female presents with a 3-month history of painful swelling in the superotemporal quadrant of the left orbit. She undergoes an incision biopsy which demonstrates glandular tubules with lumina, excess basement membrane and mucin, and islands of anaplastic cells without squamous differentiation. Which of the following is the most likely diagnosis?
   A. Adenoid cystic carcinoma
   B. Dacryoadenitis
   C. Pleomorphic adenoma
   D. Sarcoidosis

44. A 62-year-old patient is listed for post-Mohs reconstruction of the lower lid following Mohs excision of a basal cell carcinoma (BCC). The original tumour size measured 8 mm diameter but was clinically well circumscribed. Which best describes the likely choice of reconstruction for an anticipated full thickness lid defect?
   A. Direct closure
   B. Full thickness skin graft
   C. Hughes tarsoconjunctival flap
   D. Mustarde cheek rotation flap

45. What is the most common cause of unilateral axial proptosis in a 45-year-old man?
   A. Cavernous haemangioma
   B. Lymphoproliferative disease
   C. Orbital inflammatory disease
   D. Thyroid eye disease

46. An MRI is done for investigation of headaches in an otherwise fit and healthy 52-year-old female. A well circumscribed intraconal 20 mm round lesion is noted in the orbits. It is homogenous, high signal on T2. Which of the following is the most likely diagnosis?
   A. Cavernous haemangioma
   B. Metastasis from a breast primary
   C. Pleomorphic adenoma
   D. Solitary fibrous tumour

47. Which of the following is **NOT** currently recommended for 7 mm superficial BCC located in the upper lid?
   A. Mohs micrographical surgical excision
   B. Radiotherapy
   C. Surgical excision with 3–4 mm margin
   D. Topical imiquimod

48. In a patient with an isolated lacrimal gland mass, what test would be the most sensitive to differentiate between lymphoma and orbital inflammatory disease (OID)?
   A. Contrast enhanced MRI
   B. Orbital biopsy
   C. Serum LDH
   D. Steroid response

49. Which of the following statements about orbital rhabdomyosarcoma is correct?
   A. Most commonly occurs between first and second decade of life
   B. Most commonly located in the superotemporal quadrant
   C. Most commonly of embryonal cell type
   D. Most commonly arises from extraocular muscles

50. Which of the following is recommended for 6-monthly follow-up of patients who have had enucleation for ocular melanoma?
   A. CT abdomen
   B. PET CT
   C. Serological liver function tests
   D. Ultrasound of the liver

51. A 30-year-old male patient has a history of treated unilateral retinoblastoma. What is the chance of his children developing retinoblastoma?
   A. 1%
   B. 7%
   C. 15%
   D. 40%

52. Which of the following features of choroidal naevus is associated with increased risk of transformation to choroidal melanoma?
   A. Absence of ultrasonographic hollowness
   B. Absence of halo
   C. Tumour thickness of 1 mm
   D. Presence of drusen

53. A 26-year-old female presents with an acute unilateral visual loss. The visual acuity in the affected eye is 6/30 with a relative afferent pupillary defect (RAPD), numerous grey/white retinal lesions at the posterior pole (<100 μm in size), and optic disc swelling. There are no anterior chamber or vitreous cells. The fellow eye is normal. The patient is systemically well but describes a flu-type illness prior to the onset of visual symptoms. What is the most likely diagnosis?
   A. Acute posterior multifocal placoid pigment epitheliopathy (APMPPE)
   B. Birdshot chorioretinopathy
   C. Multiple evanescent white dot syndrome (MEWDS)
   D. Punctate inner choroidopathy (PIC)

54. A 28-year old male presents with a history of recurrent unilateral anterior uveitis. He has evidence of posterior synechiae and an irregular, large pupil. Iris retroillumination demonstrates marked sectoral iris atrophy. The vitreous is clear. The other eye is normal. What is the most likely diagnosis?
    A. Fuchs' heterochromic uveitis
    B. Herpetic uveitis
    C. Human leukocyte antigen-B27 (HLA-B27)-related uveitis
    D. Ocular sarcoidosis

55. The Standardization of Uveitis Nomenclature (SUN) grading system includes which of the following criteria?
    A. Granulomatous keratitic precipitates
    B. Macular oedema
    C. Vitreous cells
    D. Vitreous haze

56. A 28-year-old Caucasian male presents with his first episode of uveitis. He is found to have unilateral panuveitis with a mobile hypopyon and a focus of retinitis associated with vasculitis. His past medical history includes deep vein thrombosis and pustular skin lesions. What is the most likely diagnosis?
    A. Behçet's disease
    B. Herpetic uveitis
    C. HLA-B27 related uveitis
    D. Syphilis

57. Which of the following HLA types is associated with birdshot chorioretinopathy?
    A. HLA-A29
    B. HLA-B27
    C. HLA-B51
    D. HLA-DR1

58. A 68-year-old female patient presents with severe bilateral necrotizing anterior scleritis and has a history of chronic sinusitis. There is no evidence of intraocular inflammation. She describes recent onset weight loss, epistaxis, arthralgia, haemoptysis, and chronic cough. A CT chest shows evidence of a cavitating pulmonary lesion. Routine inflammatory markers are elevated and renal impairment is detected. Quantiferon test is negative. What is the most likely diagnosis?
    A. Granulomatosis with polyangiitis
    B. Lupus-associated scleritis
    C. Rheumatoid arthritis-associated scleritis
    D. Tuberculosis-associated scleritis

59. The following are appropriate treatment regimes in toxoplasma uveitis, **EXCEPT**:
    A. Observation alone for a peripheral focus of toxoplasma retinitis
    B. Oral clindamycin plus oral corticosteroid
    C. Oral spiramycin during pregnancy
    D. Oral steroid alone in a patient with allergy to co-trimoxazole

60. A 36-year-old male presents with a 5-day history of ocular pain, redness, and photophobia affecting his left eye. He reports generalized malaise of several months' duration, abdominal discomfort, oral and perianal ulceration, and has had to give up running as this causes pain under the ball of his right foot. Examination reveals an acute left anterior uveitis complicated by hypopyon and posterior synechiae. His erythrocyte sedimentation rate (ESR) and C-reactive protein (CRP) are both elevated. Which of the following is the most likely diagnosis?
    A. Behçet's disease
    B. Crohn's disease
    C. Infectious endogenous endophthalmitis
    D. Ulcerative colitis

61. Which of the following features is characteristic of Fuchs' heterochromic cyclitis?
    A. Absence of vitritis
    B. Inferiorly located stellate keratic precipitates
    C. Presence of posterior synechiae
    D. Usually asymptomatic

62. A 58-year-old gentleman underwent retinal detachment repair to the right eye 4 months previously. Unfortunately, this was complicated by severe postoperative inflammation, requiring medication with high-dose systemic corticosteroids. Following the tapering of the steroids, he developed sympathetic ophthalmia of the left eye. He is now established on immunosuppression and attends for regular follow-up visit. He has developed gastrointestinal (GI) upset on mycophenolate mofetil and feels nauseous. The left anterior segment is quiet and there is no vitritis. The OCT of his left eye is shown in Figure 3.1A.
   A. He will need to increase his oral immunosuppressive medication
   B. He will need to be treated with pulsed intravenous methylprednisolone or equivalent
   C. His systemic symptoms will subside as he perseveres with his medication; his ocular inflammation is well controlled
   D. The inflammation affecting the left eye will settle once the right eye is enucleated

63. A 65-year-old type 1 diabetic female inpatient is referred to the eye clinic for 2 days' history of right eye pain with worsening blurred vision. She is currently being treated for a liver abscess. She denied past ocular history of trauma or surgery. Examination confirms vision 6/60 in the right eye with hypopyon anterior uveitis. There are no granulomatous features. Mydriatic examination reveals intense vitritis through which fundus haemorrhages in the macular area are just visible in the macular area. The asymptomatic left eye is normal. Which of the following statement is correct about this condition?
   A. *Streptococcus pneumonia* is likely to be the main culprit
   B. Bilateral involvement is rare
   C. The mortality can be as high as 50% in the presence of sepsis
   D. Approximately 20% cases end up with vision of no light perception (NPL) or evisceration

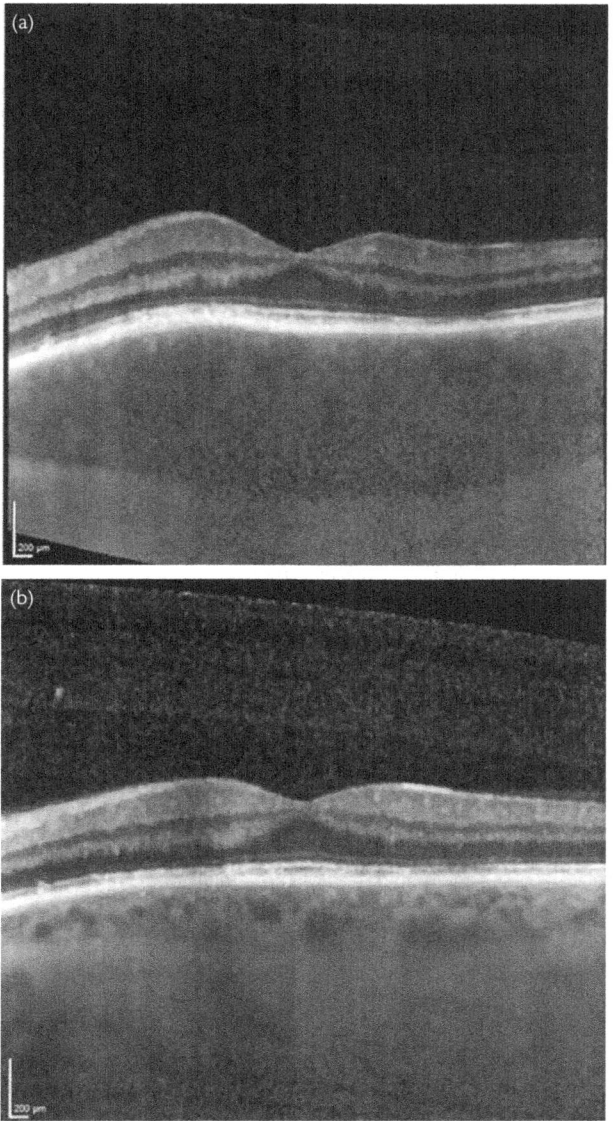

Figure 3.1

chapter 3
CLINICAL OPHTHALMOLOGY 3
ANSWERS

1. Answer: C

The prevalence of childhood amblyopia with acuity worse than LogMAR 0.3 is 1%. The mortality rate among children in the year following diagnosis of severe visual impairment is 10%, when compared with the total child population. Annual age group specific incidence of childhood visual impairment was reported to be highest in the first year of life at 4.0 per 10 000. Congenital cataract remains an important cause of severe visual impairment in the developing world.

According to the most recent UK study (2007–2010), cerebral visual impairment (21–31%) and optic nerve disorders (16%) have emerged as the most common causes for severe sight impairment, whereas congenital globe anomalies (18%) and retinal dystrophy (17%) are the two most common causes for sight impairment.

Mitry D, et al. Causes of certifications for severe sight impairment (blind) and sight impairment (partial sight) in children in England and Wales. *Br J Ophthalmol* 2013;97:1431–6.

Rahi JS, Cable N, British Childhood Visual Impairment Study Group. Severe visual impairment and blindness in children in the UK. *Lancet* 2003;362:1359–65.

2. Answer: B

Sturge–Weber syndrome (SWS) is a type of phakomatoses that is characterized by hamartomas involving the brain, eye, and skin. It affects approximately 1:50 000 babies, with no gender predilection. It is related to **sporadic** mutation of the *GNAQ* gene, which leads to stimulation of cell proliferation and inhibition of apoptosis.

Pathological ocular changes are seen in up to 50% of patients ipsilateral to the Prader–Willi syndrome (PWS) in SWS. The risk of glaucoma in SWS ranged between 30% and 70% and is related to anterior chamber malformation, high episcleral venous pressure, and changes in ocular haemodynamics. Over 75% have bilateral PWS, however only upper eyelid PWS is seen in 20%. Of those with glaucoma, 60% cases are of early onset and 40% manifest glaucoma in later life. Choroidal haemangiomas may be present up to 70% of patients with SWS and typically exist in diffuse form, which gives rise to a bright red or red-orange colour appearance of the fundus ('tomato ketchup appearance'). The incidence of SWS and central nervous system manifestations without a PWS or ocular abnormality is between 5% and 15%. This group is referred as type III or encephalofacial angiomatosis

Mantelli F, et al. Ocular manifestations of Sturge–Weber syndrome: pathogenesis, diagnosis, and management. *Clin Ophthalmol* 2016;10:871–8.

Sullivan TJ, et al. The ocular manifestations of Sturge–Weber syndrome. *J Pediatr Ophthalmol Strabismus* 1992;29:349–56.

3. Answer: C

The current recommended treatment technique by RCOphth is transpupillary diode laser to give near-confluent laser burn to the entire avascular retina when prethreshold criteria is met. A summary of treatment criteria is given in Table 3.1.

Table 3.1 Treatment criteria for retinopathy of prematurity

Zone	Plus disease	Stage	Treatment
I	+	Any stage	Treat
I	−	≥3	Treat
II	+	≥3	Treat
II	+	2	Consider

Data from Cryotherapy for Retinopathy of Prematurity Cooperative Group. Multicenter Trial of Cryotherapy for Retinopathy of Prematurity: ophthalmological outcomes at 10 years. Arch Ophthalmol 2001;119:1110–8; and The Early Treatment for Retinopathy of Prematurity Cooperative Group Revised indications for treatment of retinopathy of prematurity: results of the early treatment for retinopathy of prematurity randomized trial. Arch Ophthalmol 2003;121:1684–6.

To answer this question, the candidates should be familiar with three main studies concerning the treatment of retinopathy of prematurity, namely CRYO-ROP, ETROP, and BEAT-ROP.

Cryotherapy for Retinopathy of Prematurity (CRYO-ROP) study
- A randomized controlled trial evaluating the efficacy and safety of cryotherapy versus observation for threshold ROP
- Defines threshold ROP (all criteria required):
  - Zone I/II
  - Plus disease
  - Stage 3
  - 5 continuous clock hour or 8 non-continuous, cumulative clock hours
- **Conclusion:** Cryotherapy in 'threshold ROP' reduces the risk of adverse outcome (defined as retinal detachment, macular fold, or retrolental mass) by 50% compared to no treatment

Early Treatment of Retinopathy of Prematurity (ETROP) study
- A randomized controlled trial evaluating the efficacy and safety of early laser therapy versus observation for prethreshold ROP
- Defines prethreshold ROP into type 1 and type 2 (not important)
- Type 1 prethreshold ROP is defined as:
  - Zone 1, any stage of ROP with Plus
  - Zone 1, Stage 3 without Plus
  - Zone 2, Stage 2, or Stage 3 with plus disease
- Results supports the use of early laser for **type 1 ROP** and 'watch and wait' strategy for type 2 ROP, which is similar to the management of mild ROP.
- Unfavourable visual outcome at 9 months: 14% vs. 20% (reduced by 30%)
- Unfavourable structural outcome at 9 months: 9% vs. 16% (reduced by 40%)
- **Conclusion:** Early laser therapy in high-risk prethreshold ROP reduced unfavourable visual and structural outcomes.

Cryotherapy for Retinopathy of Prematurity Cooperative Group. Multicenter Trial of Cryotherapy for Retinopathy of Prematurity: ophthalmological outcomes at 10 years. Arch Ophthalmol 2001;119:1110–8.

The Early Treatment for Retinopathy of Prematurity Cooperative Group Revised indications for treatment of retinopathy of prematurity: results of the early treatment for retinopathy of prematurity randomized trial. *Arch Ophthalmol* 2003;121:1684–6.

4. Answer: D

The minimum required findings for diagnosis of congenital (infantile) esotropia according to the Pediatric Eye Disease Investigator Group, are:

1. Esotropia—usually 40–50 dioptres, but with a range of 10–90 PD
2. Normal neurologic status (except for strabismus)
3. Refractive error expected for age (usually low to moderate hyperopia), correction of which does not eliminate esotropia
4. Asymmetric optokinetic nystagmus characterized by robust temporal to nasal response and erratic nasal to temporal response

Other common clinical findings often present but not essential to the diagnosis are:
- Manifest nystagmus
- Oblique muscle dysfunction
- Dissociated strabismus either vertical deviation or a horizontal deviation primarily an exodeviation of one eye (DHD)
- Variable angle
- Latent nystagmus/manifest latent nystagmus
- Torticollis

American Academy of Ophthalmology. *Strabismus: Infantile Esotropia*. Available at: https://www.aao.org/disease-review/strabismus-infantile-esotropia

5. Answer: B

Stickler syndrome type I (STL1) is responsible for approximately 70% of reported cases and presents with a wide variety of symptoms affecting the eye, ear, facial appearance, palate, and musculoskeletal system and occurs due to mutations over the entire *COL2A1* gene on chromosome 12q13.11.

Type I has the highest risk of retinal detachment. Type II also includes eye abnormalities, but type III does not (and is often called non-ocular Stickler syndrome). Types IV, V, and VI are very rare and have each been diagnosed in only a few individuals.

Stickler syndrome type III (STL3) has been described as the non-ocular form of Stickler syndrome, affecting the joints and hearing without involving the eyes. Stickler syndrome type III is caused by mutations of the *COL11A2* gene on chromosome 6p21.3.

Some patients will exhibit congenital abnormalities of the anterior chamber drainage angle, which may predispose them to a higher risk of glaucoma. Experience suggests, however, that this is a relatively uncommon finding and that in most patients with glaucoma, this is a chronically progressive angle closure phenomenon resulting from retinal detachment and proliferative vitreoretinopathy causing secondary angle closure.

Alshahrani ST, et al. Rhegmatogenous retinal detachments associated to Stickler syndrome in a tertiary eye care center in Saudi Arabia. *Clin Ophthalmol* 2016;10:1–6.

Snead MP, et al. Stickler syndrome, ocular-only variants and a key diagnostic role for the ophthalmologist. *Eye (Lond)* 2011;25:1389–400.

6. Answer: A

The opacity of posterior polar cataract is in the capsule itself. Posterior polar cataracts are genetically determined with autosomal dominant inheritance and some have been associated with mutations in *PITX3*. The lens opacities in patients with persistent fetal vasculature are generally capsular and can be associated with shrinkage, thickening, and vascularization of the capsule. There may be a posterior plaque outside or involving the lens capsule with a clear lens that nonetheless must be treated as a cataract. Posterior subcapsular cataract can be congenital but are more commonly acquired as a result of injury or steroid use. The opacities are cortical and do not involve the capsule proper.

Posterior lenticonus, the central and sometimes paracentral posterior capsule, is thin and bulges posteriorly. This usually occurs at the location where the hyaloid system attaches to the eye. The distortion can cause a localized area of extreme myopic refraction. There may or may not be subcapsular cortical opacification. Interference with vision can be the result of optical distortion or of capsular opacification. Most cases are unilateral, although bilateral and familial cases have been reported. Surgery is associated with good visual outcomes in most cases. Spontaneous rupture of the lens can rarely occur, leading to abrupt progression to total cataract.

Gillespie RL, et al. Personalized diagnosis and management of congenital cataract by next-generation sequencing. *Ophthalmology* 2014;121:2124–37.

Xu LT, Traboulsi EI. Genetics of congenital cataracts. In: Wilson ME, Trivedi RH (eds). *Pediatric Cataract Surgery: Techniques, Complications and Management*. Philadelphia, PA: Lippincott Williams & Wilkins, 2014.

7. Answer: B

Variable angle of strabismus include:
- Uncorrected refractive error
- Anisometropia
- Nystagmus compensation (blockage) syndrome
- Convergence excess esotropia

Microtropia is associated with Inconspicuous shift or no shift on cover test, stable alignment, the fixation is central or parafoveal in one eye. Mild amblyopia is frequent with reduced or absent stereopsis. Microtropia may exist in two forms, with and without identity. Studies have shown that microtropia with identity is a reliable indicator of presence of amblyopia and possible need for occlusion therapy.

Lysons D, Tapley J. Is microtropia a reliable indicator of the presence of amblyopia in anisometropic patients? *Strabismus* 2018;26:118–21.

8. Answer: B

Standard management of Duane syndrome (DS) may involve surgery. The indications for surgery include:
- Elimination or improvement of an unacceptable head turn
- Elimination or reduction of significant misalignment of the eyes
- Reduction of severe retraction
- Improvement of upshoots and downshoots

Surgery does not eliminate the fundamental abnormality of innervation and no surgical technique has been completely successful in eliminating the abnormal eye movements. Simple horizontal muscle recession procedures, vertical transposition of the rectus muscle, or combinations of the two may be successful in improving or eliminating head turns and misalignment of the eyes. The choice of procedure must be individualized. A prism can be placed on the patient's glasses to correct for the face turn (though this is not commonly used). The success rate in eliminating an abnormal head position is 79–100%. Surgery does not improve motility or stereopsis/fusion. A risk of diplopia may be present with or without surgery.

Merino P, et al. Horizontal rectus surgery in Duane syndrome. *Eur J Ophthalmol* 2012;22:125–30.

Pressman SH, Scott WE. Surgical treatment of Duane's syndrome. *Ophthalmology* 1986;93:29–38.

9. Answer: B

In X-linked recessive juvenile retinoschisis (XLRS), foveal changes are seen in all cases and peripheral retinoschisis in one-half of cases. Maculopathy is characterized by stellate spoke-like appearance with microcysts. Vitreous veils are a common feature of X-linked juvenile retinoschisis. The mutation in RS1 can be detected in 90–95% of patients who have a clinical diagnosis. It not only helps confirm the diagnosis but also provides useful genetic information of the patient and offspring.

In juvenile X-linked retinoschisis (XLR), ERG findings show electronegative ERG responses (i.e. normal a-wave, reduced b-wave). ERG dysfunction is found throughout the retina and is not limited to schitic areas. Therefore, both focal and macular ERG and full-field ERG yield similar results. OCT reveals cystic spaces primarily in the inner nuclear and outer plexiform layers of the retina. Although there are cystic changes at the macula, there is no sign of leakage at the cystic areas on fundus fluorescein angiography, which is in contrast to the usual cystoid macular oedema.

Indocyanine green angiography (ICGA) performed on patients with XLRS shows a distinct hyperfluorescence in the macular region that is associated with radial lines of hypofluorescence centred on the foveola in the early phase. This feature disappears in the late phase of the ICGA.

Sikkink SK, et al. X-linked retinoschisis: an update. *J Med Genet* 2007;44:225–32.

Souied EH, et al. Indocyanine green angiography of juvenile X-linked retinoschisis. *Am J Ophthalmol* 2005;140:558–61.

10. Answer: B

Most primary congenital glaucoma (PCG) cases occur sporadically. They are familial in 10–40% of cases, usually with autosomal recessive inheritance and variable penetrance. The classic triad of symptoms in PCG is epiphora, photophobia, and blepharospasm, but could be absent in rare occasions. In fact, photophobia and blepharospasm are found in only 7.5% of patients at first presentation, while epiphora is only present in 3.3%. Cloudy cornea and buphthalmos account for the most common presenting sign, found in over 40% of patients.

In PCG, the glaucomatous cup enlarges circumferentially, as the scleral canal is uniformly stretched in all directions. In adult onset glaucoma, rim thinning preferentially occurs at the inferior and superior rim due to the abundance of nerve fibre layer in that area. Most general anaesthetics and central nervous system depressants decrease the intraocular pressure (IOP), except for ketamine which increases the muscle tone of the extraocular muscles, paradoxically increasing the IOP. Chloral hydrate has the least effect on IOP, followed by ketamine.

Tamcelik N, et al. Demographic features of subjects with congenital glaucoma. *Indian J Ophthalmol* 2014;62:565–9.

Wadia S, et al. Ketamine and intraocular pressure in children. *Ann Emerg Med* 2014;64:385–8.

Yu Chan JY, et al. Review on the management of primary congenital glaucoma. *J Curr Glaucoma Pract* 2015;9:92–9.

11. Answer: D

Acute onset of concomitant esotropia is an uncommon form of strabismus. In the clear majority of cases it will have no obvious underlying neurological cause.
- Check for history of previous strabismus, occlusion therapy or monocular visual loss, or myopia cause little worry
- No apparent cause for the acute concomitant esotropia—the possibility of an underlying neurological disease should at least be considered
- Presence of nystagmus or the inability to restore binocularity in any of these patients should be considered sufficiently abnormal and warrants neurological investigation

Indications for and specific types of treatment need to be individualized for each patient.
- Optical correction: cycloplegic refraction and prescription of glasses
- Prisms to eliminate diplopia and to re-establish binocular vision: base out prisms in the ipsilateral eye
- Chemodenervation: botox of the ipsilateral medial rectus muscle to reduce medial rectus contracture
- Extraocular muscle surgery in stable deviations that are too large to allow spontaneous binocular fusion

Chen J, et al. Acute acquired concomitant esotropia: clinical features, classification, and etiology. *Medicine (Baltimore)* 2015;94:e2273.

12. Answer: B

Congenital MED or known as double elevator palsy can be caused by:
- Paralysis of the superior rectus (SR) muscle without any involvement of the inferior oblique muscle.
- Primary inferior rectus (IR) restriction or secondary restriction due to long-standing SR palsy
- Lesion in the supranuclear pathway of upgaze located in the pretectum

MED features include:
- Inability to elevate the eye above midline in abduction, adduction, or from primary position of gaze
- Hypotropia of the affected eye on the affected side present as orthophoria in primary gaze. Rarely the affected eye may fixate
- Ptosis of the affected eye or sometimes pseudoptosis may be seen
- Chin-up as compensatory head position

Indications for surgery are:
- Vertical deviation in primary gaze
- Deviation-induced amblyopia
- Diplopia in primary gaze
- Restricted binocular fields

The goal of surgery is to:
- Improve the position of the affected eye in primary gaze
- Increase the field of binocular vision

If restriction to upgaze is demonstrated on the forced duction test (FDT), IR restriction is present. An IR recession with conjunctival recession should be done in such patients. If the FDT is non-restrictive, the affected patient has either SR paresis or supranuclear MED, and the Knapp procedure should be performed.

Bagheri A, et al. Double elevator palsy, subtypes and outcomes of surgery. *J Ophthal Vis Res* 2008;3:108–13.

Kim JH, Hwang JM. Congenital monocular elevation deficiency. *Ophthalmology* 2009; 116:580–4.

13. Answer: B

Thyroid eye disease (TED) affects extraocular muscles in a predictable manner:
- The IR and medial rectus are most commonly involved
- This presents as hypotropia and/or esotropia
- Pain with eye movement, characterized as dull, deep orbital pain affects 30% of patients
- 40% of patients are affected by restrictive extraocular myopathy

Most TED patients with diplopia due to strabismus will not require surgical intervention, as most can be effectively managed with prism spectacles. Indications for strabismus surgery include:
- Intractable diplopia in primary gaze or with reading
- Abnormal head posture
- Cosmetically unacceptable globe position

Following surgical approach is recommended in TED patients affected by proptosis, strabismus, and lid retraction: orbital decompression → strabismus surgery → lid surgery. This is because orbital decompression can alter/cause strabismus. Sometimes extraocular muscle recession may worsen proptosis. In addition, strabismus surgery can affect eyelid position; therefore, it should be undertaken prior to any corrective eyelid procedures:
- Large IR muscle recession can result in lower eyelid retraction, which is largely due to adherence between the IR muscle and the capsulopalpebral fascia of the lower eyelid.
- With SR recession, connection points between the SR and upper eyelid elevators may worsen upper eyelid retraction.

Bartley GB, et al. Clinical features of Graves' ophthalmopathy in an incidence cohort. *Am J Ophthalmol* 1996;121:284–90.

14. Answer: A

Intermittent exotropia (IXT) is classified into three types: basic exotropia (BE), distance exotropia (DE), and convergence insufficiency (CI). In BE, the distance deviation is within 10 PD of the near deviation. In DE, the distance deviation is greater than nearby 10 PD. DE can be further classified intro true vs. simulated divergence excess. In true divergence excess, the near deviation remains less than the distance deviation after a brief period of occlusion. In simulated divergence excess, however, the near deviation approaches distance deviation after occlusion. In CI type IXT, the near deviation is greater than distance by 10 PD.

Exam findings in intermittent exotropia typically reveal normal visual acuities at distance and near, good stereopsis at near (during phoric phase), no diplopia, suppression, or anomalous correspondence, or a combination of latter two. Proportion of time the deviation is manifest is as important as the magnitude of deviation as it gives information about the 'quality' of control. True fusion experienced during the phoric phase or anomalous fusion during the tropic phase. Evidence of fusion in the presence of a manifest deviation is indicative of anomalous correspondence.

Clarke MP. Intermittent exotropia. *J Pediatr Ophthalmol Strabismus* 2007;44:153–7.

Kushner BJ, Morton GV. Distance/near differences in intermittent exotropia. *Arch Ophthalmol* 1998;116:478–86.

15. Answer: C

The most important objective in the management of a child with retinoblastoma is survival of the patient, and the second most important goal is preservation of the globe. The focus on visual acuity comes later, after safety of the patient and globe is established. Therapy is tailored to each individual case and based on the overall situation, including threat of metastatic disease, risks for second cancers, systemic status, laterality of the disease, size and location of the tumour, and estimated visual prognosis.

In recent years, eyes with unilateral retinoblastoma are generally managed with enucleation if the eye is classified as Reese–Ellsworth group V; for those eyes in groups I to IV, chemoreduction or focal measures are used. For bilateral retinoblastoma, chemoreduction is utilized in most cases unless there is an extreme asymmetric involvement, with one eye having advanced disease necessitating enucleation while the other eye has minimal disease, treatable with focal methods. Most children with bilateral retinoblastoma are treated with chemoreduction for at least one of their two involved eyes. Selective ophthalmic arterial injection therapy has been shown to be a promising treatment for intraocular retinoblastoma, with eye preservation rate ranging from 100% (group A) to 30% in group E according to International Classification of Intraocular Retinoblastoma.

Focal therapies include laser photocoagulation, thermotherapy, cryotherapy, and plaque radiotherapy. Most of these therapies are employed for small tumours, especially those that have been reduced by chemoreduction. Commonly, focal therapies are applied to an eye while the child is receiving chemoreduction, and they are repeated to each tumour at each chemotherapy session. Plaque radiotherapy is generally reserved for tumours that fail other focal therapies, even those that reach a moderate size, up to 8 or 10 mm in thickness. The remainder of the focal therapies are reserved for small tumours, generally those under 3 mm in greatest dimension.

Shields CL, Shields JA. Recent developments in the management of retinoblastoma. *J Pediatr Ophthalmol Strabismus* 1999;36:8–18.

Shields CL, et al. Chemoreduction plus focal therapy for retinoblastoma: factors predictive of need for treatment with external beam radiotherapy or enucleation. *Am J Ophthalmol* 2002;133:657–64.

Suzuki S, et al. Selective ophthalmic arterial injection therapy for intraocular retinoblastoma: the long-term prognosis. *Ophthalmology* 2011;118:2081–7.

16. Answer: B

Rhabdomyosarcoma (RMS) is the most common soft-tissue sarcoma of childhood. After neuroblastoma and Wilms' tumour, it is the third most common extracranial childhood solid tumour. Orbital tumours being characterized by embryonal histology in most cases. On the other hand, extremity tumours are more commonly found in adolescents and are more likely to have an alveolar histologic subtype.

It is the most common cause of primary malignant orbital tumour in childhood (around 4%). It usually begins around 8 years of age with slight male predilection. It can be extraconal (35%), intraconal (15%), or both (50%). It preferentially affects the superior nasal quadrant and the main signs include non-axial unilateral exophthalmos, often with inflammatory character, rapid progressive ptosis, and may mimic orbital cellulitis.

The two histologic subtypes of RMS, embryonal and alveolar, have been found to have distinct genetic alterations that may play a role in the pathogenesis of these tumours. Alveolar RMS has been demonstrated to have a characteristic translocation between the long arm of chromosome 2 and the long arm of chromosome 13, referred to as t(2;13)(q35;q14). Embryonal RMS is known to have loss of heterozygosity at the 11p15 locus with loss of maternal genetic information and duplication of paternal genetic information. Orbital tumours produce proptosis, and, occasionally, ophthalmoplegia. Embryonal RMS is the most common subtype (50%; can be remembered as Everyone has it), whereas alveolar RMS has a worse outcome (which can be remembered as awful outcome).

Malempati S, Hawkins DS. Rhabdomyosarcoma: review of the Children's Oncology Group (COG) Soft-Tissue Sarcoma Committee experience and rationale for current COG studies. *Pediatr Blood Cancer* 2012;59:5–10.

Pater LE, et al. *Rhabdomyosarcoma Review 2017*. Children's Oncology Group. Available at: https://www.qarc.org/COG/Rhabdomyosarcoma_.pdf

17. Answer: B

Kearns-Sayers syndrome (KSS) is a type of mitochondrial myopathy that demonstrates the following: (a) chronic progressive external ophthalmoplegia, onset before age 20 years, and (b) pigmentary retinopathy. KSS also has at least one of the following: (a) cardiac conduction defects; (b) cerebrospinal fluid (CSF); (c) protein level greater than 100 mg/dL; and (d) cerebellar syndrome. Other abnormalities in KSS can include mental retardation, Babinski sign, hearing loss, seizures, short stature, delayed puberty, and various endocrine disorders, such as diabetes mellitus, hypoparathyroidism, and hearing loss.

Chinnery PF. *Mitochondrial Disorders Overview*. GeneReviews® [Internet] 2014. Available at: http://www.ncbi.nlm.nih.gov/books/NBK1224/

18. Answer: D

Patients with acquired Brown syndrome in late childhood or adulthood experience diplopia when tropic. Diplopia may occur when the patient looks up and to the contralateral side of the affected eye. Patients with congenital Brown syndrome rarely complain of diplopia, because most patients have developed suppression. Limited elevation in adduction, an invariable sign, is the hallmark of Brown syndrome. Even in severe cases of congenital Brown syndrome, there is minimal hypotropia in primary position and no hypotropia in downgaze. In contrast, much larger hypotropias have been observed in cases of Brown syndrome associated with trauma or periorbital surgery. Patients often present with compensatory head-posturing, their chin up, and a contralateral face turn to avoid the hypotropia that increases in upgaze and gaze to the contralateral side of the affected eye. A feature that often is associated with acquired Brown syndrome is an audible or palpable superior nasal click on ocular rotations up and nasal ward; sometimes, the pain is associated with this ocular movement.

Parks MM, Brown M. Superior oblique tendon sheath syndrome of Brown. *Am J Ophthalmol* 1975;79:82–6.

Suh SY, et al. Size of the oblique extraocular muscles and superior oblique muscle contractility in Brown syndrome. *Invest Ophthalmol Vis Sci* 2015;56:6114–20.

19. Answer: A

Neurofibromatosis type 1 (NF1), also known as von Recklinghausen NF or peripheral NF, is characterized by multiple café au lait spots (patches of tan or light brown skin) and neurofibromas (soft, fleshy growths) on or under the skin. Enlargement and deformation of bones and curvature of the spine (scoliosis) may also occur. Occasionally, tumours may develop in the brain, on cranial nerves, or on the spinal cord. About 50–75% of people with NF1 also have learning disabilities.

Lisch nodules are the most common ocular clinical finding in adults older than 20 years with NF-1. Hamartomas of the choroid are usually in the posterior pole and are flat, ill-defined lesions. No laboratory tests are pertinent in evaluating ophthalmologic manifestations of NF-1. However, tissue biopsy of skin lesions is occasionally necessary to confirm the diagnosis of NF-1.

Savar A, Cestari DM. Neurofibromatosis type I: genetics and clinical manifestations. *Semin Ophthalmol* 2008;23:45–51.

20. Answer: D

Leber's hereditary optic neuropathy (LHON) carriers remain asymptomatic until they experience blurring or clouding of vision in one eye. In the vast majority of cases, visual dysfunction is bilateral, the fellow eye becoming affected either simultaneously (25%) or sequentially (75%), with a median intereye delay of 8 weeks. Visual acuity usually reaches low in 4–6 weeks after the first start of symptoms and is severely reduced to 6/60 or less. The characteristic field defect in LHON is a centrocaecal scotoma.

Other clinical features include the early impairment of colour perception but, more importantly, pupillary reflexes are preserved and patients usually report no pain on eye movement. Fundoscopy provides other diagnostic clues and in classical cases the following abnormalities can be observed: vascular tortuosity of the central retinal vessels, a circumpapillary telangiectatic microangiopathy, and swelling of the retinal nerve fibre layer. However, it must be stressed that in ~20% of LHON cases, the optic disc looks entirely normal in the acute phase.

Yu-Wai-Man P, et al. Leber hereditary optic neuropathy. *J Med Genet* 2002;39:162–9.

21. Answer: A

The standard management of CFEOM may involve surgery. The goal of surgery is the elimination or improvement of an unacceptable head position, the reduction of ptosis, and the elimination or reduction of significant misalignment of the eyes. Successful surgery at a young age may avoid loss of vision in one or both eyes. However, surgery does not eliminate the fundamental abnormality, and no surgical technique has been completely successful in eliminating the abnormal eye movements. These patients require a stepwise surgical approach to correct strabismus and eyelid position. The vertical and horizontal misalignments are addressed first followed by the ptosis repair, as extraocular muscle surgery can alter eyelid position. FDT is useful in differentiating other causes of non-restrictive misalignment of the eyes.

Whitman M, et al. *Congenital Fibrosis of the Extraocular Muscles.* In: GeneReveiws at GeneTests: Medical Genetics Information Resource; Seattle, WA: University of Washington, 1993–2018. Available at: https://www.ncbi.nlm.nih.gov/books/NBK1348/

22. Answer: B

Accommodative esotropia is defined as a convergent deviation of the eyes associated with activation of the accommodation reflex. It comprises more than 50% of all childhood esotropias and can be classified into three forms: (1) refractive; (2) non-refractive; and (3) partially accommodative or decompensated. All three forms possess the following characteristics:

- Onset usually between 6 months and 7 years of age, averaging 2.5 years
- Intermittent at onset, then becoming constant over time
- Often initiated by trauma or illness
- Frequently associated with amblyopia
- May be associated with diplopia in older children, but later disappears as a suppression scotoma develops
- Often has a hereditary basis

Early onset esotropia normally presents before the age of 6 months, with a constant, large angle of strabismus (>30 PD), no or mild amblyopia, small to moderate hyperopia, latent nystagmus, dissociated vertical deviation, limitation of abduction (although the patients in fact have normal abduction, they appear to have limitation due to cross fixation), and absent or reduced binocular vision, in the absence of nervous system disorders. Refractive accommodative esotropia usually occurs in a child between 2 and 3 years of age. The average cycloplegic refractive error in refractive accommodative esotropia is +4.75 D. The angle of deviation is typically the same for distance and near, averaging between 20 and 40 PD. Despite full spectacle correction, if the distance esotropia is still noted to be high, the patient has a partially accommodative esotropia. A subgroup of patients with accommodative esotropia have significantly larger esotropia at near, that is, non-refractive or high accommodative convergence (AC:A) ratio accommodative esotropia. They usually present between 2 and 3 years of age. The refractive error in this condition may be hyperopic, emmetropic, or myopic. The average refractive error is +2.25 D.

Rutstein RP. Update on accommodative esotropia. *Optometry* 2008;79:422–31.

23. Answer: B

In most individuals with X-linked ocular albinism (XLOA), the best corrected visual acuity is between 20/40 (6/12) and 20/200 (6/60). XLOA is a non-progressive disorder and the visual acuity typically slowly improves until mid-to-late teens and then remains stable throughout life. Hypersensitivity to light, often called 'photophobia', is present in most affected individuals but varies in intensity and significance from one individual to another. Substantial refractive errors are common, most often as hypermetropia with oblique astigmatism. High myopia or compound myopic astigmatism may occur in some affected individuals. Most affected individuals have reduced or absent binocular functions as a consequence of misrouted optic pathway projections, and ocular misalignment (strabismus). A positive angle Kappa is often found in individuals with albinism.

Brodsky MC, Fray KJ. Positive angle Kappa: a sign of albinism in patients with congenital nystagmus. *Am J Ophthalmol* 2004;137:625–9.

Lewis RA. Ocular albinism, X-linked. In: Adam MP, et al. (eds). *GeneReviews*. Seattle, WA: University of Washington, Seattle, 1993–2018.

24. Answer: B

A dacryocystocele usually presents with tense, blue, non-pulsatile swelling BELOW the medial canthus that is evident at or shortly after birth. The clinical appearance is classic, but if in doubt organize MRI scan to exclude meningocele and meningomyelocele, in which the lesions typically present ABOVE the medial canthus. Treatment is observation for 2 weeks, during which most spontaneously get better and surgery is only indicated if it does not settle in 2 weeks, acute dacryocystitis sets in, or respiratory difficulties develop.

Sullivan TJ, et al. Management of congenital dacryocystocoele. *Aust N Z J Ophthalmol* 1992;20:105–8.

Wong RK, VanderVeen DK. Presentation and management of congenital dacryocystocele. *Pediatrics* 2008;122:e1108–12.

25. Answer: B

A 'green-stick' floor fracture is also known as a 'white eye blow-out fracture' where the force of the injury has been transmitted via the bony orbital floor, causing the bone to fracture then snap back into place often causing entrapment of the IR or associated soft tissues. This can result in a restrictive vertical gaze palsy and secondary oculo-cardiac reflex when attempting upgaze from the entrapped muscle, resulting in vomiting and vasovagal syncope. Severe fibrosis and restricted eye movement can result due to muscle ischaemia if not surgically released.

Lane K, et al. Evaluation and management of pediatric orbital fractures in a primary care setting. *Orbit* 2007;26:183–91.

26. Answer: D

Most commonly TON is due to direct or vascular injury to the optic nerve within the optic canal. Fracture through the optic canal is less common, and the fundus examination is normal acutely unless there is an optic nerve avulsion or a very anterior nerve injury. High-dose steroids have been shown to worsen prognosis in severe head injury.

Timlin H, et al. RCOphth FOCUS article: *Traumatic Orbital Emergencies*. Available at: https://www.rcophth.ac.uk/wp-content/uploads/2015/02/Focus-Autumn-2015.pdf

27. Answer: B

The clinical findings of the indirect fistulas are almost always less dramatic than those of a direct carotid cavernous fistula, although over time the low-flow state of an indirect dural sinus fistula may become a greater flow as new arterial connections develop. Other than by the tell-tale symptom of a cranial bruit, differentiating high flow from low flow is best determined by angiographic studies.

Chaudhry IA, et al. Carotid cavernous fistula: ophthalmological implications. *Middle East Afr J Ophthalmol* 2009;16:57–63.

28. Answer: D

The higher the raw score sum, the better probability of achieving higher visual acuity at 6 months. Visual acuity at presentation represents the biggest single variable in calculating the OTS score (see Table 3.2).

Computational method for deriving the OTS score:

Raw score sum = sum of raw points

Table 3.2 Calculation of the OTS score

Initial visual factor		Raw points
A. Initial raw score (based on initial VA)	NPL	60
	PL or HM	70
	1/200 to 19/200	80
	20/200 to 20/50	90
	≥ 20/40	100
B. Globe rupture		−23
C. Endophthalmitis		−17
D. Perforating injury		−14
E. Retinal detachment		−11
F. Relative afferent pupillary defect		−10

Reproduced from Scott, R. (2016). The ocular trauma score. *Community Eye Health*, 28(91):44-5. CC BY-NC 4.0.

29. Answer: D

There are a number of characteristic ocular fundus findings reported in abusive head trauma or shaken baby syndrome; however, none of them are pathognomonic. Characteristic features include severe retinal haemorrhages (preretinal, intraretinal, and subretinal), perimacular folds, and haemorrhagic retinal cysts and retinoschisis. Optic nerve sheath haemorrhages are more common in abuse than in other conditions in autopsy studies.

The Royal College of Paediatrics and Child Health and The Royal College of Ophthalmologists. *Abusive Head Trauma and the Eye in Infancy*, 2013. Available at: https://www.rcophth.ac.uk/wp-content/uploads/2014/12/2013-SCI-292-ABUSIVE-HEAD-TRAUMA-AND-THE-EYE-FINAL-at-June-2013.pdf

30. Answer: C

A lamellar laceration is a closed globe injury. A ruptured globe is caused by a blunt force where the eye will rupture at the weakest point, often an old surgical wound site or just behind the muscle insertions. A penetrating injury requires an entrance wound and a perforating injury requires both entrance and exit wound. See Figure 3.2.

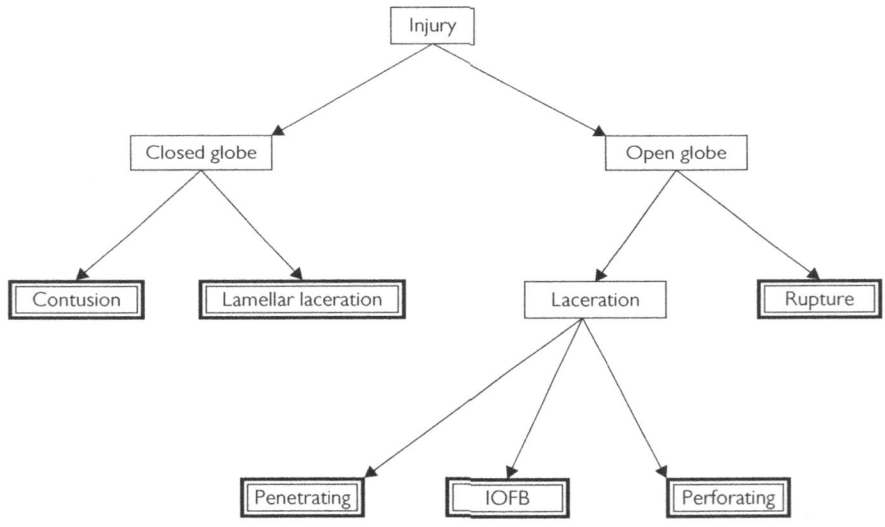

Figure 3.2

This figure was published in *Ophthalmology Clinics of North America*, 15, 2, Kuhn F, et al., Birmingham Eye Trauma Terminology (BETT): Terminology and classification of mechanical eye injuries, pp. 139–43, Copyright Elsevier 2002.

31. Answer: C

Both full blood count and temperature are essential to establish a likelihood of infective orbital cellulitis, the commonest cause of acute paediatric unilateral proptosis. A weight is required to calculate the dosage of both antibiotics and analgesia which are required for emergency treatment. Neoplastic causes such as orbital rhabdomyosarcoma should be considered in the differential, but CT or MRI imaging would be required; plain film X-ray is non-diagnostic and unnecessary exposure to radiation. The other important differential diagnosis to be considered in this situation is orbital neuroblastoma, which usually occurs in patients less than 2 years old. It typically presents as unilateral or bilateral periorbital ecchymosis (or known as 'raccoon eyes'). Other ophthalmic features include proptosis, periorbital swelling, Horner's syndrome, opsoclonus, optic neuropathy, and strabismus.

Sindhu K, et al. Aetiology of childhood proptosis. *J Paediatr Child Health* 1998;34:374–6.

32. Answer: B

Features of aponeurotic dehiscence include high skin crease, normal levator function, reduced MRD1, unaffected Bell's phenomenon, and normal orbicularis function.

Low skin crease is found in congenital ptosis. Reduced Bell's phenomenon and limited upgaze are associated with chronic progressive external ophthalmoplegia. Reduced MRD2 means the lower lid is higher than normal, which is not related to the upper lid. Important features of various types of ptosis are summarized in Table 3.3, next. It is noteworthy to mention that all the elements in the first column should be examined for during the clinical examination of ptosis.

Table 3.3 Important features of various types of ptosis

	Aponeurotic	Myogenic	Myasthenic	Congenital
MRD1	Low	Low	Low	Low
Levator function	Normal	Reduced	Variable	Reduced
Skin crease	High/lost	Normal	Normal	Low/absent
Orbicularis function	Normal	Weak	Weak	Normal
Bell's phenomenon	Normal	Poor	Normal unless significant upgaze restriction	Normal unless associated elevator palsy
Other features	Deep superior sulcus	May have significant ocular motility restriction	Improvement in MRD1 after rest/ice	Lid lag in down gaze

Leatherbarrow B. *Oculoplastic Surgery*, 2nd edition. Chapter 7: Blepharoptosis. London, UK: Informa Healthcare, 2011.

33. Answer: D

Trichiasis is defined as misdirected lashes arising from a lid margin of normal position. Entropion is pseudotrichiasis. OCP and SJS are rare. Trachoma is the seventh most prevalent cause of blindness worldwide according to the World Health Organization Global data on visual impairment in the year 2002.

Resnikoff S, et al. *Global Data on Visual Empairment in the Year 2020*. Available at: http://www.who.int/bulletin/volumes/82/11/en/844.pdf?ua=1

34. Answer: A

Churg–Strauss syndrome (CSS), or currently known as eosinophilic granulomatosis with polyangiitis (EGPA), is a small- and medium-vessel vasculitis characterized by asthma, hypereosinophilia, and multisystem vasculitis. There are usually distinct clinical phases of CSS. The disease begins with asthma and atopic allergies that may begin in childhood before progression to the eosinophilic phase, which is characterized by eosinophilic infiltration with granulomatous inflammation and can have an array of clinical presentations including orbital inflammation. A vasculitic phase usually follows this. Presentation of sarcoid and GPA are usually much less acute; sarcoid usually affecting the lacrimal gland and GPA almost invariably involves sinus or respiratory tract symptoms.

Akella SS, et al. Ophthalmic eosinophilic granulomatosis with polyangiitis (Churg-Strauss syndrome): a systematic review of the literature. *Ophthalmic Plast Reconstr Surg* 2019;35(1):7–16.

35. Answer: B

Blepharophimosis, ptosis, and epicanthus inversus syndrome (BPES) is a rare autosomal dominant disease that mainly affects the development of the eyelids. People with this condition have Blepharophimosis (narrowing of the eye opening), Ptosis, and Epicanthus inversus (an upward fold of the skin of the lower eyelid near the inner canthus) but not epicanthus tarsalis (fold more prominent in upper eyelid). In addition, there is an increased distance between the inner corners of the eyes (telecanthus) but not the interpupillary distance. Type 1 BPES is also associated with primary ovarian failure which can lead to subfertility and type 2 BPES has no systemic association. *FOXL2* gene mutation is implicated in both type 1 and 2 BPES.

Yang L, et al. Identification of a novel *FOXL2* mutation in a single family with both types of blepharophimosis—ptosis-epicanthus inversus syndrome. *Mol Med Rep* 2017;16:5529–32.

36. Answer: A

DON can be treated by systemic glucocorticoids, surgery, or both. Orbital radiotherapy is not recommended in the case of DON unless as an adjunct to proven therapies. High-dose intravenous steroids administered in pulses are more efficacious and associated with fewer adverse effects than oral or retrobulbar steroids. Selenium has only been shown to be beneficial in mild TED.

Bartalena L, et al. Consensus statement of the European Group on Graves' orbitopathy (EUGOGO) on management of GO. *Eur J Endocrinol* 2008;158:273–85.

Marcocci C, et al. Selenium and the course of mild Graves' orbitopathy. *N Engl J Med* 2011;364:1920–31.

37. Answer: C

NF1 is an autosomal dominant condition that can cause a range of ophthalmic manifestations. Plexiform neurofibromas may involve the eyelid, orbit/periorbital, and facial structures (termed OPPN) and could cause visual loss in children. Most OPPN track along the distribution of trigeminal nerve and can be categorized into three types:

a. Isolated upper eyelid (~33%)—usually assumes a characteristic 'S'-shaped deformity, ptosis is usually mild, and progression into orbit is unlikely. Rarely a ptosis may be secondary to an encephalocoele due to an absent sphenoid wing.

b. Eyelid and periorbital region—affecting V1 and V2 distribution of trigeminal nerve. Ptosis may be severe, which can cause amblyopia, and progression to orbit is possible.

c. Orbit with/without lid involvement—invades lateral orbit and potentially cavernous sinus.

There are no clotting abnormalities associated with NF, although surgery of plexiform neurofibroma can be complicated by difficulty controlling haemostasis due to the vascularity of the lesion; however, there is no role for routine clotting testing. CT can be used to assess the bony orbits to look for absent sphenoid wing, but radiation should be avoided in children and the bony deformities can be detected by MRI. MRI is useful for delineating soft-tissue abnormalities, the extent of plexiform neurofibroma (including orbital involvement), and bony deformities (figures are available in the reference). VFT can be used to examine any visual field obstruction and is helpful in supporting the need for ptosis surgery but is not essential.

Avery RA, et al. Orbital/periorbital plexiform neurofibromas in children with neurofibromatosis type 1: multidisciplinary recommendations for care. *Ophthalmology* 2017;124:123–32.

38. Answer: D

It is essential to provide extra glucocorticoid cover for patients on long-term steroid treatment because of their acquired adrenal insufficiency. Ptosis correction would be classified as 'minor' surgery. Intramuscular hydrocortisone is preferred to intravenous injection for its more sustained duration.

Addison's Disease Self-Help Group. *ADSHG Surgical Guidelines*, 2017. Available at: https://www.addisons.org.uk/surgery

39. Answer: A

A patient with OID should only have a therapeutic trial of steroids if they have specific features consistent with myositis. All other presentations of inflammatory orbital disease should be investigated further to exclude underlying causes before they can be labelled as idiopathic and treated accordingly.

Mombaerts I, et al. Consensus on diagnostic criteria of idiopathic orbital inflammation using a modified Delphi approach. *JAMA Ophthalmol* 2017;135:769–76.

40. Answer: B

Surgical decompression for optic neuropathy would involve removal of the medial orbital wall, predominantly towards the apex in order to expand the space around the optic nerve. This necessitates access into the ethmoid and sphenoid sinuses. Maxillary sinus is commonly opened inferoposteriorly for drainage and to aid decompression. The frontal sinus being superiorly aids neither.

Rootman DB. Orbital decompression of thyroid eye disease. *Surv Ophthalmol* 2018;63:86–104.

41. Answer: D

Muir–Torre syndrome is an uncommon autosomal dominant condition characterized by sebaceous carcinomas of the skin and visceral malignancies (most commonly colorectal carcinoma). It is a phenotypic variant of hereditary non-polyposis colorectal cancer. Some autosomal recessive cases have been documented. The median age of onset is 53 years of age and most cases were reported in Caucasian patients. Bazex syndrome is characterized by skin disorders with underlying malignancies, most commonly squamous cell carcinoma of the head and neck. Gardner syndrome is an autosomal dominant disorder characterized by familial adenomatous polyposis and it is associated with congenital hypertrophy of retinal pigment epithelium. Gorlin–Golz syndrome, also known as naevoid BCC syndrome, is a rare autosomal dominant disease characterized by multiple BCC, hypertelorism, strabismus, myelinated nerve fibres, retinal abnormalities, and other systemic features such as palmar and plantar pits and ectopic calcification of the brain.

Chen JJ, et al. Review of ocular manifestations of nevoid basal cell carcinoma syndrome: what an ophthalmologist needs to know. *Middle East Afr J Ophthalmol* 2015;22:421–7.

Gay JT, Gross GP. *Muir-Torre Syndrome*. StatPearls [Internet]. Treasure Iland, FL: StatPearls Publishing, 2018. Available at: https://www.ncbi.nlm.nih.gov/books/NBK513271/

42. Answer: B

Activity is characterized by the inflammatory phase of the disease. It can be graded by clinical assessment using tools such as the clinical activity severity score; with a score >3 suggesting activity.

Some features of activity can persist when the acute inflammation has settled, such as pain due to congestion or diplopia due to muscle fibrosis. Reduced colour vision is a sign of optic neuropathy, which is a sign of severity, not activity. Upper lid oedema is secondary to inflammation which resolves in the inactive phase.

Mourits MP, et al. Clinical activity score as a guide in the management of patients with Graves' ophthalmopathy. *Clin Endocrinol (Oxf)* 1997;47:9–14.

43. Answer: A

Painful mass in the region of the lacrimal gland suggests either inflammation or neoplasm with perineural invasion. The histological features given are those of a biopsy from glandular tissue, but a benign lesion would not contain anaplastic cells. A pleomorphic adenoma would usually present with a longer duration of painless growth and there would be squamous metaplasia on the biopsy.

Gunduz AK, et al. Overview of benign and malignant lacrimal gland tumors. *Curr Opin Ophthalmol* 2018;29:458–68.

44. Answer: C

A full thickness lid defect needs to have posterior lamella reconstruction with tissue to replace the rigidity of the tarsus lined with a mucosal surface. Ideally this is done with like-for-like donor tarsal plate, either from the ipsilateral upper lid with a Hughes flap or a free tarsal graft. It would not be possible to close a 10–12 mm full-thickness defect in the lower lid by direct closure. Both a full thickness skin graft and a Mustarde flap would only reconstruct the anterior lamella. For an elderly patient, the size of skin defect can be classified into small (30%), moderate (30–60%), and large (>60%). The following table (Table 3.4) provides a very good summary on the methods of reconstruction of upper and lower eyelid defects based on the size of the defect.

Subramanian N. Reconstructions of eyelid defect. *Indian J Plast Surg* 2011;44:5–13.

Table 3.4 Reconstruction methods for upper and lower eyelid defects, based on the size of the defect

Size of defect	Upper eyelid defect	Lower eyelid defect
Small	- DC with lateral cantholysis or Tenzel's semicircular flap	- DC with or without lateral cantholysis or Tenzel's semicircular flap
Moderate	- Mustarde's lid switch flap - Cutler–Beard method	- AL: Advancement of cheek skin, full thickness skin graft, Tripier flap unipedicle - PL: Hughes' tarsoconjunctival flap
Large	- Mustarde's lid switch flap - Cutler–Beard method	- AL: Mustarde's cheek rotation flap, nasolabial flap, median forehead flap, lateral temporal flap - PL: Chondromucous graft nasal septum - AL + PL: Full thickness skin graft or Tripier bipedicle flap with Hughes' flap
Other	- AL: Fricke's flap, lateral temporal flap, midline forehead flap - PL: Free mucous membrane graft, tarsoconjunctival flap	

Data from Subramanian N. Reconstructions of eyelid defect. *Indian J Plast Surg* 2011;44:5–13.

45. Answer: D

TED or Grave's disease is the most common cause for unilateral or bilateral proptosis (whether or not axial or non-axial) among adults. The differential diagnosis of unilateral proptosis can be remembered as '**VEIN**':

Vascular—CCF, arteriovenous malformation, lymphangiectasia

Endocrine—TED

Infective—orbital cellulitis

Inflammatory—OID, myositis, sarcoidosis, granulomatosis with polyangiitis, etc.

Neoplasms—cavernous haemangioma, lymphoma, etc.

Kamminga N, et al. Unilateral proptosis: the role of medical history. *Br J Ophthalmol* 2003;87:370–1.

46. Answer: A

Cavernous haemangioma is the most common primary benign orbital tumours in adults, commonly affecting women at fourth and fifth decades of life. It is a slow growing and often asymptomatic lesion; therefore, it is commonly an incidental finding. The most common sign is axial proptosis due to intraconal location.

Orbital metastases usually present late in multisystem disease but may manifest as the first sign in 15% cases. The lesions are usually located at superior lateral extraconal quadrant. Common primary sites include breast, skin (melanoma), and prostate. Radiographic features are variable, ranging from well-defined round lesions to infiltrating lesions. Pain and diplopia are common symptoms.

Pleomorphic adenomas arise from the lacrimal gland which is an extraconal structure. Solitary fibrous tumour is heterogeneous in signal with low intensity areas which correspond to dense acellular collagen, and is relatively less common.

Calandriello L, et al. Cavernous venous malformation (cavernous hemangioma) of the orbit: Current concepts and a review of the literature. *Surv Ophthalmol* 2017;62:393–403.

Valenzuela AA, et al. Orbital metastasis: clinical features, management and outcome. *Orbit* 2009;28:153–9.

47. Answer: B

Radiotherapy is not advisable in the upper lid due to collateral damage to the conjunctiva, which can result in keratinization. All the other treatments have been recommended for superficial BCC.

The Royal College of Ophthalmologists. *Focus Article: Periocular Basal Cell Carcinoma.* Winter 2011. Available at: https://www.rcophth.ac.uk/wp-content/uploads/2014/08/Focus-Winter-2011.pdf

48. Answer: B

Lymphoma and OID are indistinguishable on clinical and radiological examination, and both improve with steroid treatment. Orbital lymphoma is not reliably associated with serological markers, unlike more disseminated lymphoma which can be associated with a rise in serum lactate dehydrogenase.

Mombaerts I, et al. Consensus on diagnostic criteria of idiopathic orbital inflammation using a modified Delphi approach. *JAMA Ophthalmol* 2017;135:769–76.

49. Answer: C

Rhabdomyosarcoma (RMS) is a highly malignant tumour and is one of the few life-threatening diseases that present first to the ophthalmologist. It is the most common soft-tissue sarcoma of the head and neck in childhood and comprises 4% of all paediatric malignancies, with 10% of all cases occurring in the orbit. Most of these tumours occur in the first decade of life; however, RMS has been reported from birth to the eighth decade. Patients with orbital RMS usually present with proptosis developing rapidly over weeks (80–100%), or globe displacement (80%) which is usually downward and outward because two-thirds of these tumours are superonasal. The mass is usually close to extraocular muscles, but there is no enlargement of the muscle belly. Previously, RMS was believed to arise from extraocular muscles, but now it is thought that it originates from pluripotent mesenchymal cells that have the ability to differentiate into skeletal muscle. The embryonal type comprises 50–70% of orbital RMS.

Jurdy L, et al. Orbital rhabdomyosarcomas: a review. *Saudi J Ophthalmol* 2013;27:167–75.

50. Answer: D

Patients judged at high risk of developing metastases should have 6-monthly lifelong surveillance incorporating a clinical review, nurse specialist support, and liver-specific imaging by a non-ionizing modality such as ultrasound. Liver function tests alone are an inadequate tool for surveillance.

Nathan P, et al. *Uveal Melanoma National Guidelines—Melanoma Focus*, 2015. Available at: http://melanomafocus.com/wp-content/uploads/2015/01/Uveal-Melanoma-National-Guidelines-Full-v5.3.pdf

51. Answer: B

The genetic mechanism of retinoblastoma is governed by the Knudson's two-hit hypothesis whereby both Rb1 tumour suppressor genes need to be mutated for the development of retinoblastoma. The pattern of inheritance is autosomal dominant, but phenotypically it is recessive at cellular level. It can exist in either hereditary/germline or somatic/sporadic form (whereby there is only unilateral involvement). Hereditary form usually results in bilateral and multifocal retinoblastoma and is associated with an increased risk of secondary tumours, notably pinealoma (or known as trilateral retinoblastoma). It has a 90% penetrance, which means the offspring of the affected patients will have a 45% chance of developing retinoblastoma (50% inheriting the gene × 90% penetrance). It is also important to remember that around 10–15% of the unilateral cases have hereditary form of mutation; therefore, in a parent who has unilateral retinoblastoma, there is up to 7% chance of his/her children developing retinoblastoma [15% (hereditary) × 50% (dominant inheritance) × 90% (incomplete penetrance) = around 7%]. If the parent has a unilateral disease and the first child develops retinoblastoma (indicative of germ line mutation), the second child has a 45% risk of developing retinoblastoma. If there is no family history and a child develops retinoblastoma, the risk of sibling developing retinoblastoma is 2% (if the first child has bilateral disease) or 1% (if the first child has unilateral disease).

Draper GJ, et al. Patterns of risk of hereditary retinoblastoma and applications to genetic counselling. *Br J Cancer* 1992;66:211–9.

52. Answer: B

Choroidal naevus is the most common benign intraocular tumour, occurring in about 1 in 10 people. In view of its high prevalence, it is important to familiarize with the risk factors for transformation into melanoma from clinicians' and patients' perspective. Shields et al. have conducted an analysis on 2514 consecutive cases of choroidal naevi and have found the following risk factors based on multivariate analysis. This can be memorized by a mnemonic: '**T**o **F**ind **S**mall **O**cular **M**elanoma **U**sing **H**elpful **H**ints **D**aily'. Patients with three or more of these factors are likely to develop melanoma.

T—Thickness > 2 mm

F—Fluid (subretinal)

S—Symptoms

O—Orange pigment

M—Margin of tumour within 3 mm of the optic disc

UH—Ultrasonographic hollowness

H—Halo absent

D—Drusen absent

Shields CL, et al. Melanoma of the eye: revealing hidden secrets, one at a time. *Clin Dermatol* 2015;33:183–96.

53. Answer: C

MEWDS is usually a self-limiting condition, typically affecting young females (F:M = 4:1) and often preceded by a viral-type illness. It is almost always unilateral with no or very little vitritis, small subtle white-grey lesions (100–200 μm) at the posterior pole to midperiphery and a granular fovea appearance. A RAPD and swollen optic disc may be observed. The other diseases have different features and lesion morphology to that described. In APMPPE, larger white-creamy placoid retinal pigment epithelium lesions are seen acutely followed by chorioretinal scarring. Birdshot is a chronic disease with multiple creamy chorioretinal lesions (often oval), vitritis, and retinal vasculitis, and depigmentation. In birdshot, anterior uveitis is mild or absent, but disc swelling can be observed. PIC usually affects young myopic patients, typically female, with no-mild vitritis and multiple white chorioretinal lesions (usually 50–100 μm) which become atrophic +/− pigmented in time. PIC may present with secondary choroidal neovascularization (CNV) as a complication. RAPD and granular macular appearance would not be observed in typical PIC and are key features of MEWDS.

Salvatore S, et al. Multimodal imaging in acute posterior multifocal placoid pigment epitheliopathy demonstrating obstruction of the choriocapillaris. *Ophthalmic Surg Lasers Imaging Retina* 2016;47:677–81.

Tavallali A, Yannuzzi LA. MEWDS, common cold of the retina. *J Ophthalmic Vis Res* 2017;12:132–4.

54. Answer: B

Understanding the features of anterior uveitis syndromes is important for answering such questions, with need to focus on the disease course, iris involvement, type of keratitic precipitates, and posterior synechiae. The description of sectoral iris atrophy, large irregular pupil, and posterior synechiae are typical descriptors of herpetic uveitis, alongside raised pressure and/or corneal disease. Fuchs' uveitis typically causes heterochromia, diffuse rather than sectoral iris atrophy, vitreous opacity is common, and posterior synechiae are absent. HLA-B27 uveitis is typically recurrent non-granulomatous fibrinous uveitis with risk of posterior synechiae. Similarly, ocular sarcoidosis can present with unilateral or bilateral anterior uveitis (granulomatous or non-granulomatous) and synechiae.

Tay-Kearney ML, et al. Clinical features and associated systemic diseases of HLA-B27 uveitis. *Am J Ophthalmol* 1996;121:47–56.

Van der Lelij A, et al. Anterior uveitis with sectoral iris atrophy in the absence of keratitis: a distinct clinical entity among herpetic eye diseases. *Ophthalmology* 2000;107:1164–70.

55. Answer: D

Systems for classification of uveitis have been assessed in FRCOphth examinations. The SUN grading system is an internationally accepted system for standardization of reporting clinical data in uveitis. This includes anatomical classification (anterior, intermediate, posterior, or panuveitis) based on the site(s) of uveitis and not on the presence of complications (such as cystoid macular oedema (CMO)). Criteria for the onset, duration, and course of the uveitis were also established. Standardized grading schemes for grading anterior chamber cells, anterior chamber flare, and vitreous haze were developed. Although presence of vitreous cells is an important feature, the grading system does not include vitreous cells. Macular oedema can be reported as present or absent but is not part of the grading criteria. Similarly the type of keratitic precipitates is not graded.

Jabs DA, et al. Standardization of Uveitis Nomenclature (SUN) Working Group. Standardization of uveitis nomenclature for reporting clinical data. Results of the First International Workshop. *Am J Ophthalmol* 2005;140:509–16.

56. Answer: A

Both the ocular features and systemic manifestations described are typical of Behçet's disease. Behçet's disease is a chronic, multisystem inflammatory disease characterized by orogenital ulceration. The ocular disease can involve all segments of the eye with non-granulomatous anterior uveitis with a mobile hypopyon and retinitis and occlusive vasculitis (arterial or venous) described. The systemic disease spectrum can be diverse including neurological (headache, venous sinus thrombosis, cranial nerve palsies, vasculitis), intestinal, cutaneous (pustular folliculitis, erythema nodosum), vascular (venous thrombosis), and urogenital (epididymitis, orchitis) manifestations.

Sakane T, et al. Behçet's disease. *N Engl J Med* 1999;341:1284–91.

57. Answer: A

HLA disease associations are an important list to compile for the exam, with particular focus on diseases with ophthalmic involvement. Birdshot chorioretinopathy is strongly associated with HLA-A29. HLA-A29 is found in up to 7% of the Caucasian population and >95% of patients with birdshot chorioretinopathy. HLA-B51 is associated with Behçet's disease but is not part of the diagnostic criteria. HLA-B27 is associated with multiple inflammatory conditions including spondyloarthropathy, inflammatory bowel disease, psoriatic arthropathy, and non-granulomatous anterior uveitis. HLA-DR1 is associated with rheumatoid arthritis.

Suarez-Almazor ME, et al. HLA-DR1, DR4, and DRB1 disease-related subtypes in rheumatoid arthritis. Association with susceptibility but not severity in a city wide community based study. *J Rheumatol* 1995;22:2027–33.

Wee R, Papaliodis G. Genetics of birdshot chorioretinopathy. *Semin Ophthalmol* 2008;23:53–7.

58. Answer: A

The aetiology of scleritis includes inflammatory, infective (e.g. syphilis, tuberculosis, and herpetic) and masquerade conditions (lymphoma and myeloma). Important inflammatory systemic associations are rheumatoid arthritis, granulomatosis with polyangiitis (GPA), and less commonly sarcoidosis. GPA (formerly known as Wegener's granulomatosis) is characterized by presence of antineutrophil cytoplasmic antibodies (ANCA). Around 80–95% of cases are associated with cytoplasmic-ANCA (c-ANCA) directed against proteinase 3 antibodies (PR3) the remainder are perinuclear antibodies (pANCA) against myeloperoxidase (MPO).

The features described are typical features of GPA. GPA has a spectrum of manifestations especially ear, nose, and throat (ENT) and respiratory plus renal, rheumatological, cutaneous, and neurological disease. Peak incidence is 64–75 years old. Typical upper and lower respiratory complications are epistaxis, nasal congestion, chronic sinusitis, haemoptysis, and cough.

Constitutional symptoms include weight loss, fatigue, and night sweats. The age of onset of joint problems in this patient is very atypical for rheumatoid arthritis. Gamma-interferon assay testing (Quantiferon®) is used for tuberculosis testing and a negative result indicates no previous exposure to *Mycobacterium Tuberculosis*.

Kubaisi B, et al. Granulomatosis with polyangiitis (Wegener's disease): An updated review of ocular disease manifestations. *Intractable Rare Dis Res* 2016;5:61–9.

Schonermarck U, et al. Prevalence and spectrum of rheumatic diseases associated with proteinase 3-antineutrophil cytoplasmic antibodies (ANCA) and myeloperoxidase-ANCA. *Rheumatology (Oxford)* 2001;40:178–84.

59. Answer: D

The indications for treatment of toxoplasma retinochoroiditis are: lesions involving/threatening a major vessel, the disc, or macula; significant vitritis and immunocompromised status. Observation may be appropriate for non-sight threatening peripheral lesions in immunocompetent patients. Oral spiramycin is used for treatment of toxoplasmosis pregnancy (on a named patient basis). Oral steroids must NOT be used without antitoxoplasmosis therapy and can cause significant worsening of inflammation. Treatment regimes include co-trimoxazole, clindamycin, azithromycin, atovaquone, and sulfadiazine/pyrimethamine/folinic acid (not folate) with oral corticosteroid therapy. There is no definite consensus on the best treatment regimen.

Lima GS, et al. Current therapy of acquired ocular toxoplasmosis: a review. *J Ocul Pharmacol Ther* 2015;31:511–7.

Ozgonul C, Besirli CG. Recent developments in the diagnosis and treatment of ocular toxoplasmosis. *Ophthalmic Res* 2017;57:1–12.

60. Answer: B

The differential of acute anterior uveitis associated with oral and anal ulceration is between Behçet's disease and Crohn's disease. No mention is made of genital ulceration or other systemic features of Behçet's disease. Ulceration in ulcerative colitis (UC) is mostly restricted to the large bowel. However, UC is associated with HLA-B27 which is frequently associated with enthesitis such as plantar fasciitis or Achilles tendonitis. Crohn's disease is associated with both HLA-B27 and oral and perianal ulceration unlike infectious endogenous endophthalmitis, which should always be in the differential of hypopyon but is not easily linked to either of the other features. All of these conditions would be expected to elevate ESR and CRP.

Chang JH, et al. Acute anterior uveitis and HLA-B27. *Surv Ophthalmol* 2005;50:364–88.

61. Answer: D

Fuchs' heterochromic cyclitis (FHC) is a chronic, low-grade anterior segment uveitis that accounts for around 3% of all uveitis cases. Affected patients are usually asymptomatic and may sometimes complain of mild blurry vision or floaters. It is commonly unilateral (90%) and typical ocular findings include widespread stellate keratic precipitates (cf. inferiorly located keratic precipitates in HLA-related anterior uveitis), mild anterior chamber reaction with mild but persistent cells and flare, absence of posterior synechiae, iris nodules (around 20%), presence of abnormal vessels in iris and trabecular meshwork which may lead to spontaneous or surgical-induced haemorrhage (Amsler's sign), and presence of vitritis. The cause of FHC is unknown but rubella virus has been implicated in the pathogenesis.

Bonfioli AA, et al. Fuchs' heterochromic cyclitis. *Semin Ophthalmol* 2005;20:143–6.

62. Answer: B

The notable feature shown in Figure 3.1A is the marked thickening of the choroid, in the range of 500 microns, suggestive of active choroiditis. The absence of obvious anterior chamber or vitreous inflammation or subretinal fluid should not lull the clinician into a false sense of security. This is an only eye situation that requires urgent rescue with high-dose systemic corticosteroids. Further options may then be considered. These include introduction of a calcineurin inhibitor or an antitumour necrosis factor (TNF) agent. He will also likely need to reduce the dose of mycophenolate mofetil in the face of GI upset. Following the high-dose intravenous methylprednisolone, the choroidal thickening significantly improved (shown in Figure 3.1B).

Arevalo JF, et al. Update on sympathetic ophthalmia. *Middle East Afr J Ophthalmol* 2012;19:13–21.

63. Answer: C

This is a clinical vignette suggestive of endogenous endophthalmitis and the most likely culprit in this case is *Klebsiella pneumonia* in view of the underlying liver abscess and diabetes. Around 95–100% patients with *Klebsiella* endophthalmitis are associated with underlying pyogenic liver abscess and 50–70% of them also have diabetes. The mortality is around 0–20% but can be as high as 50% in patients with septic shock. Around 67–80% of the affected patients end up with vision of NPL or evisceration. Poor visual prognostic factors include diabetes, presence of hypopyon, diffuse posterior involvement, and delayed treatment for more than 24 hours from the onset.

Sheu SJ, et al. Risk factors for endogenous endophthalmitis secondary to Klebsiella pneumonia liver abscess: 20-year experience in Southern Taiwan. *Retina* 2011;31:2026–31.

Tan YM, et al. Ocular manifestations and complications of pyogenic liver abscess. *World J Surg* 2004;28:38–42.

chapter 4

PHARMACOLOGY, THERAPEUTICS, AND INVESTIGATIONS

QUESTIONS

1. A 34-year-old female with a history of severe active bilateral panuveitis is being counselled on systemic immunosuppression therapies. She is keen to start a family and has expressed that she wishes to become pregnant. Which of the following drugs is absolutely contraindicated in pregnancy?
   A. Azathioprine
   B. Ciclosporin
   C. Methotrexate
   D. Prednisolone

2. A 1-year-old boy with congenital glaucoma requires treatment for raised intraocular pressure (IOP). Which of the following topical treatments is contraindicated?
   A. Brimonidine
   B. Brinzolamide
   C. Latanoprost
   D. Timolol

3. In a patient with a history of allergy to sulphonamide antibiotic therapy there is a possibility of cross-reactivity to which of the following drugs?
   A. Azathioprine
   B. Clarithromycin
   C. Co-trimoxazole
   D. Trimethoprim

4. An assay for thiopurine methyltransferase (TPMT) is recommended before starting which immunosuppressive agent?
   A. Azathioprine
   B. Mycophenolate mofetil
   C. Mycophenolate sodium
   D. Tacrolimus

5. In the management of acute anterior uveitis associated with **HLA B27**, subconjunctival 'mydricaine' is often used to break posterior synechiae. Which of the following statement about mydricaine preparation is true?
   A. It contains phenylephrine, procaine, and atropine
   B. It contains adrenaline, procaine, and atropine
   C. It should not be used in the second trimester of pregnancy
   D. It is licensed for use in the treatment of uveitis in the United Kingdom

6. **What is the mechanism of action of vigabatrin (Sabril)?**
   A. Selective irreversible inhibitor of gamma-aminobutyric acid (GABA)-transaminase
   B. Non-selective irreversible inhibitor of GABA-transaminase
   C. Selective reversible inhibitor of GABA-transaminase
   D. Non-selective reversible inhibitor of GABA-transaminase

7. **Tocilizumab, an anti-interleukin 6 receptor antibody, is approved by the National Institute for Health and Care Excellence (NICE) for treatment of which of the following conditions?**
   A. Giant cell arteritis
   B. Granulomatosis with polyangiitis
   C. Multiple sclerosis
   D. Thyroid eye disease

8. **Which of the following mechanisms of action best describes aflibercept?**
   A. Inhibits vascular endothelial growth factor (VEGF)-A
   B. Inhibits VEGF-B
   C. Inhibits VEGF-A and -B
   D. Inhibits VEGF-A and -B and placental growth factor

9. **A 27-year-old male presented to casualty with a one-week history of bilateral reduced vision. An optical coherence tomography (OCT) performed in casualty revealed bilateral retinal striae. Which of the following is a possibility?**
   A. He had seen his neurologist 10 days earlier who had increased his topiramate from 75 mg to 100 mg
   B. He had seen his neurologist 10 days earlier who had increased his sodium valproate from 500 mg OD to BD
   C. He had seen his neurologist 10 days earlier who had stopped his phenytoin
   D. He had seen his neurologist 10 days earlier who had stopped his vigabatrin

10. **What is the mechanism of action of the commonly used fusidic acid (or fucithalmic acid)?**
    A. Inhibits cell wall synthesis
    B. Inhibits DNA replication
    C. Inhibits folic acid metabolism
    D. Inhibits protein synthesis

11. **Tacrolimus and cyclosporine have similar mechanisms of action. However, which of the following is correct?**
    A. Tacrolimus is ten times more potent than cyclosporine
    B. Tacrolimus is 100 times more potent than cyclosporine
    C. Cyclosporine is ten times more potent than tacrolimus
    D. Cyclosporine is 100 times more potent than tacrolimus

12. **A 45-year-old male presented to the corneal clinic with severe keratitis, which had not improved despite treatment with tear substitutes. He was prescribed topical cyclosporine (1 mg/ml or 0.1%). He was particularly concerned about the main adverse events. Which is the commonest investigator-related adverse event?**
    A. Blurred vision
    B. Erythema of the eyelid
    C. Instillation site pain
    D. Ocular hyperaemia

13. **What is the mechanism of action of vismodegib—a drug that is used in basal cell carcinoma (BCC)?**
    A. Causes alkylation of DNA
    B. Inhibits Hedgehog pathway
    C. Inhibits interleukin 2
    D. Inhibits tumour necrosis factor (TNF)-alpha

14. **A 79-year-old keen gardener with age-related macular degeneration attends the clinic after purchasing a box of MacuShield, which contains the ingredient of meso-zeaxanthin. He asks which plant is used:**
    A. *Allium tricoccum*
    B. *Allium tuberosum*
    C. Daffodil
    D. Marigold

15. A 45-year-old Caucasian patient attends eye casualty. He reports distorted vision. On examination he has evidence of 1 mm punched out yellow spots, a macular choroidal neovascular membrane (CNVM) seen on optical coherence tomography angiography with scarring adjacent to the optic disc. He reports a recent sabbatical to the Ohio-Mississippi River Valley. Which of the following is the correct treatment?

    A. Oral terbinafine 250 mg daily for six weeks
    B. Oral terbinafine 500 mg daily for four weeks
    C. Oral tetracycline 500 mg daily for two days
    D. Focal laser

16. Which of the following is not a known side effect of gefitinib—an epidermal growth factor receptor (EGFR) inhibitor?

    A. Blepharoconjunctivitis
    B. Corneal erosion
    C. Metamorphopsia
    D. Trichomegaly

17. A 63-year-old female patient presents to the eye clinic with chronic conjunctivitis. Examination reveals cicatricial conjunctival conjunctivitis with symblepharon and subtarsal conjunctival scarring. She also discloses a history of glucose-6-phosphate dehydrogenase (G6PD) deficiency. Which of the following medications is contraindicated?

    A. Dapsone
    B. Mycophenolate mofetil
    C. Rituximab
    D. Tacrolimus

18. What is the mechanism of action of imiquimod, a drug that is approved for treating superficial BCC?

    A. Anti-interleukin (IL)-2
    B. Anti-IL-12
    C. Interferon β-1a antagonist
    D. Toll-like receptor 7 agonist

19. Which of the following conditions is NOT associated with the following OCT image in an adult patient (shown in Figure 4.1)?

    A. Central serous chorioretinopathy
    B. Harada's disease
    C. Macular telangiectasia
    D. Pre-eclampsia

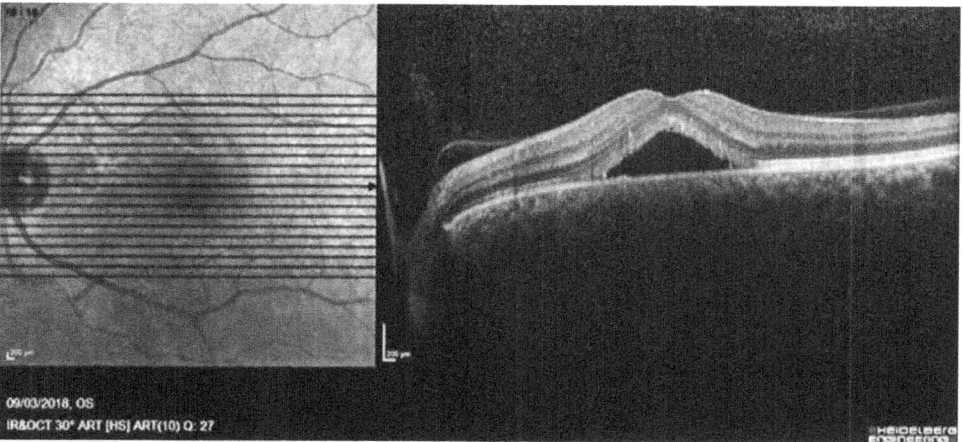

Figure 4.1

20. A patient presents with blurred vision with evidence of uveitis and multifocal serous retinal detachment. The patient has headache, tinnitus, and neck stiffness. Lumbar puncture shows evidence of pleocytosis. A wide-field fundus fluorescein angiography (FFA) is performed and shows multiple foci of pinpoint hyperfluorescence followed by pooling of fluorescein within the subretinal space. What is the most likely diagnosis?

   A. Posterior scleritis
   B. Primary central nervous system (CNS) lymphoma
   C. Sympathetic ophthalmia
   D. Vogt–Koyanagi–Harada (VKH) disease

21. If FFA of CNVM shows early lacy hyperfluorescence and late leakage, which of the following is correct?

   A. The lesion is a classic lesion
   B. The lesion is a predominantly classic lesion
   C. The lesion is a minimally classic lesion
   D. The lesion is an occult lesion with no classic features

22. In testing for *Mycobacterium tuberculosis* which statement is most true?

   A. A positive gamma-interferon test result indicates active *Mycobacterium tuberculosis* infection
   B. Gamma-interferon testing is not influenced by prior Bacillus Calmette–Guérin (BCG) vaccination
   C. Gamma-interferon testing is negative in patients who have received a full course of antituberculous therapy
   D. Gamma-interferon testing in interpreted by quantification of degree of skin induration at the site of subcutaneous injection of plasma protein derivative (PPD).

23. In FFA, what is the normal arm-eye time?
    A. 2–3 seconds
    B. 10–12 seconds
    C. 20 seconds
    D. 60 seconds

24. Which of the following medication is associated with the OCT appearance shown in Figure 4.2?
    A. Hydroxychloroquine
    B. Nicotinic acid
    C. Rifabutin
    D. Tamoxifen

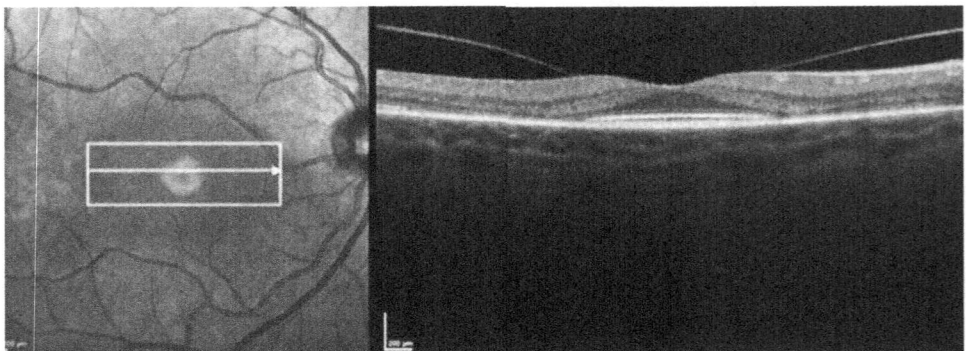

Figure 4.2

25. Which of the following statement regarding culture media for corneal scraping is true?
    A. Cooked meat broth specifically grows aerobic bacteria
    B. Blood agar grows most bacteria and fungi
    C. Chocolate agar is particularly good for meningococci and streptococci
    D. Brain heart infusion grows anaerobic bacteria

26. Which of following about ophthalmic ultrasonography is true?
    A. The use of lower frequency transducer allows generation of images with much higher resolution
    B. The use of lower frequency transducer allows greater depth penetration
    C. Orbital ultrasound uses a high frequency ultrasonic transducer
    D. B-scan can be used to measure axial length

27. **What is the following imaging technique shown in Figure 4.3 and what is the most likely diagnosis?**
    A. Fluorescein angiography; wet macular degeneration
    B. Indocyanine green angiography; wet macular degeneration
    C. Autofluorescence; adult vitelliform disease
    D. Red free imaging, adult vitelliform disease

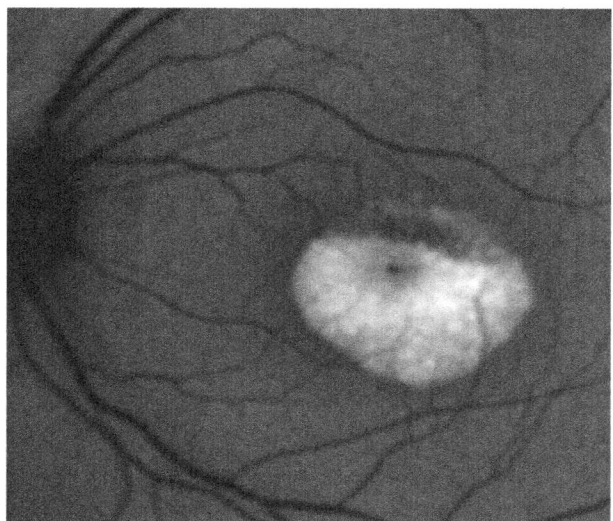

Figure 4.3

28. **Which of the following statements regarding indocyanine green angiography (ICGA) is true?**
    A. Is safer in pregnancy than fluorescein angiography
    B. Is contraindicated in patients with iodine allergy
    C. Has an excitation peak at 490 nm and emission of 530 nm
    D. Does not stain the stool

29. **Which of the following options regarding anterior segment optical coherence tomography (AS-OCT) is true?**
    A. Uses a shorter wavelength light source compared to posterior OCT
    B. Is inferior to ultrasound biomicroscopy (UBM) in visualization of the lens
    C. Does not easily allow assessment of the drainage angle
    D. Is inferior to UBM in the assessment of anterior stromal scars

30. **Which of the following statements about A-scan is true?**
    A. The axial length of the globe may be artefactually longer in the presence of silicone oil
    B. The axial length of the globe may be artefactually longer in eyes with asteroid hyalosis
    C. Can be used to locate intraocular foreign body
    D. It obtains the axial length measurement from the retinal pigment epithelium

31. **Visual evoked potential (VEP):**
    A. Is a reliable test of the optic nerve function in a patient with advanced macular degeneration
    B. Cannot detect subclinical optic nerve demyelination
    C. Shows a decreased amplitude and increased peak-time of P100 in optic neuritis
    D. Flash VEP provides more information than pattern reversal VEP

32. **What is the principle of imaging utilized by Pentacam machine?**
    A. Placido disc
    B. Placido disc and scanning slit technique
    C. Purkinje images
    D. Scheimpflug imaging

33. **The requirements to complete a Lees screen test to measure ocular deviation is:**
    A. Normal vision in at least one eye
    B. Normal colour vision in both eyes
    C. Normal retinal correspondence
    D. Normal visual field

34. **Which of the following statements about prism adaptation test (PAT) is correct?**
    A. It is effective in predicting postoperative sensory and motor fusion especially in patients with congenital esotropia
    B. The angle increase after PAT is generally smaller than diagnostic occlusion test
    C. Preoperative prism correction is not useful in the determination of the amount of surgery
    D. The increase in the squint angle after PAT is caused by an anomalous sensorial relationship between the two eyes

35. **Which of the following orthoptic tests CANNOT measure torsion?**
    A. Hess chart
    B. Maddox rod
    C. Maddox wing
    D. Synoptophore

36. **Which of the following about accommodative convergence/accommodation (AC/A) ratio is correct?**
    A. Gradient AC/A method requires measurement of interpupillary distance (IPD)
    B. Heterophoria AC/A requires a plus lens for the test
    C. The normal AC/A ratio is 3–5 degree/dioptre
    D. AC/A ratio is usually low in simulated intermittent distance exotropia (IDEX)

37. **Which of the following neuroimaging tests is shown to be best in imaging intracranial aneurysm?**
    A. Computed tomography (CT)
    B. CT angiography
    C. Magnetic resonance imaging (MRI) with no contrast
    D. MR angiography

38. **A 62-year-old man presented to clinic describing reduction in vision. He had thought it had been coming on over 3 months. He had no headaches and his recent refraction was unchanged from previous attendance at optometry. On examination his visual acuity was 6/12 in both eyes and his colour vision was reduced to 3/14 in both eyes. There was bilateral temporal pallor of both optic nerves but otherwise no relative afferent pupillary defect. OCT of each optic nerve showed loss of temporal nerve fibres bilaterally. Visual fields to confrontation showed a bitemporal hemianopia. What radiological investigations would you perform next?**
    A. Computed tomography angiogram (CTA) of circle of Willis
    B. CT head
    C. MRI of orbit
    D. MRI brain with gadolinium

39. **Which of the following features is most likely found in the condition shown in Figure 4.4?**
    A. Anterior segment dysgenesis
    B. Cataract
    C. Optic nerve hypoplasia
    D. Retinal dystrophy

40. **What is the choice of neuroimaging in patients with suspected optic neuritis?**
    A. CT head with contrast
    B. CTA of circle of Willis
    C. MRI using fluid attenuated inversion recovery (FLAIR) sequence
    D. MR head and orbit with gadolinium contrast

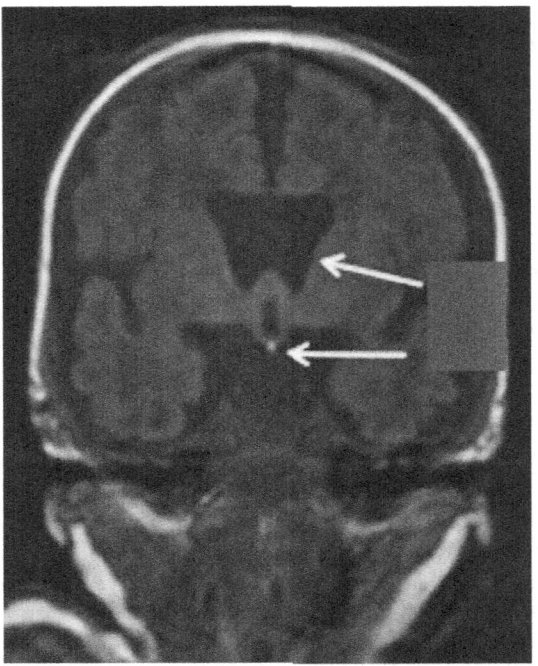

Figure 4.4

Reprinted by permission from Springer Nature: Nature, *European Journal of Human Genetics*, 18(4):393–397, Septooptic dysplasia. Webb, E., and Dattani, M. https://doi.org/10.1038/ejhg.2009.125. Copyright © 2009, Springer Nature.

41. **A 53-year-old man, a heavy smoker, presents to the eye emergency clinic with 3 days' history of significant right-sided ear pain, mild ptosis, and anisocoria, suggestive of possible Horner's syndrome. What is the most appropriate radiological investigation for this patient?**
    A. CT head and CTA head and neck
    B. MRI head and base of skull with gadolinium
    C. MRI head and magnetic resonance angiography (MRA) Circle of Willis
    D. MRI internal auditory meatus

42. **Which of the following about dacryoscintigram (DSG) is correct?**
    A. It requires injection of a radio-opaque contrast medium into the lacrimal drainage system
    B. Patient is instructed to lie flat during the procedure
    C. It is not useful for proximal obstruction
    D. It is a useful investigation for functional epiphora

chapter 4

PHARMACOLOGY, THERAPEUTICS, AND INVESTIGATIONS

ANSWERS

1. Answer: C

Methotrexate at any dose is contraindicated in pregnancy due to teratogenic effects and must be stopped at least 3 months before conception. Mycophenolate mofetil is also not safe for use in pregnancy with risk of teratogenicity and spontaneous abortion. Azathioprine, ciclosporin, and tacrolimus can be safely used in pregnancy if prescribed within recommended doses. Prednisolone is compatible with all stages of pregnancy.

Flint J, et al. BSR and BHPR guideline on prescribing drugs in pregnancy and breastfeeding—part I: standard and biologic disease modifying anti-rheumatic drugs and corticosteroids. *Rheumatology (Oxford)* 2016;55:1693–7.

2. Answer: A

This is an important safety topic in pharmacology. Brimonidine can cause Central nervous system (CNS) depression in children including drowsiness or lethargy. The drug is contraindicated in neonates and infants (<2 years old). Alternative IOP lowering therapy should be considered in children under 12 years and used with caution and close monitoring. There are no apparent contraindications to β-blocker therapy in this patient (namely asthma, chronic obstructive pulmonary disease (COPD), bradycardia, and heart block) and topical brinzolamide is effective and safe to use in children. Prostaglandin therapy is also safe in children.

Al-Shahwan S, et al. Side-effect profile of brimonidine tartrate in children. *Ophthalmology* 2005;112:2143.

Coppens G, et al. The safety and efficacy of glaucoma medication in the pediatric population. *J Pediatr Ophthalmol Strabismus* 2009;46:12–18.

3. Answer: C

Co-trimoxazole is a combined antibiotic of trimethoprim and sulfamethoxazole, which contains the sulfonamide chemical group. It is usually used for the treatment of toxoplasma uveitis. In the context of ophthalmology, it is noteworthy to mention about acetazolamide, which is a sulfonamide derivative. The British National Formulary (BNF) highlights that acetazolamide is contraindicated if there is confirmed sulfonamide hypersensitivity.

Mayo Clinic. Sulfa allergy: Which medications should I avoid? Available at: https://www.mayoclinic.org/diseases-conditions/drug-allergy/expert-answers/sulfa-allergy/faq-20057970

4. Answer: A

Azathioprine (AZA) is metabolized to its active metabolite by a series of enzyme steps, including TPMT. TPMT enzyme activity is highly variable: 90% of individuals have high/normal activity, 10% have intermediate activity, and 0.3% low/absent activity. The British Society of Rheumatology disease-modifying antirheumatic drug (DMARD) guidelines recommend performing TPMT assay before starting AZA. The assay provides additional risk of toxicity but does not replace routine monitoring. Patients with low enzyme activity are at potential risk of profound neutropenia (which may be delayed by several months). Reduced dosing or an alternative drug should be considered. Baseline laboratory organ function (FBC, U&E, LFTs) are mandatory before starting all the medications but no specific enzyme assay is required for the other medications.

Ledingham J, et al. BSR and BHPR guideline for the prescription and monitoring of non-biologic disease-modifying anti-rheumatic drugs. *Rheumatology (Oxford)* 2017;56:865–68.

McLeod HL, et al. Analysis of thiopurine methyltransferase variant alleles in childhood acute lymphoblastic leukaemia. *Br J Haematol* 1999;105:696–700.

5. Answer: B

Mydricaine for subconjunctival injection is marketed by Moorfields Pharmaceuticals in 0.3 ml vials, indicated for use in acute anterior uveitis to achieve maximal mydriasis. Caution is advised in pregnancy but use of mydricaine is not contraindicated. The product is not licensed for use in the United Kingdom but is routinely used on an off-license basis in the absence of a licensed alternative. It comes in two preparations; mydricaine No.1 is used in paediatric or elderly patients and it contains procaine 3 mg, atropine 0.5 mg, and adrenaline 108 µg, whereas mydricaine No. 2 is used in adult patients and it contains procaine 6 mg, atropine 1 mg, and adrenaline 216 µg (effectively double the dose of the No. 1 preparation).

Steel DH, Thorn J. The incidence of systemic side-effects following subconjunctival mydricaine no. 1 injection. *Eye (Lond)* 1999;13:720–2.

6. Answer: A

Vigabatrin acts as a selective irreversible inhibitor of GABA-transaminase. The drug is water soluble and rapidly absorbed by the gastrointestinal tract. Maximal efficacy is usually seen in the 2–3 g/day range (children 50–100 mg/kg/day). It is predominantly used in partial epilepsy, with or without secondary generalization. It is the one of the main treatments for West syndrome (infantile spasms). Dr West first described the condition in his 4-month-old son in 1841.

The Royal College of Ophthalmologists. *The Ocular Side-Effects of Vigabatrin (Sabril) Information and Guidance for Screening.* 2008. Available at: https://www.rcophth.ac.uk/wp-content/uploads/2015/01/2008-SCI-020-The-Ocular-Side-Effects-of-Vigabatrin-Sabril.pdf

7. Answer: A

Tocilizumab (RoActemra) is an immunosuppressive drug. It is a humanized monoclonal antibody that targets against the interleukin-6 receptor (IL-6R). Tocilizumab is approved by NICE for the treatment of rheumatoid arthritis and giant cell arteritis. It can be used in combination with a tapering course of glucocorticoid or alone following discontinuation of glucocorticoid. It is given every week via subcutaneous injection (162 mg). The main clinical evidence for the use of tocilizumab came from GiACTA, a multicentre, double-blind, randomized controlled trial.

National Institute for Health and Care Excellence (NICE). *Tocilizumab for Treating Giant Cell Arteritis [TA518].* Available at: https://www.nice.org.uk/guidance/ta518

8. Answer: D

Aflibercept, also known as Eylea or VEGF Trap, is a novel soluble decoy receptor which utilizes the fusion of components from multiple endogenous receptors. It inhibits VEGF-A, VEGF-B, and placental growth factor (PlGF). It has a much higher affinity to VEGF-A than ranibizumab and bevacizumab. More importantly it is the only anti-VEGF agent that targets VEGF-B and PlGF.

Papadopoulos N, et al. Binding and neutralization of vascular endothelial growth factor (VEGF) and related ligands by VEGF Trap, ranibizumab and bevacizumab. *Angiogenesis* 2012;15:171–85.

9. Answer: A

The use of topiramate is becoming increasingly popular for the management of epilepsy, migraine, trigeminal neuralgia, and depression. The anterior segment ocular side effects have been extensively reported but the documentation and mechanism of a pure topiramate maculopathy is less well understood. This is highlighted by the omission of any reference of a pure maculopathy in the RCOphth guidelines. A thorough drug history including any recent change in dosage when faced with a similar clinical scenario is required. It is imperative the underlying diagnosis behind the use of topiramate is established and changes in dosage or discontinuation must be carried out in consultation with the patient's GP and/or neurologist. Topiramate maculopathy is not a life-threatening condition, whereas status epilepticus is.

Severn P, et al. Topiramate maculopathy secondary to dose titration: first reported case. *Eye (Lond)* 2015;29:982–4.

10. Answer: D

Fusidic acid is a bacteriostatic antibiotic that inhibits protein synthesis by preventing the turnover of elongation factor G (EF-G) from the ribosome. It primarily works on Gram-positive bacteria. Following is a summary table of the mechanisms of action (MOA) of commonly used antibiotics (Table 4.1).

Table 4.1 Mechanisms of action for commonly used antibiotics

MOA	Antibiotics
Inhibit cell wall synthesis (therefore effective against Gram-positive bacteria)	Penicillin, cephalosporin, vancomycin
Inhibit protein synthesis: - Inhibit 30 S subunits of ribosome - Inhibit 50 S subunits of ribosome - Inhibits EF-G of ribosome	Aminoglycoside, tetracycline Chloramphenicol, macrolide Fusidic acid
Inhibit DNA synthesis	Fluoroquinolone
Inhibit folic acid metabolism	Sulfonamide, trimethoprim

Kapoor S, et al. Action and resistance mechanisms of antibiotics: a guide for clinicians. *J Anaesthesiol Clin Pharmacol* 2017;33:300–5.

11. Answer: B

Tacrolimus and cyclosporine are both immunosuppressive agents that inhibit calcineurin, which then subsequently inactivates nuclear factor of activated T cells (NFAT) and inhibits IL-2. Tacrolimus, or also known as fujimycin or FK506, is used mainly after allogenic transplants to decrease the risk of organ rejection. It was first described in 1987 from the fermentation broth of a Japanese soil that contained the bacterium *Streptomyces tsukubaensis*. The main enzyme responsible for its metabolism is CYP3A5. Tacrolimus is 50–100 times more potent than cyclosporine and has been shown to be effective in the treatment of immune-mediated diseases such as corneal graft rejection, ocular inflammation, ocular pemphigoid, and uveitis.

PHARMGKB. *Tacrolimus/Cyclosporine Pathway, Pharmacodynamics*. Available at: https://www.pharmgkb.org/pathway/PA165985892

12. Answer: C

Topical ciclosprorin drops (Ikervis) are indicated for severe keratitis in adult patients with dry eye disease that has not improved despite treatment with tear substitutes. The main adverse events with ciclosporin eye drops appear to be related to ocular discomfort when administering the medicine. Pooled data from SANSIKA, SICCANOVE, and two phase II studies indicate that the most common ocular adverse events considered by the investigator as possibly related to ciclosporin were: instillation site pain (16%), instillation site irritation (9%), eye irritation (8.8%), eye pain (3.5%), instillation site lacrimation (2.9%), lacrimation increased (2.1%), instillation site erythema (1.9%), ocular hyperaemia (1.9%), conjunctival hyperaemia (1.7%), erythema of eyelid (1.7%), eyelid oedema (1.3%), and blurred vision (1.2%).

Scottish Medicines Consortium. Cyclosporin (Ikervis). SMC No. (1089/15). Available at: https://www.scottishmedicines.org.uk/medicines-advice/ciclosporin-ikervis-fullsubmission-108915/

13. Answer: B

Vismodegib is an approved medication for locally advanced or metastatic BCC. It works by inhibiting the Hedgehog pathway, which is important for cell growth and differentiation during embryogenesis. A dysregulated Hedgehog signalling pathway has been implicated in the pathogenesis of BCC. Mitomycin-C is an immunosuppressant commonly used in glaucoma surgery and its primary mechanism of action is alkylation of DNA. Tacrolimus and cyclosporine inhibit interleukin-2, whereas infliximab and adalimumab are the common anti-TNF-alpha treatment.

Aditya S, Rattan A. Vismodegib: a smoothened inhibitor for the treatment of advanced basal cell carcinoma. *Indian Dermatol Online J* 2013;4:365–68.

14. Answer: D

Macushield is a food supplement containing the antioxidant carotenoids, zeaxanthin, and meso-zeaxanthin. Meso-zeaxanthin is extracted from marigolds. It is a xanthophyll carotenoid and contains three stereoisomers of zeaxanthin. In 2013, the Age-Related Eye Disease Study 2 (AREDS2) reported a reduced risk of visual loss and a reduced risk of disease progression in patients with non-advanced age-related macular degeneration. However, the AREDS2 preparation did not contain meso-zeaxanthin, which is the dominant carotenoid at the very centre of the macula, and the presence of which is essential for maximum collective antioxidant effect.

Nolan JM, et al. What is meso-zeaxanthin, and where does it come from? *Eye (Lond)* 2013;27:899–905.

15. Answer: D

The patient is suffering from presumed ocular histoplasmosis syndrome (POHS) and has the classical triad of yellow spots, a macular CNVM, and atrophy/scarring adjacent to the optic disc. In addition, linear rows of histo-spots might be visible in the peripheral fundus. POHS is a type of multifocal chorioretinitis caused by *Histoplasma capsulatum* and is endemic in Ohio and Mississippi river valleys. It is likened to HLA DRw2 and B7. There is a common misconception that the condition is treated with oral antifungal treatment, which is not the case. For a well-defined lesion, the patient can be offered focal or photodynamic therapy laser. Surgical removal of the lesion could be considered if the lesion remains too central. In addition, antivascular endothelial growth factor (VEGF) treatment and intravitreal triamcinolone (4 mg) steroids have also been tried with varying degrees of success.

Iyengar SS, Dyer DS. Diagnosing and treating histoplasmosis. 2019. Available at: https://www.aao.org/eyenet/article/diagnosing-treating-histoplasmosis

16. Answer: C

EGFR inhibitors are used for the treatment of many solid tumours, including non-small cell bronchial carcinoma, pancreatic carcinoma, colorectal carcinoma, and BCC. EGFR is one of the key receptors in wound healing of the cornea. Epidermal growth factor (EGF) stimulates proliferation of the epithelial cells of the meibomian glands in the eyelids. If the effect of EGF is inhibited, corneal wound healing is delayed and meibomian glands become inflamed.

Hager T, Seitz B. Ocular side effects of biological agents in oncology: what should the clinician be aware of? *Onco Targets Ther* 2014;7:69–77.

17. Answer: A

Dapsone is an antibiotic which also possess anti-inflammatory and immunosuppressive properties. It has been shown to be effective in treating mild ocular cicatricial pemphigoid. However, it should not be used in patients with G6PD deficiency as it increases the risk of haemolysis. In addition, systemic treatment needs to be escalated to either azathioprine, methotrexate, mycophenolate, or cyclophosphamide if the condition is not adequately controlled with dapsone within 3 months.

Neff AG, et al. Treatment strategies in mucous membrane pemphigoid. *Ther Clin Risk Manag* 2008;4:617–26.

18. Answer: D

Imiquimod is an approved topical medication for treating superficial BCC. It acts as a toll-like receptor 7 agonist and it modifies the immune response through upregulation of the cytokines. While surgery is the gold standard for treating BCC, imiquimod has been shown to be a relatively effective, less invasive, and cheaper treatment option for superficial BCC.

Kamath P, et al. A review on imiquimod therapy and discussion on optimal management of basal cell carcinomas. *Clin Drug Investig* 2018;38:883–9.

19. Answer: C

All these conditions are associated with serous retinal detachments, except macular telangiectasia. The image shown in Figure 4.1 is a case of central serous chorioretinopathy (CSCR). Candidates for the Fellowship of the Royal College of Ophthalmologists (FRCOphth) Part 2 exam should be aware of the differential diagnosis for serous retinal detachments at the macula. These include:

- Vascular: Age-related macular degeneration (including idiopathic polypoidal choroidal vasculopathy), retinal macroaneurysm
- Idiopathic—CSCR
- Ischaemia (choroidal hypoperfusion): Pre-eclampsia, malignant hypertension
- Inflammation: Harada's disease
- Neoplasia: Choroidal tumours

Hikichi T, et al. Causes of macular serous retinal detachment in Japanese patients 40 years and older. *Retina* 2009;29:395–404.

20. Answer: D

The diseases listed are all differential diagnoses for serous retinal detachment. VKH is a bilateral granulomatous uveitis disorder associated with serous detachments, vitritis, and disc oedema. VKH presents in four different phases: prodrome, acute, convalescent, and recurrent. Associated systemic manifestations include headache, meningism, tinnitus, poliosis, and vitiligo. The FFA findings described are highly-characteristic of this condition. Ultrasound B-scan is useful for differentiating from posterior scleritis as there will be absence of T-sign, which is due to sub-Tenon's fluid. Lymphoma is a masquerade disease but the cerebrospinal fluid (CSF) findings and systemic features exclude this answer. Sympathetic ophthalmia is also a bilateral granulomatous disorder but is not associated with systemic disease and a history of trauma or intraocular surgery/procedure is necessary for diagnosis.

O'Keefe GA, Rao NA. Vogt-Koyanagi-Harada disease. *Surv Ophthalmol* 2017;62:1–25.

21. Answer: A

The FFA features of CNVM are important, including features differentiating between different subtypes. Classic CNVMs are described as early bright or lacy hyperfluorescence followed by late leakage. Predominantly classic lesions are where classic choroidal neovascularization (CNV) forms at least 50% of the lesion and minimally classic where this is less than 50%.

Occult membranes are classified as fibrovascular pigment epithelial detachments (PED) or late leakage of undetermined origin. The former shows stippled or irregular hyperfluorescence followed by leakage in the later stages of the angiogram. Classic membranes are located in the subretinal space and are type 2 membranes, whereas occult membranes are subretinal pigment epithelium and termed type 1 membranes.

Arias L, Mones J. Fluorescein angiography. Last revision October 2011. Available at: http://www.amdbook.org/content/fluorescein-angiography-0

22. Answer: B

NICE published UK guidelines for the diagnosis and management of active and latent tuberculosis in 2016. Testing for tuberculosis involves Mantoux skin testing (if available) and gamma-interferon assay ((G-IFN) Quantiferon®) blood test. G-IFN is a quantitative analysis of G-IFN release by T cells on exposure to *M. tuberculosis* antigen. Mantoux test is a subcutaneous injection of PPD of *M. tuberculosis* and the degree of reaction is quantified in mm of reaction at 48–72 hours. G-IFN is not influenced by prior BCG, whereas Mantoux testing is and therefore must be interpreted according to history of previous BCG. G-IFN is NOT useful for distinguishing between active and latent disease; it indicates prior exposure and not activity. G-IFN therefore remains positive after a full course of antituberculous therapy.

National Institute for Health and Care Excellence (NICE). *Tuberculosis. NICE Guideline [NG33]*. January 2016. Available at: https://www.nice.org.uk/guidance/ng33

23. Answer: B

FFA progresses through stages: (a) choroidal flush; (b) arterial; (c) arteriovenous; (c) venous; and (d) late re-circulation. The time from injection in the arm to appearance in the central retinal artery (arm–eye time) is 10–12 seconds, 1–2 seconds after the initial choroidal flush. A delay in the arm–eye time can reflect cardiovascular disease, such as carotid disease and is seen in ocular ischaemic syndrome. The venous stage is maximal at 30 seconds.

American Academy of Ophthalmology. Fluorescein angiography. 2019. Available at: https://eyewiki.aao.org/Fluorescein_Angiography

24. Answer: A

The OCT appearance in Figure 4.2 is consistent with hydroxychloroquine maculopathy. It demonstrates the 'flying saucer' sign. An ovoid appearance of the central fovea created by preservation of central foveal outer retinal structures surrounded by perifoveal loss of the photoreceptor inner segment/outer segment (IS/OS) junction, and perifoveal outer retinal thinning. The RCOphth had recently released

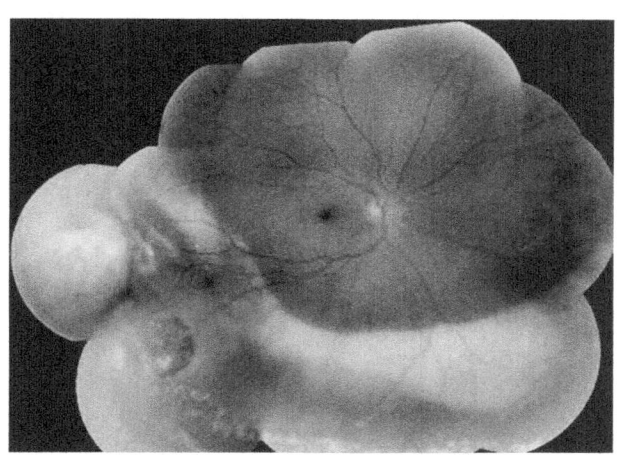

Figure 2.4

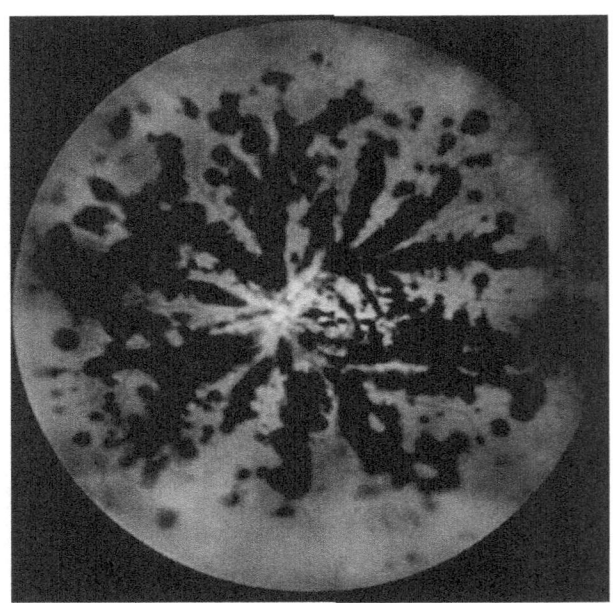

Figure 6.1

the screening guidelines for hydroxychloroquine retinopathy. It is also important that candidates for the FRCOphth Part 2 examination are similar with causes of drug-induced maculopathy.

American Academy of Ophthalmology. Talk: drug-induced maculopathy. 2018. Available at: http://eyewiki.aao.org/Talk%3ADrug_induced_maculopathy

Royal College of Ophthalmologists. *Clinical Guidelines: Hydroxychloroquine and Chloroquine Retinopathy: Recommendations*. February 2018. Available at: https://www.rcophth.ac.uk/wp-content/uploads/2018/03/Hydroxychloroquine-and-Chloroquine-Retinopathy-Screening-Guideline-and-Recommendations.pdf

25. Answer: B

Following is a summary table of culture media for various microorganisms (Table 4.2).

Microbeonline. Bacterial Culture Media: classification, types and uses. 2010. Available at: https://microbeonline.com/types-of-bacteriological-culture-medium/

Table 4.2 Culture media and their corresponding microorganisms

Culture media	Intended microorganisms
Blood agar	Most bacteria and fungi
Brain heart infusion	Streptococci and meningococci
Chocolate agar	*Haemophilus influenza*, *Neisseria* spp., and *Moraxella* spp.
Cooked meat broth	Anaerobic and fastidious bacteria
Non-nutrient agar with *E. coli* overlay	*Acanthamoeba* spp.
Sabouraud dextrose agar	Fungi

26. Answer: B

Higher frequency and shorter wavelength are usually associated with higher resolution of images but poorer penetration. For example, ultrasound biomicroscopy (UBM) for anterior segment imaging uses ultrasound frequencies in the 50–100 MHz range, whereas the commonly used diagnostic B-scan uses frequencies of 8–10 MHz and orbital ultrasound uses 4–5 MHz. A-scan can be used to measure the axial length.

Kendall CJ, et al. Diagnostic ophthalmic ultrasound for radiologists. *Neuroimaging Clin N Am* 2015;25:327–65.

27. Answer: C

Fundus autofluorescence (FAF) is a novel imaging technique to examine the distribution of lipofuscin deposition in the retina. Hyper-FAF indicates dysfunctional retinal pigment epithelium. In Figure 4.3 the optic disc shows hypo-FAF and the deposit in adult vitelliform, which is usually rich in lipofuscin, hyperfluoresces on atrial fibrillation (AF). In red free imaging, the disc appears white and not dark.

Schmitz-Valckenberg S, et al. Fundus autofluorescence imaging: review and perspectives. *Retina* 2008;28:385–409.

28. Answer: B

Safety data on the use of indocyanine green (ICG) in pregnancy is scarce and generally considered a relative contraindication. ICG contains 5% iodine hence it is contraindicated in patients with iodine allergy. It has an excitation peak at 810 nm and emission of 830 nm. The longer wavelength light enhances depth penetration, especially in cases of retinal haemorrhage. Side effects of ICG include nausea/vomiting, sneezing, pruritus, staining of stool, backache, syncope, and anaphylaxis.

Lim JI. Recent developments in indocyanine green angiography. *Curr Opin Ophthalmol* 1996;7:46–50.

29. Answer: B

Anterior segment OCT uses a longer wavelength light compared to posterior segment OCT (1310 nm vs. 800 nm). UBM allows better visualization of the lens due to greater depth penetration. It is superior in assessment of the cornea, including post-graft position, post-LASIK graft thickness, and thickness of anterior stromal scars.

Konstantopoulos A, et al. Recent advances in ophthalmic anterior segment imaging: a new era for ophthalmic diagnosis? *Br J Ophthalmol* 2007;91:551–7.

30. Answer: A

Ultrasound travels slower in silicone oil compared to vitreous, hence the axial length can be artefactually longer if the correct setting is not used. In contrast, ultrasound travels faster with asteroid hyalosis and the axial length can be measured shorter than the true axial length. B-scan rather than A-scan is used to locate intraocular foreign body and detect calcification on optic disc drusen. It is also important to remember that, unlike optical biometry (e.g. IOLMaster) which uses partial coherence intereferometry, A-scan or acoustic biometry measure the axial length from inner limiting membrane and not retinal pigment epithelium.

Silverman RH. Focused ultrasound in ophthalmology. *Clin Ophthalmol* 2016;10:1865–75.

31. Answer: C

VEP records gross electrical response from the visual cortex in response to a changing visual stimulus such as multiple flash or changing pattern stimuli. It requires relatively normal retinal/macular function to be a reliable test. It is often used to detect subclinical optic nerve demyelination, chiasmal and retrochiasmal dysfunction, and non-organic visual loss. Pattern reversal VEP provides more information than flash VEP but flash VEP is useful in poorly cooperative patients.

Creel D. Visually evoked potentials (2012). In: Kolb H, et al. (eds). *Webvision: The Organization of the Retina and Visual System [Internet]*. Salt Lake City, UT: University of Utah Health Sciences Center, 1995. Available at: https://www.ncbi.nlm.nih.gov/books/NBK107218/

32. Answer: D

Various anterior segment imaging systems are currently used in clinical practice. Orbscan utilizes the principle of slit-scanning and Placido disc technology, whereas Pentacam uses a single rotating Scheimpflug camera and a static camera in combination with a monochromatic slit-light source around the optical axis to obtain multiple slit images.

Oliveira CM, et al. Corneal imaging with slit-scanning and Scheimpflug imaging techniques. *Clin Exp Optom* 2011;94:33–42.

33. Answer: C

In Hess tests, both eyes are dissociated using lenses of different colours. In the Lees screen test, the eyes are dissociated using two opalescent glass screens at right angles to each other, bisected by a two-sided plane mirror. A Hess screen test requires a decent visual acuity and normal colour vision of each eye to be useful. It also requires a normal retinal correspondence since the results will be inaccurate if the patient cannot superimpose two macular images. The fovea of each eye should have a common visual direction or else the deviation that shall be mapped out will not be the right one.

The success of the Lees screen test 50 years ago is due to the fact that this method did not need the complementary red-green colours—hence normal colour vision is not necessary in this test. The Lees screen test, such as the red-green screen tests, requires a decent visual acuity, normal retinal correspondence, and adequate dimming of the room. There should not be a large visual field defect.

Timms C. Lees screen test. *Am Orthopt J* 2006;56:180–3.

34. Answer: D

PAT is effective in predicting postoperative sensory and motor fusion in patients with acquired esotropia. During PAT, the patients are given prisms of adequate power to re-align the visual axis. This sometimes stimulates the restoration of some form of binocular vision. Other patients may also benefit from prism adaptation. The angle change is generally smaller after diagnostic occlusion of one eye than after prism adaptation. Preoperative prism correction allows a more accurate determination of the amount of surgery, prevents the risk of undue overcorrection, and promotes the development of binocularity. The increase in the squint angle after prism adaptation is caused by an anomalous sensorial relationship between the two eyes. Surgery tailored to the squint angle after prism adaptation seems advisable in patients with normosensoric esotropia.

Kiyak Yilmaz A, et al. The impact of prism adaptation test on surgical outcomes in patients with primary exotropia. *Clin Exp Optom* 2015;98:224–7.

35. Answer: B

Torsion can be measured by various orthoptic tests, including Hess chart, double Maddox rod, Maddox wing, Bagolini glasses, and synaptophore. Maddox rod only measures latent/manifest horizontal and vertical deviation. Maddox wing measures heterophoria at near fixation and allows the measurement of horizontal, vertical, and cyclo-deviation.

Guyton DL. Clinical assessment of ocular torsion. *Am Orthop J* 1983;33:7–15.

36. Answer: C

AC/A ratio is the measurement of the convergence induced by accommodation for every dioptre of accommodation. The normal AC/A ratio is around 3–5 degree/dioptre. It is important in the diagnosis and/or treatment of some types of strabismus, including IDEX. In simulated IDEX, the AC/A ratio is usually high, masking the near exotropia. This can be unmasked by a patch test or a +3.0 D lens. It can be measured either gradient or heterophoria method. Gradient method is measured using a minus or a plus lens and the change in phoria with the additional lens compared to without the lens yields the AC/A ratio. The heterophoria method is calculated by the following formula:

AC/A=IPD+near fixation distance in metres × (near phoria–distance phoria)

Wybar K. Relevance of the AC/A ratio. *Br J Ophthalmol* 1974;58:248–54.

37. Answer: B

Both CT and MR angiogram have been shown to be good in detecting intracranial aneurysms. However, CTA is more sensitive than MRA in detecting small unruptured aneurysms.

Numminen J, et al. Detection of unruptured cerebral artery aneurysms by MRA at 3.0 tesla: comparison with multislice helical computed tomography angiography. *Acta Radiol* 2011;52:670–4.

38. Answer: D

This is a clinical scenario suggestive of pituitary adenoma. Lesions of the chiasm are usually slow growing and therefore cause chronic progressive visual loss. Many patents do not describe definite visual field loss but a gradual reduction in bilateral visual function. Bitemporal hemianopia is most commonly caused by a pituitary adenoma but there are many causes of this visual field defect including craniopharyngioma, meningiomas, and a suprasellar aneurysm of the carotid artery.

Patients who are found to have this field defect need imaging sequences, most commonly MRI with contrast, as this will show a hypodense region in T1 imaging and they are solid tumours with homogenous enhancement with contrast on T2. There is occasionally a cystic component. They most commonly compress the inferior chiasm, so the superior visual field on the temporal side will be affected first before progressing to bitemporal hemianopia.

Lucas JW, Zada G. Imaging of the pituitary and parasellar region. *Semin Neurol* 2012;32:320–31.

39. Answer: C

The coronal MRI scan shown in Figure 4.4 demonstrates the absence of septum pellucidum, which is a diagnostic feature of septo-optic dysplasia (SOD), or also known as De Morsier's syndrome. SOD is a neurological disorder characterized by a classic triad of optic nerve hypoplasia, pituitary hormone abnormalities, and midline brain defect, including agenesis of septum pellucidum and/or corpus callosum. The diagnosis is made when there is present of two features. Around 60% of the patients have hypopituitarism and absent septum pellucidum. Significant visual impairment is found in around 20–30% of the patients. The affected child may present with strabismus, nystagmus, or other visual abnormalities. Multidisciplinary teamwork, involving ophthalmologist, endocrinologist, paediatricians, and neurodevelopmental team, is essential in the management of these patients.

Webb EA, Dattani MT. Septo-optic dysplasia. *Eur J Hum Genet* 2010;18:393–7.

40. Answer: C

MRI FLAIR sequence is similar to a T2-weighted image but the former has the ability to suppress signals from cerebrospinal fluid (CSF), highlighting periventricular hyperintense lesions such as multiple sclerosis-associated plaques. The following references provide good neuroimaging pictures demonstrating the distinguishing features of MRI T1, T2, and FLAIR sequences.

Rovira A, et al. Recommendations for using and interpreting magnetic resonance imaging in multiple sclerosis. *Neurologia* 2010;25:248–65.

Trip SA, Miller DH. Imaging in multiple sclerosis. *J Neurol Neurosurg Psychiatry* 2005;76:iii11–18.

41. Answer: A

Most patients that have developed a new onset Horner's, in particular a painful Horner's, must have imaging performed. The course of the sympathetic fibres supplying the iris dilator muscle is very long and therefore any interruption of the sympathetic pathway could cause a Horner's lesion. Therefore, the imaging protocol must reflect the course of the pathway. In this case the likely diagnosis is a carotid artery dissection and the imaging of choice would be a study to evaluate the entire sympathetic pathway of head, neck, and upper chest to a level of T2 with contrast. This is followed by an MRA of the head and neck. This extensive imaging is time-consuming in the emergency setting and in this patient CT and CTA is the best option.

Gao Z, Crompton JL. Horner syndrome: a practical approach to investigation and management. *Asia Pac J Ophthalmol (Phila)* 2012;1:175–9.

42. Answer: D

DSG is a useful test for diagnosing functional epiphora. The patient is instructed to sit upright during the procedure while a drop of radioactive tracer isotope (usually technetium-99m) is administered to the inferior fornix of both eyes. The patient then blinks normally and images are taken at regular intervals. It is useful for proximal obstruction and distal obstruction of nasolacrimal drainage system. In contrast dacryocystogram requires the injection of a radio-opaque contrast via the puncta, which may mask the proximal obstruction. The patient is instructed to lie supine during the procedure.

Peter NM, Pearson AR. Comparison of dacryocystography and lacrimal scintigraphy in the investigation of epiphora in patients with patent but nonfunctioning lacrimal systems. *Ophthalmic Plast Reconstr Surg* 2009;25:201–5.

chapter 5

BASIC SCIENCE AND MISCELLANEOUS

QUESTIONS

1. **Bruch's membrane is a:**
   A. Bilaminar structure
   B. Trilaminar structure
   C. Pentalaminar structure
   D. Hexalaminar structure

2. **Which of the following statements about the superior orbital fissure (SOF) is true?**
   A. It communicates with the cavernous sinus
   B. It transmits the ophthalmic artery
   C. The oculomotor nerve travels via the SOF outside the tendinous ring
   D. The trochlear nerve travels via the SOF within the tendinous ring

3. **Which of the following muscles is supplied by the contralateral oculomotor nucleus?**
   A. Inferior rectus
   B. Inferior oblique
   C. Medial rectus
   D. Superior rectus

4. **Which of the following statement regarding the lens is true?**
   A. Contains an anterior Y-shaped suture and a posterior inverted Y-shaped suture
   B. Has a thinner anterior lens capsule than the posterior capsule
   C. The anterior-posterior diameter of lens does not change with age
   D. Contains lens epithelium at the posterior but not the anterior lens capsule

5. **All of the following are pathologic characteristics of retinoblastoma, EXCEPT:**
   A. Calcification
   B. Fleurettes
   C. Flexner–Wintersteiner rosettes
   D. Psammoma bodies

6. **Which glucose receptor is found in adipose tissues and striated muscle (skeletal muscle and cardiac muscle)?**
   A. Glut 1
   B. Glut 2
   C. Glut 3
   D. Glut 4

7. **Which of the following structures derives from neural crest cells?**
   A. Conjunctival epithelium
   B. Lacrimal glands
   C. Retinal pigment epithelium
   D. Trabecular meshwork

8. **Which of the following phakomatoses conditions has a different inheritance mode among the others?**
   A. Neurofibromatosis-1 (NF-1)
   B. Sturge–Weber syndrome
   C. Tuberous sclerosis
   D. Von Hippel–Lindau (VHL) syndrome

9. **The retinoblastoma protein (protein name abbreviated pRb; gene name abbreviated RB or RB1) is a tumour suppressor protein. It is located on:**
   A. Chromosome 13
   B. Chromosome 14
   C. Chromosome 15
   D. Chromosome 16

10. **The following genes have been associated with primary open angle glaucoma, EXCEPT:**
    A. *LAMA1*
    B. *MYOC*
    C. *OPTN*
    D. *WDR36*

11. **Following is a family tree (Figure 5.1) with a Disease A running in the family. What is the most likely inheritance pattern of Disease A?**
    A. Autosomal dominant
    B. Autosomal recessive
    C. Mitochondrial
    D. X-linked recessive

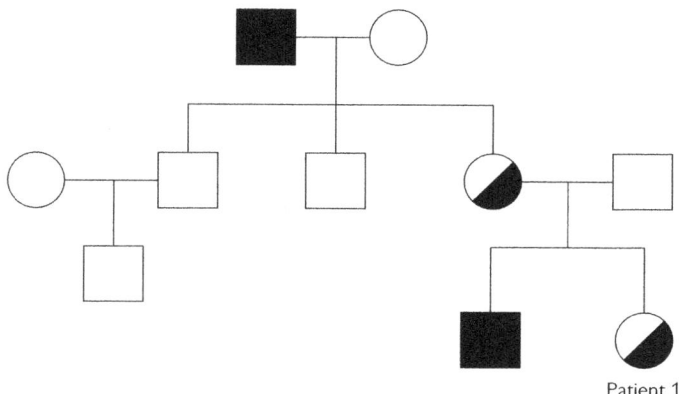

Patient 1

Figure 5.1

12. Which of the following has a similar spherical equivalent as −2.00/+3.50 × 90?
    A. −1.00/+4.50 × 90
    B. −3.00/+2.50 × 180
    C. +1.00/−2.50 × 90
    D. +2.00/−3.50 × 180

13. A glaucoma consultant asks you to analyse his data. The excel spreadsheet contains 120 observations of intraocular pressure (IOP); 60 of which were made after using drug A and 60 of which were made after using drug B. This is an example of:
    A. Unit of analysis issue
    B. Unilateral analysis bias
    C. Bilateral analysis
    D. Bilateral bias

14. Ten trainees are operating in ten different theatres during the week. The number of surgeries performed by each trainee is different. Following is the number of cases performed by each trainee:

    1, 2, 3, 3, 3, 4, 4, 7, 8, 10

    Based on the information given, what is the mean, median, mode, and skew in terms of the number of cases being performed by the trainees?
    A. 4.5, 3, 3.5, positive skew
    B. 4.5, 3, 4, negative skew
    C. 4.5, 3.5, 3, positive skew
    D. 4.5, 4, 3, negative skew

15. **Incorrect rejection of the null hypothesis. This is an example of:**
    A. Type 1 error
    B. Type 2 error
    C. Type 3 error
    D. Type 4 error

16. **Which of the following is true about the incidence and progression of age-related macular degeneration (AMD) in the Blue Mountains Eye Study?**
    A. Male sex was independently associated with early AMD incidence
    B. The presence of complement factor D was independently associated with early AMD incidence
    C. Current smoking was associated with early AMD incidence
    D. Fish consumption was inversely associated with late AMD incidence

17. **When there is no information about a study population, which of the following statistical tests can be employed to test differences between two groups?**
    A. Wilcoxon signed-rank test
    B. Paired sample T-test
    C. One-way analysis of variance (ANOVA)
    D. Independent sample T-test

18. **A 50-year-old type 2 diabetic attends the eye clinic and asks about cholesterol management and eye disease. Which combination is evidence based?**
    A. Simvastatin 40 mg + atorvastatin 80 mg
    B. Simvastatin 40 mg + ezetimibe 10 mg
    C. Simvastatin 40 mg + fenofibrate 160 mg
    D. Simvastatin 40 mg + pravastatin 40 mg

19. **Which of the following is correct about the Collaborative Ocular Melanoma Study (COMS)?**
    A. 10% of the small sized choroidal melanoma demonstrated evidence of tumour growth at 5 years
    B. Brachytherapy was as effective as enucleation for medium sized choroidal melanoma in terms of tumour-related and all-cause mortality at 5 years
    C. Addition of preoperative external beam radiotherapy to enucleation significantly reduced the tumour-related mortality at 5 years compared to enucleation alone
    D. Younger age was shown to be a poor prognostic factors for mortality

20. **Which of the following about Herpetic Eye Disease Study (HEDS) is correct?**
    A. Steroid treatment led to worse outcomes in patients with stromal keratitis
    B. There was no apparent benefit in the addition of oral aciclovir to the treatment regime of topical corticosteroids and topical antiviral treatment in patients with acute stromal keratitis
    C. There was no benefit in adding oral aciclovir to the treatment of herpes simplex virus (HSV) iridocyclitis in patients receiving topical corticosteroids and trifluridine prophylaxis
    D. Psychological stress appears to be a trigger of recurrences of ocular HSV disease

21. **Based on the findings of Optic Neuritis Treatment Trial (ONTT), which is the best treatment option for acute optic neuritis?**
    A. 3 days of IV methylprednisolone 250 mg QID alone
    B. 3 days of IV methylprednisolone 250 mg QID then 11 days of oral prednisolone 1 mg/kg
    C. 7 days of oral methylprednisolone 500 mg
    D. 14 days of oral prednisolone 1 mg/kg

22. **According to the North America Symptomatic Carotid Endarterectomy (NASCET) study, which of the following regarding carotid endarterectomy (CEA) is correct?**
    A. CEA has been shown to significantly reduce the risk of stroke in symptomatic patients with mild (<50%) to severe (70–99%) carotid stenosis
    B. CEA is recommended in patients with asymptomatic severe carotid stenosis
    C. In patients with severe carotid stenosis, the risk of ipsilateral stroke at 2 years after combined CEA and aspirin is 10%
    D. There is a twofold increase risk of perioperative severe stroke or death in patients who have CEA compared to medical treatment only

23. **Which of following nutritional supplements was NOT found to be beneficial in reducing the risk of developing advanced AMD?**
    A. Copper
    B. Lutein
    C. Omega-3
    D. Vitamin C

24. **A 15-year-old boy has asked for surgery to correct a cosmetic squint. His parents refuse to give their consent. He is deemed Gillick competent. Can he have the surgery?**
    A. Gillick competence requires one parent to consent if both alive
    B. Gillick competence requires the child to be older than 16 years
    C. The Fraser clause overrules consent in cosmetic procedures
    D. He can have the surgery

25. **A Lithuanian taxi driver who speaks no English attends the eye clinic with cataract. He does not understand any English and his friend translates in broken English. He wants to have the cataract surgery but is anxious about procedure. Which consent form would be most appropriate for cataract surgery with sedation?**
   A. Consent 1
   B. Consent 2
   C. Consent 3
   D. Consent 4

26. **The four principles used as a common framework for the analysis of medical ethics are:**
   A. Autonomy, beneficence, justice, and non-maleficence
   B. Autonomy, beneficence, capacity, and non-maleficence
   C. Autonomy, beneficence, justice, and maleficence
   D. Autonomy, beneficence, capacity, and maleficence

27. **A female patient comes to your clinic wearing revealing clothes. She then comes up very close to you and starts asking personal questions in a seductive tone. What would be the appropriate response?**
   A. Continue to examine her with the door open
   B. Refer her to another doctor
   C. Call in a nurse as a chaperon
   D. Refuse to examine her

28. **A 40-year-old patient attends the glaucoma clinic for the first time. Which of the following is most likely to be TRUE regarding the implications of visual field loss on his current licence?**
   A. If he holds a group 1 licence, he needs to inform the Driver and Vehicle Licensing Agency (DVLA) if his horizontal field does not extend to 160°, with extension of at least 70° to left and right
   B. If he holds a group 1 licence, he needs to inform the DVLA if he has blepharospasm
   C. If he holds a group 2 licence, he needs to inform the DVLA only when there is a defect within 20° of fixation above or below the horizontal meridian
   D. If he holds a group 2 licence he needs to inform the DVLA if he has any defect in the central 30° in either eye

29. A 70-year-old patient presents to the eye casualty with a transient episode history of decreased vision, described as a curtain coming down. The symptom has fully resolved by the time he arrives at the eye casualty. His past medical history includes hypertension and type 2 diabetes. The presenting vision is 6/6 in both eyes and confrontational visual field is full in both eyes. Slit-lamp examination shows mild non-proliferative diabetic retinopathy and silver wiring of the retinal arterioles. What advice should be given in terms of driving?
    A. The patient can continue to drive but stop if notices another similar episode of visual disturbance
    B. The patient should stop driving for at least 1 week
    C. The patient should stop driving for at least 2 weeks
    D. The patient should stop driving for at least 1 month

30. Which of the following analytic methods refers to analysis of all the costs and consequences of an intervention in monetary term?
    A. Cost-benefit analysis
    B. Cost-effectiveness analysis
    C. Cost-minimization analysis
    D. Cost-utility analysis

31. There have been a number of cases of bacterial endophthalmitis in your unit over the past month. Which of the following statements should raise particular concern?
    A. An incidence of 1.0%
    B. Each case has arisen from a different theatre list
    C. Microbiological analysis indicating a different organism in each case
    D. The finding that each case has been operated on by a different member of staff

32. The majority of vigabatrin related defects:
    A. Extend to within 5° of fixation
    B. Extend to within 10° of fixation
    C. Extend to within 20° of fixation
    D. Extend to within 30° of fixation

33. Which of the following is true about the NHS Diabetic Eye Screening Programme (NDESP)?
    A. All patients with treated proliferative diabetic retinopathy will need to be reviewed at least once a year in the hospital eye service
    B. 10% of the patients with negative primary grading results need to undergo internal quality assurance process via secondary grading
    C. The screening service may screen diabetic patients up to every 6-monthly
    D. Digital surveillance could only provide annual screening

34. **A 65-year old type 2 insulin-dependent diabetic of 10 years was found to have reduced vision by his optician. On examination, his visual acuity was 6/15. There were multiple areas of microaneurysm on the macula and an area of hard exudates 500 microns from the fovea. Optical coherence tomography showed a central retinal thickness (CRT) of 402 mm. He has no other past ocular history otherwise. He runs his own company and tells you that he is a very busy man. What is the most appropriate management plan?**
    A. Offer the patient focal laser to the area of hard exudates
    B. Offer the patient intravitreal aflibercept every month for 3 months, then 2 monthly
    C. Offer the patient intravitreal aflibercept every month for 5 months, then 2 monthly
    D. Offer the patient illuvien injection

35. **Based on the Royal College of Ophthalmologists' (RCOphth) guideline on instrument decontamination, which of the following is true?**
    A. 70% alcohol wipes have been shown to be sufficient to disinfect diagnostic contact lenses
    B. Diagnostic contact lenses should be soaked in 1% sodium hypochlorite solution for 10 minutes between patients
    C. Tonometer prisms should be soaked in 1% sodium hypochlorite solution for 5 minutes between patients
    D. Single-use instruments have bene shown to be cost-effective in reducing the possible transmission risk of Creutzfeldt–Jakob disease (CJD)

36. **Which of the following options regarding the UK eye retrieval and eye bank services is correct?**
    A. The death-to-retrieval time should be 18 hours or less
    B. The use of demented patients' ocular tissues for transplantation is considered a contraindication in most cases
    C. Hypothermic storage is the common method used in UK eye bank due to the advantage of longer storage time
    D. The endothelial cell count needs to be more than 2500 cells/mm^2 to be considered suitable for penetrating/endothelial keratoplasty

chapter 5
BASIC SCIENCE AND MISCELLANEOUS
ANSWERS

1. Answer: C

Bruch's membrane (BM) is a pentalaminar structure, which is located between the retinal pigment epithelium (RPE) and the fenestrated choroidal capillaries. From inside to outside, it is composed of basement membrane of RPE, inner collagenous zone, central band of elastic fibres, outer collagenous zone, and basement membrane of choriocapillaris. BM is a dynamic structure involved actively or passively in diseases such as the onset and progression of diseases like retinitis pigmentosa, AMD, pseudoxanthoma elasticum, Sorsby's fundus dystrophy, and Malattia Leventinese.

Booij JC, et al. The dynamic nature of Bruch's membrane. *Prog Retin Eye Res* 2010;29:1–18.

2. Answer: A

The SOF is bordered between greater and lesser wings of the sphenoid bone and it connects to cavernous sinus. The mnemonic '**SINA-LFTs**' can be used to remember the structures that transmit through SOF within or outside the tendinous ring. The optic canal transmits ophthalmic artery and optic nerve.

Structures that travel with**in** the tendinous ring include:

Superior and **I**nferior divisions of III nerve

Nasociliary nerve of V1

Abducens nerve

Structures that travel outside tendinous ring include:

Lacrimal nerve of V1

Frontal nerve of V1

Trochlear nerve

Superior ophthalmic vein.

Shumway CL, Wade M. *Anatomy, Head and Neck, Orbit Bones.* StatPearls [Internet]. Treasure Island, FL: StatPearls Publishing, 2018. Available at: https://www.ncbi.nlm.nih.gov/books/NBK531490/

3. Answer: D

Fibres to the inferior oblique, inferior rectus, and medial rectus muscles supply the ipsilateral eye whereas fibres to the superior rectus muscle decussate and supply the contralateral eye. The decussating fibres pass through the opposite superior rectus nucleus; thus, damage to the right oculomotor nucleus might have bilateral superior rectus muscle involvement.

Brazis PW. Localization of lesions of the oculomotor nerve: recent concepts. *Mayo Clin Proc* 1991;66:1029–35.

4. Answer: A

As lens fibres grow anteriorly and posteriorly, the ends of the fibres meet and interdigitate with the ends of fibres arising on the opposite side of the lens, forming a pattern of cell association known as sutures. At 8 weeks' gestation, an erect Y-suture appears anteriorly and an inverted Y-suture appears posteriorly. The anterior lens capsule is thicker than the posterior lens capsule. The lens epithelium is beneath the anterior capsule but not the posterior capsule.

Bassnett S, Sikic H. The lens growth process. *Prog Retin Eye Res* 2017;60:181–200.

5. Answer: D

There are various pathologic characteristics of retinoblastoma, depending on the extent of retinal differentiation. These included Homer–Wright pseudo-rosettes (neuroblastic differentiation), Flexner–Wintersteiner rosettes (early retinal differentiation), and fleurettes (photoreceptor differentiation). Calcification is also a common feature of retinoblastoma. Psammoma bodies are associated with meningioma and other tumours, but not retinoblastoma.

Eagle RC Jr. The pathology of ocular cancer. *Eye (Lond)* 2013;27:128–36.

6. Answer: D

GLUTs are integral membrane proteins that contain 12 membrane-spanning helices with both the amino and carboxyl termini exposed on the cytoplasmic side of the plasma membrane. 14 GLUTS are encoded by the human genome. Glut 4 is the principle glucose transporter involved in regulating whole body glucose homeostasis.

Stöckli J, et al. GLUT4 exocytosis. *J Cell Sci* 2011;124:4147–59.

7. Answer: D

Following is the summary of the embryologic origin of various ocular structures:

Surface ectoderm: epidermis of the eyelids, conjunctiva, corneal epithelium, lens, and lacrimal glands

Neuroectoderm: epithelial lining of iris and ciliary body, RPE, and optic nerve

Neural crest cells: corneal stroma, Descemet membrane and endothelium, sclera, iris stroma, ciliary body stroma and muscles, and trabecular meshwork

Mesoderm: vitreous, choroid, sclera, endothelial lining of ocular blood vessels and extraocular muscles

Graw J. Eye development. *Curr Top Dev Biol* 2010;90:343–86.

Williams AL, Bohnsack BL. Neural crest derivatives in ocular development: discerning the eye of the storm. *Birth Defects Res C Embryo Today* 2015;105:87–95.

8. Answer: B

Phakomatoses is a group of conditions that affects brain, eye, and skin. These include NF-1, NF-2, tuberous sclerosis, and VHL. They all have autosomal dominant inheritance. Sturge–Weber syndrome and Wyburn–Mason syndrome are different from 'true phakomatoses' where they occurred sporadically.

Rosser T. Neurocutaneous disorders. *Continuum (Minneap Minn)* 2018;24:96–129.

9. Answer: A

The protein is encoded by the RB1 gene located on chromosome 13 (13q14.1-q14.2). If both alleles of this gene are mutated early in life, the protein is inactivated and results in development of retinoblastoma cancer, hence the name Rb. Two forms of retinoblastoma were noticed: a bilateral, familial form, and a unilateral, sporadic form. Sufferers of the former were six times more likely to develop other types of cancer later in life. This highlights the fact that mutated Rb could be inherited and supported the two-hit hypothesis.

Kleinerman RA, et al. Risk of new cancers after radiotherapy in long-term survivors of retinoblastoma: an extended follow-up. *J Clin Oncol* 2015;23: 2272–9.

10. Answer: A

All the genes have been implicated in primary open angle glaucoma except LAMA1, which encodes one of the alpha 1 subunits of laminin. It is associated with Poretti-Boltshauser syndrome, which is characterized by cerebellar dysplasia, cerebellar cyst, high myopia, variable retinal dystrophy, and eye movement abnormalities.

Sakurada Y, Mabuchi F. Advances in glaucoma genetics. *Prog Brain Res* 2015;220:107–26.

11. Answer: D

This is a common genetic question presented in a family tree fashion, which should be familiarized by all candidates. Generally speaking, square refers to male and circle refers to female; fully shaded shape refers to having the disease, non-shaded shape refers to no disease and half shaded refers to carrier of the disease. In this question, there are three generations involved. The grandfather of patient 1 has Disease A and only his female children is affected. This disease is not possible to have an autosomal recessive inheritance pattern because all the children of the grandfather should be a carrier instead of being fully affected. Similarly autosomal dominant inheritance pattern is unlikely because the male and female children of the grandfather should have 50% chance of being affected, though it is still possible for both male children to be unaffected. Mitochondrial inheritance is not possible in this case because mitochondria is only inheritable exclusively from the mother. Therefore, none of the children or grandchildren should be affected. Patient 1 is a carrier and her mother is a carrier and her brother is affected. Therefore, the condition is an X-linked recessive disease because the affected females are all carriers and the males are fully affected.

NHS. *Genetic and Genomic Testing*. Available at: https://www.nhs.uk/conditions/genetics/inheritance/

12. Answer: C

This is a simple question examining the candidates' knowledge on calculation of the mean refractive spherical equivalent (MRSE). Following is the equation: MRSE (dioptre) = sphere + cylinder/2 (regardless of the axis)

The given refraction has a MRSE of –0.25, which is the same as Option C.

Wilkinson ME. *Introduction to Optics and Refractive Errors of the Eye*, 2015. Available at: https://webeye.ophth.uiowa.edu/eyeforum/video/Refraction/Intro-Optics-Refract-Errors/index.htm

13. Answer: A

This scenario illustrates what is known as the 'unit of analysis' issue. The patient is the sampling unit and should be the unit of analysis. Multiple observations may be made on patients, but the statistical analysis must not ignore the fact that these observations are made on individuals. Failure to do so violates the assumption made by the majority of statistical tests that each data value is independent. Multiple observations from the same patient falsely inflate your sample size, sometimes dramatically so, leading to spurious statistical significance.

Altman DG, Bland JM. Statistics notes. Units of analysis. *BMJ* 1997;314:1874.

Bunce C, et al. Ophthalmic statistics note 1: unit of analysis. *Br J Ophthalmol* 2014;98:408–12.

14. Answer: C

The total amount of cases performed is 45 cases. 'Mean' refers to the average of the total amount; in this case is 45 cases/10 trainees = 4.5. 'Median' refers to the middle value of a set of ordered data; in this case there are ten numbers, so the value will be the average between fifth and sixth, which is (3 + 4)/2 = 3.5. Mode refers to the number that occurs most often, so in this case is 3. Positive skew has a longer right tail whereas negative skew has a longer left tail; in this case there are more lower numbers (compared to the mean value of 4.5) in this 10-data set, so it has a positive skew. The other way to interpret is that if the mean value is larger (i.e. on the right side of the horizontal axis) than the median value, it is positively skewed and *vice versa*. Refer to the following useful website for graphical explanation.

[No authors]. *A Look at Skewed Distributions*. Available at: http://www.cvgs.k12.va.us/digstats/main/descriptv/d_skewd.html

15. Answer: A

Type I error:
- Incorrect rejection of the true null hypothesis
- Maximum probability is set in advance as alpha
- Is not affected by sample size as it is set in advance
- Increases with the number of tests or end points

Type II error:
- Failure to reject false null hypothesis
- Probability is beta
- Beta depends upon sample size and alpha
- Cannot be estimated except as a function of the true population effect
- Beta gets smaller as the sample size gets larger, the number of tests or end points increases

Banerjee A, et al. Hypothesis testing, type I and type II errors. *Ind Psychiatry J* 2009;18:127–31.

16. Answer: D

The Blue Mountains Study is a large population-based cohort study to assess the 15-year incidence and progression of AMD in an older Australian population. The following are the main results of this study: 'Age was strongly associated with early and late AMD incidence. Female sex and the presence of both risk alleles of CFH-rs1061170 or ARMS2-rs10490924 were independently associated with early AMD incidence whereas current smoking and presence of ≥1 risk allele of CFH-rs1061170 or ARMS2-rs10490924 were associated with late AMD incidence. Fish consumption was inversely associated with late but not early AMD incidence. Severity of early AMD lesion characteristics was a strong predictor of progression to late AMD.'

Joachim N, et al. The incidence and progression of age-related macular degeneration over 15 years: the Blue Mountains Eye Study. *Ophthalmology* 2015;122:2482–9.

17. Answer: A

A statistical test is a formal technique used to reach conclusion concerning the reasonableness of the hypothesis by relying on the probability distribution. This hypothetical testing related to differences can be classified into parametric and non-parametric tests. Parametric tests (sample T-tests, one-way analysis of variance, etc.) are used when there is complete information about the population whereas non-parametric tests (Wilcoxon signed-rank tests, Chi-square test,

Mann–Whitney, Kruskal–Wallis test, etc.) are used when information about the population is unavailable.

Ali Z, Bhaskar SB. Basic statistical tools in research and data analysis. *Indian J Anaesth* 2016;60:662–9.

18. Answer: C

In the ACCORD Eye study, fenofibrate (160 mg daily) with simvastatin resulted in a 40% reduction in the odds of retinopathy progressing over 4 years, compared with simvastatin alone. In the FIELD (Fenofibrate Intervention and Event Lowering in Diabetes study) fenofibrate reduced the requirements for laser therapy in patients with pre-existing retinopathy (numbers need to treat (NNT) to avoid first laser = 17) and prevented disease progression (NNT = 9) in patients with pre-existing retinopathy.

ACCORD Study Group; ACCORD Eye Study Group, Chew EY, et al. Effects of medical therapies on retinopathy progression in type 2 diabetes. *N Engl J Med* 2010;363:233–44.

Keech AC, et al. Effect of fenofibrate on the need for laser treatment for diabetic retinopathy (FIELD study): a randomised controlled trial. *Lancet* 2007;370:1687–97.

19. Answer: B

The Collaborative Ocular Melanoma Study is a three-arm study, including an observational study of small choroidal melanomas, a randomized controlled trial comparing the effectiveness of brachytherapy to enucleation for medium sized choroidal melanomas, and a randomized controlled trial to examine the additional benefit of preoperative external beam radiotherapy for large choroidal melanomas. The size of choroidal melanoma was defined as small (1.5–2.4 mm height and 5–16 mm diameter), medium (2.5–10 mm apical height and ≤16 mm diameter) and large (>10 mm apical height and >16 mm diameter). The primary outcomes measures were tumour-related and all-cause mortality at 5 years. In conclusion brachytherapy serves as an effective alternative treatment to enucleation for medium sized choroidal melanomas and preoperative radiotherapy does not improve the survival. Older age, instead of younger age, at presentation is a poor prognostic factor for mortality. Following is a summary table of the main findings (Table 5.1).

Table 5.1 The main findings of the Collaborative Ocular Melanoma Study

	Small*	Medium size	Large size
5-year tumour-related mortality	1%	9% (B) vs. 11% (E)	28% (E only) vs. 26% (E + B)
5-year all-cause mortality	6%	18% (B) vs. 19% (E)	43% (E only) vs. 38% (E + B)

*31% of the small sized choroidal melanomas demonstrated evidence of tumour growth at 5 years.
B, brachytherapy; E, enucleation.
Adapted with permission from Margo, C. E. (2004) 'The Collaborative Ocular Melanoma Study: An Overview', *Cancer Control*, pp. 304–309. doi: 10.1177/107327480401100504. Copyright © 2004, © SAGE Publications.

20. Answer: B

There are two parts to the HEDS:

Conclusions from HEDS 1 (consisting of three randomized controlled trials (RCTs)):

1. Patients with acute stromal herpes simplex keratitis (HSK) who received prednisolone phosphate drops had faster resolution and fewer treatment failures (reduced by 68%)

2. There was also no apparent benefit in the addition of oral acyclovir of therapeutic dose (400 mg five times a day) to the treatment regimen of a topical corticosteroid and a topical antiviral for acute stromal keratitis
3. For patients with HSV iridocyclitis, adding oral acyclovir of therapeutic dose in addition to topical corticosteroids and trifluridine prophylaxis might be beneficial, thought the sample size was too small to achieve statistical significance

Conclusions from HEDS 2 (consisting of two RCTs and one observational study):
1. There was no benefit from the addition of oral acyclovir to treatment with topical Trifluridine in preventing the development of stromal keratitis or iritis in patients with epithelial HSK
2. It was found that oral acyclovir (400 mg BD), reduced the probability that any form of herpes of the eye would return in patients who had the infection in the previous year by 41%, particularly stromal keratitis
3. Psychological stress does not appear to be a trigger of recurrences of ocular HSV disease

Kalezic T, et al. Herpetic eye disease study: lessons learned. *Curr Opin Ophthalmol* 2013;29:340–6.

21. Answer: B

The ONTT enrolled 457 patients between 1988 and 1991 in order to study the use of corticosteroids to treat acute optic neuritis as there was no consensus on the best treatment regime. As part of the study's further analysis, the long-term risk of developing MS was also analysed, and the patients were followed up for 15 years post recruitment. All patients had an unenhanced MRI at recruitment and yearly follow-up scans until 1997, then at 10 years and then 15 years follow-up. The patients were randomized into three groups:

1. IVMP 250 mg QID 3/7 followed by OP 1 mg/kg for 11 days (group 1)
2. OP 1 mg/kg for 14 days (group 2)
3. Placebo (group 3)

Following are the main results of ONTT, which can be memorized as V-RRR (see also Table 5.2).

(a) **V**isual outcome: Neither treatment regime influenced the visual outcome at any time point up to 15 years 94% have VA ≥6/12 at 5 years; 3% have ≤6/60 at 5 years
(b) **R**ecovery of vision: Group 1 has more rapid improvement in symptoms vs. other 2 groups but no effect on final visual outcome at 6 months or 15 years
(c) **R**ecurrence of optic neuritis: Group 2 has twofold increased risk of recurrence (28%) vs. other two groups
(d) **R**isk of MS: IVMP reduced the rate of clinically definite multiple sclerosis during the first 2 years, but similar to other two groups by the third year

Table 5.2 The main findings of the Optic Neuritis Treatment Trial (ONTT)

Risk of MS	5-year	10-year	15-year
Overall	30%	38%	50%
No lesion on MRI	16%	22%	25%
1 or more lesions on MRI	33%*	56%	72%

* 51% if three or more lesions on MRI. MS, multiple sclerosis.

Optic Neuritis Study Group. Multiple sclerosis risk after optic neuritis final Optic Neuritis Treatment Trial follow-up. *Arch Neurol* 2008;65:727–32.

22. Answer: D

NASCET study is a landmark randomized controlled trial comparing the benefit and safety of CEA and aspirin (Group 1) to aspirin alone (Group 2) in symptomatic and asymptomatic patients with mild (<50%), moderate (50–69%) and severe (70–99%) carotid stenosis. Following are the main results:

- Mild stenosis: No significant difference of treatment failure rate between surgical (15%) and medical treatment (19%) at 5 years
- Moderate stenosis: 5-year rate of ipsilateral stroke = 16% vs. 22% (NNT was 15). Marginal beneficial effect in reducing risk of stroke at 2 years
- Severe stenosis:
  - Absolute risk reduction of ipsilateral stroke was 17% (NNT was 6)
  - Risk of perioperative (within 30 days) severe complication (severe stroke/death): 2.1% vs. 0.9%
  - Risk of ipsilateral stroke at 2 years: 1.6% vs. 12.2%

In summary, CEA is recommended for:

- Symptomatic stenosis of 50–99% if perioperative risk of stroke or death is <6%
- Asymptomatic stenosis of 60–99% if perioperative risk of stroke or death is <3%

Barnett HJ, et al. Benefit of carotid endarterectomy in patients with symptomatic moderate or severe stenosis. North American Symptomatic Carotid Endarterectomy Trial Collaborators. *N Engl J Med* 1998;339:1415–25.

Cina CS, et al. Carotid endarterectomy for symptomatic carotid stenosis. *Cochrane Database Syst Rev* 2000;2:CD001081.

23. Answer: C

The original Age-related Eye Disease Study (AREDS) 1 formulation contained vitamin C, vitamin E, zinc, copper, and b-carotene. AREDS 2 looked at improving the original formulation. Omega-3 fatty acids as well as the antioxidants, lutein, and zeaxanthin, which are in the same family of nutrients as β-carotene, were tried as β-carotene was found to be associated with an increased risk of lung cancer in smokers in previous study. AREDS 2 found that while omega-3 fatty acids had no effect on the formulation, lutein and zeaxanthin together appeared to be a safe and effective alternative to β-carotene.

Age-related Eye Disease Study 2 Research Group. Lutein + zeaxanthin and omega-3 fatty acids for age-related macular degeneration: the Age-related Eye Disease Study 2 (AREDS2) randomized clinical trial. *JAMA* 2013;309:2005–15.

24. Answer: D

Children under 16 years of age can consent to medical treatment if they understand what is being proposed. It is up to the doctor to decide whether the child has the maturity and intelligence to fully understand the nature of the treatment, the options, the risks involved, and the benefits. A child who has such understanding is considered Gillick competent (or Fraser competent). The parents cannot overrule the child's consent when the child is judged to be Gillick competent. Children under 16 who are not Gillick competent and very young children cannot either give or withhold consent. Those with parental responsibility need to make the decision on their behalf. The 'Fraser guideline' specifically relates to contraception and sexual health.

Gillick v West Norfolk and Wisbech AHA, 1985. Available at: http://www.bailii.org/uk/cases/UKHL/1985/7.html

Lennings NJ. Forward, Gillick: Are competent children autonomous medical decision makers? New developments in Australia. *J Law Biosci* 2015;2:459–68.

25. Answer: A

The patient has full capacity. He simply does not understand English. The patient should ideally be rebooked with a medical translator and a Lithuanian consent form, which can be downloaded from the internet. Consent 1: Adult with capacity; Consent 2: Parental agreement for a child or young person; Consent 3: Procedure where consciousness is not impaired (therefore this cannot be used in this case as sedation is required); and Consent 4: Adults who are unable to consent.

Good Practice in Consent Implementation Guide: Consent to examination or treatment. Available at: http://www.wales.nhs.uk/publications/impguide-e.pdf (see p. 4)

26. Answer: A

A common framework used in the analysis of medical ethics are the 'four principles' approach postulated by Tom Beauchamp and James Childress in their textbook *Principles of Biomedical Ethics*. It recognizes four basic moral principles. Ideally, for a medical practice to be considered 'ethical', it must respect all four of these principles: autonomy, justice, beneficence, and non-maleficence.

Beauchamp J. *Principles of Biomedical Ethics*. Oxford, UK: Oxford University Press, 2013.

Pollard BJ. Autonomy and paternalism in medicine. *Med J Aust* 1993;159:797–802.

27. Answer: C

The first thing one should do in this case is to call in a nurse as a chaperon. If patient continues to behave inappropriately she can then be warned, and the doctor has the right to refuse examination.

Davies M. Crossing boundaries: dealing with amorous advances by doctors and patients. *BMJ* 2015;351:h5368.

28. Answer: D

Visual standards for driving is an extremely common exam topic. You are required to recall all of the specific details. Be aware not only of the differences between group 1 and 2 drivers, but also implications of acute monocularity, diplopia, blepharospasm, and also grandfather rights. Group 1 includes car and motorcycles and Group 2 includes large lorries and buses. Option A is incorrect as this is a Group 2 parameter. Option B is incorrect as the guidance states that this must be 'severe' blepharospasm. There are no criteria stipulated for severity, but it is noted if the condition is mild or treated, they may drive. Option C is incorrect as this is a Group 1 parameter.

Driver and Vehicle Licensing Agency (DVLA). *Assessing Fitness to Drive: A Guide for Medical Professionals*, September 2019. Available at: https://www.gov.uk/guidance/assessing-fitness-to-drive-a-guide-for-medical-professionals

29. Answer: D

This is a common clinical scenario suggestive of amaurosis fugax. These patients should be treated as ocular transient ischaemic attack (TIA) and be referred to the TIA team for further assessment and management. Affected patients should stop driving for at least 1 month.

Driver and Vehicle Licensing Agency (DVLA). *Assessing Fitness to Drive: A Guide for Medical Professionals*, September 2019. Available at: https://www.gov.uk/guidance/assessing-fitness-to-drive-a-guide-for-medical-professionals

30. Answer: A

There are several types of economic evaluation in healthcare. Following is the summary of the commonly used analytic methods (Table 5.3).

Table 5.3 Commonly used methods of economic evaluation in healthcare

Analysis	Description
Cost-benefit	Analysis of all the costs and consequence of an intervention in monetary terms
Cost-effectiveness	Comparison of different drugs or programmes which have a common health outcome. The results are usually presented as costs per life year gained
Cost-minimization	Analysis that focuses on the cost alone and the cheapest option is chosen, provided the consequences of two or more interventions being compared are similar
Cost-utility	Analysis of costs and benefits intervention and the results are usually presented as cost per quality adjusted life year (QALY)

Data from Kernick DP. Introduction of health economics for the medical practitioner. *Postgrad Med J* 2003;79:147–50.

31. Answer: A

The correct management of an outbreak of endophthalmitis within a unit is key to ensuring patient safety, both at a local and national level. The Royal College of Ophthalmologists has a document that covers this subject and gives key factors that should be taken into consideration. An incidence of >0.8% should be taken extremely seriously.

Royal College of Ophthalmologists. *Ophthalmic Services Guidance: Managing an Outbreak of Postoperative Endophthalmitis*, July 2016. Available at: https://www.rcophth.ac.uk/wp-content/uploads/2016/07/Managing-an-outbreak-of-postoperative-endophthalmitis.pdf

32. Answer: D

Vigabatrin is associated with bilateral, concentric, predominantly nasal constriction of the visual field. The majority of defects extend to within 30o of fixation, defects outside that eccentricity, and therefore not detected by standard 30° threshold tests have been reported. This finding is in accord with a study that found that peripheral rod-derived dark-adapted visual fields were also constricted in patients having visual field constriction attributable to vigabatrin (VAVFC) on light-adapted fields. Risk factors for VAVFC include male gender, treatment dose and duration, and increasing age.

The Royal College of Ophthalmologists. *The Ocular Side-Effects of Vigabatrin (Sabril) Information and Guidance for Screening*, 2008. Available at: https://www.rcophth.ac.uk/wp-content/uploads/2015/01/2008-SCI-020-The-Ocular-Side-Effects-of-Vigabatrin-Sabril.pdf

33. Answer: B

The NDESP provides specific guidance on the diabetic screening and monitoring in the United Kingdom. All patients with diabetes will be invited to the routine digital screening test where digital photograph is obtained and primary grading is performed. Patients who have primary grading result of R1, R2, M1, or non-DR lesions will have a secondary grading and further referral outcome grading. Patients who meet the referral criteria will be suspended from the routine digital screening and sent to either of the three services: (1) slit-lamp biomicroscopy surveillance;

(2) digital surveillance (where it requires monitoring more frequently than annually); and (3) referral to hospital eye services for further assessment and management. For patients who have negative primary grading result (R0M0), 10% of the cases will undergo internal quality assurance via secondary grading and the subsequent steps are similar as above. The screening service only recalls patients for annual screening and not more frequently. Digital surveillance can provide more frequent monitoring such as every 3 or 6 monthly. Stable treated proliferative diabetic retinopathy can be reviewed in digital surveillance or annual screening service. Following link provides a good summary of the flow of the NDESP service.

Gov.UK. *NHS Diabetic Eye Screening (DES) Programme*. Available at: https://www.gov.uk/health-and-social-care/population-screening-programmes-diabetic-eye

34. Answer: C

The current options for the management of diabetic macular oedema where CRT are more than 400 mm are aflibercept, ranibizumab, Ozurdex, and illuvien. Focal laser will not help in the case of diffuse macular oedema.

NICE guideline recommends aflibercept to be given as a single 2 mg intravitreal injection every month for 5 consecutive months, followed by one injection every 2 months with no requirement for monitoring between visits. After the first 12 months, the treatment interval may be extended based on visual and anatomic outcomes. Answer B is incorrect as the regime mentioned is not the recommended regime.

Ranibizumab should be given monthly and continued until maximum visual acuity is reached (until visual acuity has been stable for 3 consecutive months). Thereafter, visual acuity should be monitored monthly. Treatment is resumed if monitoring indicates a loss of visual acuity caused by diabetic macular oedema, and continued until visual acuity has remained stable for 3 consecutive months. Ozurdex and illuvien are recommended for use in pseudophakic cases which have failed to respond to non-corticosteroid treatment, or such treatment is unsuitable.

National Institute for Health and Care Excellence (NICE). *Aflibercept for Treating Diabetic Macular Oedema*, 2015. Available at: https://www.nice.org.uk/guidance/ta346

National Institute for Health and Care Excellence (NICE). *Dexamethasone Intravitreal Implant for Treating Diabetic Macular Oedema*, 2015. Available at: https://www.nice.org.uk/guidance/ta349

National Institute for Health and Care Excellence (NICE). *Fluocinolone Acetonide Intravitreal Implant for Treating Chronic Diabetic Macular Oedema After Inadequate Response to Prior Therapy*, 2013. Available at: https://www.nice.org.uk/guidance/ta301

35. Answer: B

All candidates should be familiar with the RCOphth guideline on ophthalmic instrument decontamination for multiple-choice question and VIVA purposes. The guideline advises that all non-surgical reusable instruments (such as tonometer prisms, diagnostic contact lenses, etc.) should be decontaminated with 1% sodium hypochlorite (Milton) solution for 10 minutes between patients. Approx. 70% alcohol wipes have been shown to be insufficient to inactivate adenovirus and other viruses. Single-use instruments have not been shown to be cost-effective in reducing the possible transmission of CJD.

Royal College of Ophthalmologists. *Ophthalmic Services Guidance Ophthalmic Instrument Decontamination*, 2016. Available at: https://www.rcophth.ac.uk/wp-content/uploads/2014/12/Ophthalmic-Instrument-Decontamination.pdf

36. Answer: B

All trainees should be familiar with the UK eye retrieval and eye bank services. The death-to-retrieval time should be 24 hours or less. Once the eyes are retrieved, they are stored in the eye bank using the organ culture method at 34°C, which has the advantage of longer storage time (30 days) compared to hypothermic storage method at 4°C (7–10 days), which is the method used in the United States. The minimum cut-off limit of endothelial cell density for penetrating/endothelial keratoplasty is 2200 cells/mm^2 in the United Kingdom. A list of contraindications for the use of ocular tissues for corneal transplantation can be found on the Royal College of Ophthalmologist guideline. The contraindications include blood-borne viral infections, haematological malignancies, previous ocular inflammation or corneal surgeries, and central nervous system diseases such as dementia (most cases), multiple sclerosis, and Parkinson disease, among many others.

Royal College of Ophthalmologists. RCOphth Clinical Guidelines on Standards for the Retrieval of Human Ocular Tissue Used in Transplantation, Research and Training. Available at: https://www.rcophth.ac.uk/publications/current-clinical-guidelines/

chapter 6

MOCK EXAM

QUESTIONS

1. A 23-year-old patient presents to the eye emergency department after a splash of bleach in the eye. His presenting visual acuity is 6/36 and examination showed a central corneal defect of 80% with mild corneal oedema, 20% conjunctival staining, 1 clock-hour limbal ischaemia, and raised intraocular pressure of 24 mmHg. The cornea is otherwise clear. What is the likely clinical outcome of the patient if managed appropriately?
   A. The patient is likely to recover without any long-term ocular sequelae
   B. The patient is likely to develop persistent epithelial defect that requires long-term topical treatment
   C. The patient is likely to require surgical interventions such as amniotic membrane transplant to recover good vision
   D. The patient is likely to have a poor visual outcome

2. Which of the following statements regarding corneal collagen cross-linking is correct?
   A. It has been shown to be an effective adjunct treatment for acanthamoeba keratitis
   B. It is safe to be used in patients with corneal thickness of 350 microns
   C. The treatment regime utilizes ultraviolet-A and vitamin B_2 drops
   D. Accelerated treatment protocols have been shown to be more effective than the conventional Dresden protocol (3 mW/min for 30 min)

3. A 42-year-old man has been referred to the eye clinic with dry eyes and photophobia associated with some form of corneal stromal changes. Systemic examination reveals bilateral facial nerve paresis and skin laxity. Which of the following statements best describes the condition of this patient?
   A. The ocular examination is likely to reveal multiple grey reticular opacities at the subepithelial layer
   B. This patient is at increased risk of developing cardiac and renal failures
   C. This condition is associated with mutation in transforming growth factor β-induced (*TGFBI*) gene
   D. Recurrent corneal erosion is rare in this condition

4. **Which of the following options regarding the complication of herpes zoster ophthalmicus (HZO) is correct?**
   A. Post-herpetic neuralgia is more common in younger patients with HZO
   B. Male patients are more likely to develop post-herpetic neuralgia than the female patients
   C. Abducens nerve palsy is the most common ocular motility problem reported in patients with HZO
   D. HZO increases the risk of stroke and cardiac event within a year of the diagnosis of HZO

5. **Which of the following diseases has the highest risk of recurrence in corneal graft?**
   A. Granular dystrophy
   B. Lattice dystrophy
   C. Macular dystrophy
   D. Reis-Buckler dystrophy

6. **A 35-year-old patient presented to the eye casualty with a 1-week history of right eye pain. She was a soft contact lens wearer and had recently recovered from an episode of cold sores at the mouth corner. Slit-lamp examination showed an area of dendritic-like changes on the paracentral cornea. The patient was started on topical aciclovir and was reviewed in a week's time. One week later, there was worsening of the dendritic-like changes on the corneal epithelium with new onset of stromal oedema, keratic precipitates, and anterior chamber activity. Otherwise there were no stromal or perineural infiltrates. What is the most appropriate next step in this case?**
   A. Stop topical aciclovir, perform corneal scrape, and start the patient on topical chlorhexidine
   B. Change topical aciclovir to topical ganciclovir due to lack of treatment efficacy
   C. Continue with topical aciclovir and add topical prednisolone 0.5% 4×/day
   D. Change topical aciclovir to topical ganciclovir and add topical prednisolone 0.5% 4×/day and oral aciclovir 400 mg 5×/day

7. **Which of the following statements concerning primary Sjogren's syndrome (PSS) is correct?**
   A. Male is more commonly affected than female
   B. Negative anti-SSA (or anti-Ro) and anti-SSB (or anti-La) antibodies preclude the diagnosis of PSS
   C. There is an increased risk of T-cell lymphoma in patients with PSS
   D. The classic triad of symptoms consist of dryness of the eyes and mouth, fatigue, and pain

8. **Which of the following conditions/drugs is NOT associated with vortex keratopathy?**
   A. Atovaquone
   B. Fabry's disease
   C. Lowe syndrome
   D. Tamoxifen

9. A 65-year-old gentleman presents to the eye casualty with a 5-day history of right eye pain. He has recently investigated for recurrent episodes of nosebleed. Slit-lamp examination revealed a very injected right eye with engorged conjunctival and deep episcleral vessels associated with an area of peripheral corneal thinning spanning 3 to 6 o'clock with no infiltrate. Serologic testing revealed markedly elevated antiproteinase 3 antibody level. The patient was started on high-dose systemic prednisolone but was not able to fully control the ocular disease. What is the best next step-up treatment to further control this condition?
   A. Azathioprine
   B. Methotrexate
   C. Mycophenolate mofetil
   D. Rituximab

10. Which of the following statements concerning pterygium is true?
    A. The presence of Hudson–Stahli line at the head of pterygium is an indicative sign of chronicity of pterygium
    B. Pterygium grows across the limbus and damages the Bowman's layer
    C. Ultraviolet (UV) radiation plays an important role in the cases of recurrent pterygium
    D. Evidence suggests that sutures may result in lower risk of recurrence than fibrin glue for fixing the conjunctival graft during pterygium surgery

11. Which of the following anterior segment dysgenesis should always have chromosomal analysis to exclude a WT1 deletion, which is associated with an important systemic pathology?
    A. Aniridia
    B. Axenfeld-Rieger syndrome
    C. Peter's anomaly
    D. Trabeculodysgenesis

12. A 55-year-old patient is referred to the glaucoma clinic. During the assessment you find an intraocular pressure of 28 mmHg in the right eye (OD) and 31 mmHg in the left eye (OS), and open iridocorneal angles. There is evidence of neuroretinal rim thinning and arcuate defects on perimetric testing. What treatment would be most appropriate in this case?
    A. Latanoprost
    B. Timolol
    C. Tiopex
    D. Xalatan

13. A 32-year-old female patient with glaucoma presents to your clinic with a rise in intraocular pressure and suspected further damage to the retinal nerve fibre layer/neuroretinal rim as identified on perimetry and imaging. Her current medication is topical latanoprost once at night. She informs you that she is pregnant. Your management plan is most likely to include the following:
    A. Change latanoprost to latanoprost/timolol combination
    B. Continue with latanoprost and start brimonidine
    C. Stop latanoprost and start brimonidine
    D. Stop latanoprost and observe

14. In any patient with posterior segment ischaemia, which of the following best describes the mechanism of disruption of aqueous circulation in those who develop neovascular glaucoma?
    A. Neovascular membranes grow across the angle, causing fibrosis, contraction, and synechiael closure of the iridocorneal angle
    B. Hormones released as a consequence of ischaemia causes a secondary open angle glaucoma through an unknown mechanism
    C. Mechanical blockage of the trabecular meshwork with inflammatory particles released from friable new vessels
    D. New vessels in the anterior segment cause an increase in blood supply to the ciliary body and increased aqueous production

15. A 43-year-old male with elevated intraocular pressure (IOP) at the optometrist is referred to your clinic. On examination you can see pigment on the corneal endothelium, midperipheral transillumination defects within the iris, and heavily pigmented trabecular meshwork. Which of the following is MOST accurate with regard to this gentleman's condition?
    A. Patients tend to have mild to moderate hypermetropia
    B. Trabeculectomy for these patients has a similar success rate as for primary open angle glaucoma
    C. Laser trabeculoplasty tends not to be effective in this condition
    D. Laser iridotomy may help deepen the iridocorneal angle and reduce the risk of angle closure

16. Please select the MOST ACCURATE statement from the following options with regard to the properties of intraocular lenses used during routine cataract surgery.
    A. Hydrophobic acrylic intraocular lens (IOLs) can be folded easily, have low rates of posterior capsule opacification (PCO), and a high refractive index
    B. Round edged IOLs are associated with lower rates of PCO
    C. Silicone IOLs can be folded easily and have a high refractive index
    D. Rigid polymethylmethacrylate (PMMA) lenses have a much lower rate of PCO but require a larger incision.

17. **Based on the current guidelines, the following findings would suggest repeating biometry:**
    A. Soft contact lens wearer who has not worn contact lenses for more than 1 week
    B. Mean corneal power difference greater than 0.7 D between the two eyes
    C. Axial length greater than 0.5 mm difference between the two eyes
    D. Patient has had biometry performed after dilation and tonometry

18. **All of the following conditions are linked with microspherophakia, EXCEPT:**
    A. Ehlers–Danlos syndrome
    B. Marfan's syndrome
    C. Peters anomaly
    D. Weill–Marchesani syndrome

19. **For the following clinical scenario, please select the MOST appropriate option with regard to the formation of lens opacity. A 42-year-old woman taking long-term treatment with amiodarone to control her arrhythmia has bilateral asymptomatic lens opacities.**
    A. Anterior subcapsular deposits
    B. Posterior subcapsular opacities
    C. Sunflower cataract
    D. Vossius ring

20. **With regard to congenital cataract, which of the following statements is correct?**
    A. Sealing the wound with a suture leads to more astigmatism
    B. Bilateral cataract is more amblyogenic than unilateral cataract, and therefore should be operated on sooner
    C. Galactosaemia can result in an oil drop cataract and renal failure
    D. All of the above

21. **A 53-year-old female presents with a recurrent retinal detachment secondary to inferior proliferative vitreoretinopathy (Grade C). She undergoes further vitrectomy surgery to reattach her retina. Which is the most likely choice of endotamponade?**
    A. Hexafluoroethane (C2F6)
    B. Perfluorocarbon liquid (PFCL)
    C. Silicone oil
    D. Sulphur hexafluoride (SF6) gas

22. **A 52-year-old male presents with a retinoschisis-related retinal detachment (RSRD). Which of the following statements is correct?**
    A. RSRD retinal detachments occur predominantly in a temporal location
    B. RSRD can only occur if inner and outer leaf breaks are present
    C. Surgical outcomes are equivalent to those of conventional rhegmatogenous retinal detachments
    D. At presentation RSRD are rarely associated with proliferative vitreoretinopathy

23. **A patient presents 4 days after uncomplicated cataract surgery. Vision in the operated eye is perception of light. There is a 4 mm hypopyon present, no fundal view. A diagnosis of presumed bacterial endophthalmitis is made in the eye emergency department. Which of the following management options is most appropriate?**
    A. Vitreous biopsy and intravitreal antibiotics
    B. Hourly topical steroid, with a review in 6 hours to see if there is any improvement
    C. Three port pars plana vitrectomy and intravitreal antibiotics
    D. Anterior chamber washout and topical antibiotics

24. **Which of the following is the commonest cause of sympathetic ophthalmia within the United Kingdom?**
    A. Brachytherapy
    B. Cataract surgery
    C. Ocular trauma
    D. Vitreoretinal surgery

25. **Which of the following statement regarding familial exudative vitreoretinopathy (FEVR) is correct?**
    A. It is most commonly inherited in an autosomal recessive fashion
    B. Wide-field fluorescein angiography is the gold standard in assessing FEVR
    C. A negative family history is useful in excluding the diagnosis of FEVR
    D. Early laser photocoagulation does not reduce the risk of disease progression

26. **Which of the following options about retinal arterial macroaneurysm (RAM) is correct?**
    A. RAM may result in trilaminar retinal haemorrhages
    B. Exudative RAM is usually associated with a better visual prognosis than haemorrhagic RAM
    C. It is most commonly associated with hyperlipidaemia
    D. Haemorrhagic RAM usually requires treatment compared to exudative RAM

27. **Which of the following is true with regard to the natural history of retinal vein occlusions?**
    A. In central retinal vein occlusions 30% of eyes with a visual acuity of worse than 6/60 go on to develop rubeosis
    B. 50–60% of untreated branch retinal vein occlusion cases retain a visual acuity of better than 6/12 at 1 year

C. 20% of central retinal vein occlusions present with bilateral involvement
D. 20% of branch retinal vein occlusions will have fellow eye involvement over time

28. **Which of the following steroid preparations has National Institute for Health and Care Excellence (NICE) approval for the management of macular oedema secondary to central retinal vein occlusion?**
    A. Dexamethasone intravitreal implant 0.7 mg
    B. Fluocinolone acetonide intravitreal implant 0.19 mg
    C. Methylprednisolone acetate
    D. Triamcinolone acetonide

29. **A patient presents with painless loss of vision in the left eye and the following retinal appearance (Figure 6.1) following uneventful cataract surgery. The intracameral use of which medication has been associated with this condition?**
    A. Amphotericin
    B. Bevacizumab
    C. Cefuroxime
    D. Vancomycin

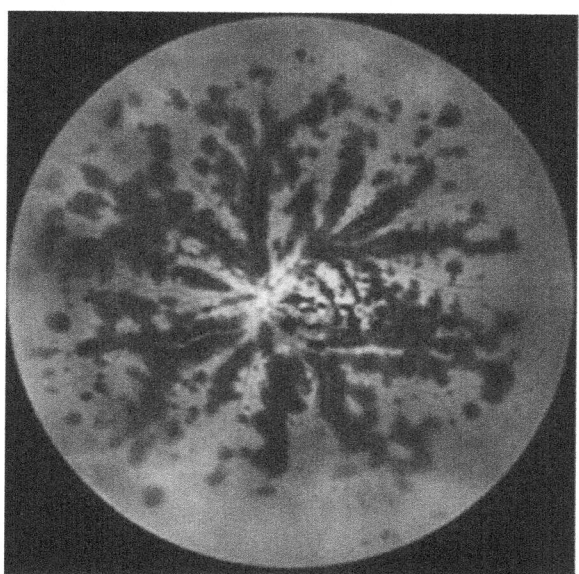

Figure 6.1

Reprinted from *Ophthalmology: Journal of the American Academy of Ophthalmology*, 124, 5, Witkin, A. et al., Vancomycin-Associated Hemorrhagic Occlusive Retinal Vasculitis: Clinical Characteristics of 36 Eyes, pp. 583–595, Copyright 2016, with permission from Elsevier. https://doi.org/10.1016/j.ophtha.2016.11.042. Published by Elsevier on behalf of the American Academy of Ophthalmology.

30. **Which of the following conditions is associated with retinitis pigmentosa and steatorrhoea?**
    A. Bardet–Biedl syndrome
    B. Bassen–Kornzweig syndrome
    C. Refsum syndrome
    D. Waardenburg syndrome

31. **Based on the ocular motility problem illustrated in Figure 6.2, where is the most likely location of the lesion?**
    A. Left medial longitudinal fasciculus
    B. Left sixth nerve nucleus
    C. Right paramedian pontine reticular formation
    D. Right parietal lobe

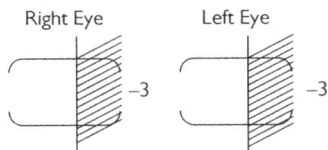

Figure 6.2

32. **A 58-year-old man presented with a 4-day history of discomfort around his right eye and new onset diplopia which he noticed when watching TV. The diplopia was worse on right gaze and on examination he was found to have an esotropia in the primary position of 10 dioptres and of 30 dioptres on right gaze. He had no other significant medical history and was on no medication. What is the most likely diagnosis?**
    A. Idiopathic intracranial hypertension
    B. Microvascular sixth nerve palsy
    C. Thyroid eye disease
    D. Traumatic injury to the eye

33. **Which of the following statements regarding Marcus-Gunn jaw-winking syndrome (MGJWS) is correct?**
    A. It represents 30% cases of congenital ptosis
    B. Amblyopia may develop in patients with MGJWS and is usually caused by the ptotic eyelid
    C. It is caused by synkinetic movement of internal pterygoid muscle and levator palpebrae superioris muscle
    D. It may present bilaterally

34. A 32-year-old man presented with a week's history of right ptosis and ear pain. Examination revealed a 2 mm ptosis of the right upper lid and he continued to describe significant ear pain. He had already received a 1-week course of oral antibiotics. In the light, his right pupil measured 2 mm and his left measured 3 mm, and in a dimly lit room his right pupil measured 2.5 mm and the left measured 4 mm. What is the most likely cause of the anisocoria?
    A. Argyll Robertson pupil
    B. Damage to oculosympathetic system
    C. Longstanding Adie pupil
    D. Physiological anisocoria

35. A 29-year-old female presented to her GP with pain around her left eye for 3 days. Her GP found her vision to be slightly reduced in the left eye so suggested she was seen in an urgent clinic in the eye department. On examination she had visual acuity of 6/6 OD and 6/12 OS. Colour vision revealed an Ishihara plate of 15/15 OD and 7/15 OS. When she was seen in the eye department she also mentioned that colours seemed washed out in her left eye compared to her right. She had a left relative afferent pupillary defect (RAPD) and on examination of her fundus, there was no sign of any abnormality. What is the most likely finding on visual field testing of this patient?
    A. Altitudinal field defect
    B. Bitemporal hemianopia
    C. Central scotoma
    D. Junctional scotoma

36. Which of the following syndromes best describes ipsilateral sixth and seventh nerve palsies with contralateral hemiparesis?
    A. Eight-and-a-half syndrome
    B. Foville syndrome
    C. Millard–Gubler syndrome
    D. Raymond-Céstan syndrome

37. Which of the following feature is most suggestive of non-arteritic anterior ischaemic optic neuropathy (NA-AION)?
    A. Altitudinal field defect
    B. Family history of visual loss
    C. Jaw claudication
    D. Recent foreign travel

38. **Which of the following statements about myotonic dystrophy (MD) is correct?**
    A. It is an autosomal recessive disease due to cytosine-thymine-guanine (CTG) trinucleotide repeat
    B. Respiratory failure is the leading cause of death in patients with MD
    C. The most common ocular motility problem is deficit in elevation of the eyes
    D. It is most commonly found in Eastern European and Asian populations

39. **A patient with a history of lupus presents with a new onset posterior uveitis and undergoes baseline investigation including syphilis testing. The following result is obtained: syphilis immunoglobulin G (IgG) with a treponemal specific antibody test is positive and rapid plasma regain result is highly positive What does this test result mean?**
    A. The patient has untreated syphilis and requires treatment
    B. The result is a false positive and no further treatment is necessary
    C. The patient appears to have previously undergone treatment for syphilis
    D. The patient has no evidence of active syphilis and no treatment is necessary

40. **A 30-year-old female is brought to the accident and emergency (A&E) department with hearing loss and altered mental state. She also mentions that her vision is blurred in both eyes. Ophthalmic examination identifies bilateral multiple branch retinal artery occlusions. Magnetic resonance imaging (MRI) of the brain demonstrates multiple lesions within the corpus callosum. What is the most likely diagnosis?**
    A. Cerebral venous thrombosis
    B. Cogan syndrome
    C. Multiple sclerosis
    D. Susac's syndrome

41. **A 44-year-old female presents with new onset polyarthralgia, including her hands, elbows, ankles, and knees. She is also noted to have a painful and tender rash affecting the shins of both legs. Inflammatory markers are high and autoantibodies were negative. Serum angiotensin-converting enzyme (ACE) was normal. A chest X-ray showed bilateral hilar lymphadenopathy. What is the most likely diagnosis?**
    A. Heerfordt's syndrome
    B. Löfgren's syndrome
    C. Rheumatoid arthritis
    D. Reactive arthritis

42. The following are features of Alport syndrome, **EXCEPT**:
    A. Anterior lenticonus
    B. Glomerulonephritis
    C. Posterior subcapsular cataract
    D. Sensorineural deafness

43. A 52-year-old lady is referred to the outpatient clinic to exclude an ocular cause for her intractable right-sided ocular pain. The pain has been ongoing for 9 months with no pain-free intervals. There is no exacerbating or relieving factor. She describes a persistent aching and occasionally stabbing behind the eye which can be associated with lid drooping and sometimes the eye can look pink. There is no movement exacerbation and the pain can make her restless. Examination of both eyes is normal as is the MRI of the brain requested from primary care. Which of the treatment is most likely to alleviate her symptoms?
    A. High-flow oxygen via venture mask with rebreathable bag
    B. Oral aciclovir
    C. Oral indomethacin
    D. Subcutaneous sumatriptan

44. A 3-month child is referred because the parents are worried about its vision. On complete eye exam no apparent cause can be found. What do you do next?
    A. Referral to a paediatrician or a paediatric neurologist and review the child at aged 6 months
    B. Referral for visual electro physiology and review the child at age 6 months
    C. Referral for a magnetic resonance image of the head and review the child with result
    D. Referral for visual electrophysiology and paediatric workup and review the child with the result

45. Which of the following is a characteristic feature of euryblepharon?
    A. Asymmetric enlargement of the horizontal palpebral fissure
    B. Elongated lid margins
    C. Upward and lateral displacement of the lateral canthus
    D. Vertical lengthening of the eyelid skin

46. A 3-month-old child is referred with a segmental capillary haemangioma of the upper eyelid more than 5 cm in size. The first line of management includes:
    A. Intralesional steroid injection as there is a risk of amblyopia
    B. MRI/MRA scan of the head and neck
    C. Pulsed-dye laser treatment to regress the lesion
    D. Surgical excision of the haemangioma

47. Which of the following statements regarding orbital cellulitis and subperiosteal abscess is correct?
A. Orbital cellulitis occurs as a secondary extension of acute or chronic bacterial sinusitis, especially the frontal sinusitis
B. Surgical intervention is more likely if the child is under 9 years of age as it is commonly polymicrobial
C. Clinical improvement correlates well with repeat computed tomography (CT) scan analysis
D. Blindness occurs in up to 11% of cases

48. A 4-month-old child was referred with features of midfacial hypoplasia, shallow orbit, proptosis, corneal exposure, finger and toe abnormality, partial syndactyly, and normal intelligence. These distinctive features are suggestive of:
A. Apert syndrome
B. Crouzon syndrome
C. Muenke syndrome
D. Pfeiffer syndrome

49. A 2-day-old unwell child was seen with bilateral red eye, non-purulent discharge, and hazy cornea. The management includes:
A. Topical aciclovir ointment five times daily and intravenous acyclovir 60 mg/kg/day in three divided doses
B. Topical cefuroxime and gentamicin drops four times daily and broad-spectrum antibiotics
C. Topical erythromycin 2-hourly and intravenous benzylpenicillin (30 mg/kg/day) in three divided doses or cefotaxime 100 mg/kg as a single dose
D. Topical tetracycline ointment four times a daily and 4-week course of oral erythromycin (50 mg/kg/day) in four divided doses

50. Which of the following statements concerning congenital megalocornea is correct?
A. It is commonly unilateral and thought to be due to defective growth of the optic cup
B. The model of inheritance is an X-linked recessive trait in more than 90%
C. It is a slowly progressive condition with a corneal diameter more than 15 mm
D. Hypermetropia is the most common refractive error associated with this condition, often accompanied with by-the-rule astigmatism

51. A 63-year gentle man presented with vertical diplopia after an injury. On examination he had a right hypertropia increasing on right gaze and left head tilt. The most likely extraocular muscle that is paretic is:
A. Right inferior rectus
B. Right superior oblique
C. Left inferior oblique
D. Left superior rectus

52. A 15-year-old patient presents to the eye emergency department complaining of double vision, with a history of blunt trauma to his right cheekbone. Which of the following signs would require urgent surgical intervention?
   A. Bradycardia in upgaze
   B. Maxillary sinus opacification
   C. 2 mm enophthalmos
   D. −2 restriction in elevation

53. All of the following facial injection sites are associated with high risk for inadvertent ophthalmic artery intra-arterial injection embolus causing central retinal artery occlusion, **EXCEPT**:
   A. Glabellar
   B. Nasal dorsum
   C. Nasojugal
   D. Temporalis

54. Which of the following signs is the best indicator of severe thyroid eye disease?
   A. RAPD
   B. Chemosis
   C. 40^ esotropia
   D. Lateral flare of the upper lid

55. A 4-year-old boy is reviewed in clinic for a congenital left upper eyelid ptosis. His unaided visual acuity is recorded as right: 0.125 and left: 0.300 LogMAR equivalent on Kay Pictures. He has normal right eye examination and a 3 mm ptosis on the left upper eyelid with levator function of 9 mm. Which of the following would be the best management option for him?
   A. Fasanella Servat
   B. Frontalis sling
   C. Levator aponeurosis advancement
   D. Patching of the right eye

56. Which of the following could cause a cicatricial ectropion?
   A. Dacryoadenitis
   B. Horizontal lid laxity
   C. Lower lid basal cell carcinoma (BCC)
   D. Ocular cicatricial pemphigoid (OCP)

57. A 45-year-old female is referred to clinic with concern regarding facial asymmetry; she thinks one eye looks sunken compared to the other. She has no significant past medical history and no history of trauma. Visual acuity and eye movements are normal, there is 3 mm of enophthalmos on the left with a deep superior sulcus but no lid malposition. Which of the following is the most likely diagnosis?
   A. Previous blow out fracture
   B. Sclerosing metastasis
   C. Scleroderma
   D. Silent sinus syndrome

58. Which of the following features is more common in squamous cell carcinoma (SCC) than BCC?
   A. Bleeding
   B. Pain
   C. Telangiectasia
   D. Ulceration

59. Which of the following is associated with an increase of choroidal melanoma metastasis?
   A. Monosomy 3
   B. Younger age at presentation
   C. Female patient
   D. Loss of chromosome 8q

60. Which of the following is the most common histopathological diagnosis for orbital malignancies in an adult?
   A. Adenoid cystic carcinoma
   B. Lymphoma
   C. Metastasis
   D. Rhabdomyosarcoma

61. Retinal astrocytoma may be associated with the following neoplasms, **EXCEPT**:
   A. Cardiac rhabdomyoma
   B. Neurofibroma
   C. Pheochromocytoma
   D. Pulmonary lymphangioleiomyoma

62. A 48-year-old male presents with a 3-month history of reduced vision in one eye. His vision is count fingers with a total retinal detachment with a large retinal tear superiorly at the ora serrata. He has evidence of 1+ anterior chamber cells and the IOP is 34 in the affected eye. The other eye is normal. He reports blunt ocular trauma prior to the onset of symptoms. What is the most likely diagnosis?
    A. Chronic uveitis complicated by exudative retinal detachment
    B. Posner–Schlossman syndrome
    C. Schwartz syndrome
    D. Sympathetic ophthalmia

63. In patients with juvenile idiopathic arthritis, which of the following has the highest risk of developing chronic anterior uveitis?
    A. ANA +ve, oligoarthritis, younger age at diagnosis
    B. ANA +ve, polyarthritis, older age at diagnosis
    C. ANA –ve, oligoarthritis, younger age at diagnosis
    D. ANA –ve, polyarthritis, older age at diagnosis

64. An 82-year-old retired engineer presents with right ocular redness and visual loss due to blurry vision and floaters over 3 weeks. His medical background is notable only for previously treated malaria. Examination reveals a right panuveitis. Through the moderately hazy vitreous a large pale patch is observed involving the macula of right fundus. There are no fundus haemorrhages and the left eye is normal. Optical coherence tomography (OCT) reveals derangement of the architecture of the outer retina. Which of the following is the most likely diagnosis?
    A. Herpes zoster
    B. Small cell carcinoma of the lung
    C. Syphilis
    D. Tuberculosis

65. Which of the following describes the method of action of adalimumab therapy in the treatment of uveitis?
    A. Anti-CD20
    B. Antitumour necrosis factor alpha
    C. Anti-vascular endothelial growth factor (VEGF)
    D. Interferon–β1a

66. **What is the recommended use of corticosteroid therapy in the United Kingdom for prevention of Jarisch–Herxheimer reaction in the treatment of neurological or ophthalmic syphilis?**
    A. A 3-day course of oral corticosteroid starting 24 hours before antibiotic therapy
    B. A 5-day course of oral corticosteroid starting concurrently with antibiotic therapy
    C. A 3-day course of oral corticosteroid starting 48 hours after initiation of antibiotic therapy
    D. A 5-day course of oral corticosteroid starting 48 hours after initiation of antibiotic therapy

67. **Which of the following best describes the mechanism of latanoprost in reducing intraocular pressure?**
    A. Increase uveoscleral outflow
    B. Reduce aqueous production
    C. Increase uveoscleral outflow and reduce aqueous production
    D. Increase conventional/trabecular outflow and reduce aqueous production

68. **Which of the following medications is associated with increased risk of tendon rupture?**
    A. Cefuroxime
    B. Ciclosporin
    C. Ciprofloxacin
    D. Cyclophosphamide

69. **Quetiapine can cause:**
    A. Corneal verticillata
    B. Dopamine maculopathy
    C. Intraoperative floppy iris syndrome (IFIS)
    D. Open angle glaucoma

70. **What is the mechanism of action of botulinum toxin?**
    A. Inhibits the presynaptic release of acetylcholine (ACh)
    B. Inhibits the postsynaptic ACh receptor
    C. Inhibits the reuptake of acetylcholinesterase
    D. Inhibits the voltage-gated calcium channels at the neuromuscular junction

71. **Which of the following statements regarding the microbiological staining technique is true?**
    A. Bacteria that allow crystal violet dye to wash off are Gram positive
    B. Giemsa stain is for bacteria, fungi, and acanthamoeba
    C. Gomori methenamine silver stains for acanthamoeba
    D. Periodic acid Schiff stain is useful for bacteria

72. **Which of the followings regarding fundus fluorescein angiography (FFA) is correct?**
    A. It incorporates a yellow green excitation filter and a blue barrier filter
    B. Sodium fluorescein is 40–50% bound to plasma albumin
    C. Sodium fluorescein is metabolized and excreted by the kidney in 24 hours
    D. Pregnancy is not an absolute contraindication

73. **In acute posterior multifocal pigment placoid epitheliopathy (APMPPE), what is the typical lesion appearance on FFA?**
    A. Persistent hypofluorescence throughout the angiogram
    B. Early hypofluorescence and late staining
    C. Early hyperfluorescence and retinal vascular leakage
    D. Early hyperfluorescence and evidence of retinal vascular occlusion

74. **Which of the following is correct about pattern electroretinogram (pERG)?**
    A. Assesses the peripheral retina
    B. Uses a reversing checkerboard to evoke small potentials that arise from the inner retina
    C. N95 is photoreceptor-driven and is key to assessing macular cone function
    D. P50 originates from the macular ganglion cells

75. **What is the clinical interpretation of the Worth four-dot (W4D) test result in the following scenario? A patient wears a green lens in front of the right eye and a red lens in front of the left eye. She sees three green lights on the W4D test.**
    A. The left eye is suppressed
    B. The right eye is suppressed
    C. The patient is likely to have diplopia
    D. The patient is likely to have binocular single vision (BSV)

76. **Which of the following orthoptic tests can be carried out without glasses?**
    A. Frisby
    B. Hess chart
    C. Titmus
    D. TNO

77. **Which of the following describes the neuroimaging shown in Figure 6.3?**
    A. MRI T1-weighted
    B. MRI T1-weighted with gadolinium enhancement
    C. MRI T2-weighted
    D. MRI T2-weighted with fluid attenuated inversion recovery (FLAIR) sequence

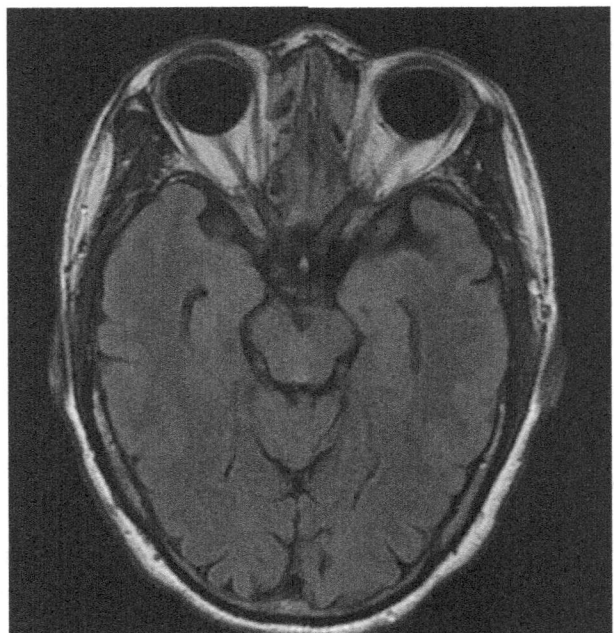

Figure 6.3

Reproduced with permission from Yau, G. et al. (2014) Neuromyelitis Optica Spectrum Disorder in a Chinese Woman with Ocular Myasthenia Gravis: First Reported Case in the Chinese Population. *Neuro-Ophthalmology*, 38(3): 140–144. https://doi.org/10.3109/01658107.2013.879903. Rights managed by Taylor & Francis.

78. **Which of the following autoantibodies is NOT implicated in myasthenia gravis?**
    A. Antiacetylcholine receptors (AChR) antibody
    B. Anticyclic citrullinated peptide (CCP)
    C. Anti-low-density lipoprotein receptor-related protein (LRP4) antibody
    D. Antityrosine kinase muscle-specific kinase (MuSK) antibody

79. **The optic vesicle is formed by day:**
    A. 12 of gestation
    B. 25 of gestation
    C. 32 of gestation
    D. 42 of gestation

80. **Which of the following cell types of choroidal melanoma is associated with the worst prognosis?**
    A. Epithelioid cell
    B. Spindle A
    C. Spindle B
    D. Mixed type

81. **Patients with gyrate atrophy result from a deficiency of:**
    A. Ornithine aminotransferase (OAT), located on chromosome 10
    B. Ornithine aminotransferase (OAT), located on chromosome 12
    C. Ornithine hexaminase (Ohex), located on chromosome 14
    D. Ornithine hexaminase (Ohex), located on chromosome 16

82. **What kind of image does slit-lamp fundus lenses (e.g. +90 D lens) produce?**
    A. Real, mirrored, and magnified
    B. Real, inverted, and magnified
    C. Virtual, mirrored, and magnified
    D. Virtual, inverted, and magnified

83. **Which of the following tests is used to compare the mean of three or more groups?**
    A. Analysis of variance (ANOVA)
    B. Contingency table
    C. Mann–Whitney U test
    D. T-tests

84. **Which of the following statements regarding the Tube Versus Trabeculectomy (TVT) study is correct?**
    A. The rate of reoperation was significantly lower in the tube group versus the trabeculectomy group
    B. The number of glaucoma medications in the tube group was significantly lower than the trabeculectomy group at 5 years
    C. The cumulative probability of failure during 5 years of follow-up was the same in both tube and trabeculectomy groups
    D. The rate of early postoperative complications was significantly higher in the tube group

85. **A 76-year-old patient attends the age-related macular degeneration clinic keen to supplement his diet in zinc. Which food has the highest content of zinc?**
    A. One cup of sliced apricots
    B. One cup of cubed avocado
    C. Three dates
    D. One of sliced kiwi

86. **A 68-year-old patient was recently diagnosed with right eye primary open angle glaucoma and left ocular hypertension. His best-corrected visual acuity is 6/6 in either eye. He is currently receiving treatment in both eyes. He normally drives a four-seater car. According to the Driver and Vehicle Licensing Agency (DVLA) driving standard, which of the following advices should be given to this patient in this circumstance?**
    A. Patient can continue to drive and does not need to inform DVLA
    B. Patient can continue to drive but needs to inform DVLA
    C. Patient should stop driving and needs to inform DVLA
    D. If patient continues to drive, you may have to breach the patient's confidentiality and inform DVLA

87. **Capacity should be assessed in a semi-structured direct interview with the patient. Capacity evaluation is assessed in a:**
    A. One-step process
    B. Two-step process
    C. Three-step process
    D. Four-step process

88. **The quality-adjusted life year or quality-adjusted-life-year (QALY) equates to:**
    A. 1 year of life × 1 year of ill health
    B. 1 year of ill health × 1 utility value
    C. 1 year of life × 1 utility value
    D. 1 year of ill health × 1 year of life

89. **A patient attends the outpatient department with a putative diagnosis of Creutzfeldt–Jakob disease (CJD). Which procedure carries the highest risk of transmission?**
    A. Brow lift
    B. Dacryocystorhinostomy
    C. Lateral rectus recession
    D. Scleral buckling

90. **Patients receiving long-term hydroxychloroquine should receive the following after 5 years of therapy:**
    A. 10–2 Humphrey visual field, spectral domain optical coherence tomography (SD-OCT), and fundus autofluorescence (FAF)
    B. 10–2 Humphrey visual field, SD-OCT, and multifocal electroretinography
    C. 30–2 Humphrey visual field and SD-OCT
    D. 30–2 Humphrey visual field and FAF

chapter 6

MOCK EXAM

ANSWERS

1. Answer: A

Chemical eye injury is a common ophthalmic emergency that requires immediate medical attention. The question is testing the candidates' knowledge on the assessment and prognostic factors of chemical eye injury, which can be based on Roper-Hall or modified Hughes classification. In this classification, limbal ischaemia—a proxy for limbal stem cell damage—and corneal haze are the two main prognostic factors for vision (Table 6.1).

Table 6.1 Limbal ischaemia and corneal haze are the two main prognostic factors for vision

Grading	Cornea	Limbal ischaemia	Prognosis
1	Clear	Nil	Good
2	Hazy; iris details visible	<1/3	Good
3	Opaque; iris details obscured	1/3–1/2	Guarded
4	Opaque; iris details obscured	>1/2	Poor

Reproduced with permission from Roper-Hall, M. (1965) Thermal and chemical burns. *Transactions of the Ophthalmological Societies of the United Kingdom*, 85:631-53. Courtesy of The Royal College of Ophthalmologists.

2. Answer: C

Corneal collagen cross-linking (CXL) was first introduced in 2003 by Wollensak et al. to treat progressive keratitis. It is a minimally, invasive procedure that combines the use of ultraviolet-A light of 365–370 nm and riboflavin/vitamin B_2 drops. The NICE guideline has recommended the use of CXL in patients with corneal ectasia with a corneal thickness of 400 micros or more to avoid corneal endothelial damage by UV irradiation. The original Dresden protocol requires a 30-minute instillation of topical riboflavin solution followed by UVA irradiation at 3 mW/cm^2 for 30 minutes (fluence of 5.4 J/cm^2). Over the recent years, various accelerated protocols, using higher UVA irradiation with shorter time span, have been proposed and examined. So far the evidence showed similar efficacy between accelerated and conventional protocols.

Photoactivated chromophore for keratitis (PACK)-CXL has been shown to be a potentially effective adjuvant treatment to topical antibiotic treatment for bacterial keratitis, but the effect on acanthamoeba keratitis has not been proven.

Berra M, et al. Treatment of Acanthamoeba keratitis by corneal cross-linking. *Cornea* 2013;32:174–8.

National Institute for Health and Care Excellence (NICE). *Photochemical Corneal Collagen Cross-Linkage Using Riboflavin and Ultraviolet A for Keratoconus and Keratectasia. Interventional Procedures Guidance [IPG466]*, 2013. Available at: https://www.nice.org.uk/guidance/ipg466

Shajari M, et al. Comparison of standard and accelerated corneal cross-linking for the treatment of keratoconus: a meta-analysis. *Acta Ophthalmol* 2019;97(1):e22–35.

3. Answer: B

This clinical scenario describes a patient suffering from a rare type of familial systemic amyloidosis called Meretoja's syndrome (or type 2 lattice corneal dystrophy). It was first described in 1969 by Dr Meretoja, a Finnish ophthalmologist. It is an autosomal dominant disease caused by mutation at the gelsolin gene at chromosome 9q, whereas type 1 lattice dystrophy is caused by gene mutation in the *BIGH3* or *TGFBI*. The symptoms/signs of Meretoja's syndrome usually starts from the third decade of life and the first sign of disease is usually corneal lattice dystrophy. The typical diagnostic triad includes corneal lattice dystrophy, progressive bilateral facial nerve palsy, and skin laxity. The affected patients are at increased risk of developing renal failure, cardiac failure, and conduction abnormalities. The amyloid stains with Congo red and demonstrates apple green birefringence and dichroism at polarizing microscopy.

Carrwik C, Stenevi U. Lattice corneal dystrophy, gelsolin type (Meretoja's syndrome). *Acta Ophthalmol* 2009;87:813–9.

Meretoja syndrome—recent articles. Available at: https://www.ncbi.nlm.nih.gov/medgen/301243

4. Answer: D

HZO is associated with a wide spectrum of ocular and non-ocular complications. Post-herpetic neuralgia (PHN) is one of the most common and debilitating complication following HZO. The risk of PHN rises significantly with age, from 4% in patients younger than 50 years old to 30–40% in patients over 80 years old. Female gender has been shown as a risk factor for PHN but the evidence is not conclusive. Third nerve palsy is the most common ocular motility disorder reported in patients with HZO but other types of ocular motility problem such as fourth, sixth, and multiple nerve palsies have been reported. HZO significantly increases the risk of stroke and cardiac events within a year of diagnosis of HZO. This is likely due to the migration of virus from neurons to the cerebral and coronary vasculatures, causing local inflammatory responses, vascular occlusion, and ischaemia.

Erskine N, et al. A systematic review and meta-analysis on herpes zoster and the risk of cardiac and cerebrovascular events. *PloS One* 2017;12:e0181565.

Marsh RJ, et al. External ocular motor palsies in ophthalmic zoster: a review. *Br J Ophthalmol* 1977;61:677–82.

Schutzer-Weissmann J, Farquhar-Smith P. Post-herpetic neuralgia—a review of current management and future directions. *Expert Opin Pharmacother* 2017;18:1739–50.

5. Answer: D

All the conditions mentioned in the answer list can be associated with recurrence of the disease in the corneal graft. The risk of recurrence can be memorized by the mnemonic of 'Rude Little Green Man' in descending order of frequency.

R—Reis-Buckler dystrophy (most common)

L—Lattice dystrophy

G—Granular dystrophy

M—Macular dystrophy (least common)

Marcon AS, et al. Recurrence of corneal stromal dystrophies after penetrating keratoplasty. *Cornea* 2003;22:19–21.

6. Answer: A

This is a clinical vignette of acanthamoeba keratitis (AK) masquerading as herpes simplex keratitis (HSK), which is a commonly encountered scenario in clinical practice. Epithelial HSK usually responds well and quickly to topical antiviral treatment. Therefore, one should always have a low threshold of suspecting AK in contact lens wearers who present with non-specific epithelial changes or 'dendritic-like' changes, especially when the condition has not improved on topical antiviral treatment. It is also noteworthy to mention that sometimes AK can coexist with HSK, therefore a positive herpes simplex virus (HSV) swab result does not exclude the diagnosis of AK. Approximately 85–90% cases of AK are related to contact lens wear. It normally progresses from epithelial to stromal disease and patients usually have disproportionate pain to clinical signs, but absence of pain does not preclude the diagnosis.

Dart JK, et al. Acanthamoeba keratitis: diagnosis and treatment update 2009. *Am J Ophthalmol* 2009;148:487–99.

7. Answer: D

PSS is a common systemic autoimmune disease that may occur in isolation or with associated organ-specific autoimmune diseases such as thyroiditis or primary biliary cirrhosis. Secondary SS is referred to when the disease occurs in association with another systemic autoimmune disease such as rheumatoid arthritis, systemic lupus erythematosus, scleroderma, or dermatomyositis. PSS has a female-to-male predominance of 9:1 with a peak incidence at around 50 years old. The classic triad of symptoms include dryness of the mouth and eyes, fatigue, and pain. PSS increases the risk of B-cell lymphoma (not T-cell lymphoma) by 15–20 times compared to the general population. The 2017 American College of Rheumatology, European League against Rheumatism (ACR-EULAR) classification specifies the diagnostic criteria for PSS, which include focus score of ≥1 on minor labial salivary gland biopsy, presence of anti-SSA (or anti-Ro) antibodies, SICCA ocular staining score of ≥5, Schirmer's test of ≤5 mm per 5 min, and unstimulated whole salivary flow of ≤0.1 ml per min. Absence of anti-SSA or anti-Ro does not exclude the diagnosis of PSS but will require the presence of focal lymphocytic sialadenitis on minor labial salivary gland biopsy to confirm the diagnosis.

Mariette X, Criswell LA. Primary Sjogren's syndrome. *N Engl J Med* 2018;378:931–9.

8. Answer: C

Vortex keratopathy, or also known as cornea verticillata, is a type of deposition keratopathy characterized by whorl-like changes at the corneal subepithelial layer. It may be associated with a wide range of drugs and conditions. Many of these drugs have cationic amphiphilic structures that allow them to cross the cell membranes, leading to intracellular phospholipid accumulation. Vortex keratopathy usually has no effect on the vision and is not an indication for discontinuing the treatment. Fabry's disease and Lowe syndrome are both metabolic disorders that can cause congenital cataract. However, Lowe syndrome does not result in vortex keratopathy.

The following mnemonic (**CAT-FANGS**) can be used to help memorize the list of drugs/condition associated with vortex keratopathy:

C—Chloroquine (common)

C—Chlorpromazine (common)

A—Amiodarone (common)

T—Tamoxifen (common)

T—Tilorone

F—Fabry's disease

A—Atovaquone

N—NSAIDs

G—Gold

G—Gentamicin

S—Suramin

Raizman MB, et al. Drug-induced corneal epithelial changes. *Surv Ophthalmol* 2017;62:286–301.

9. Answer: D

This is a clinical scenario of peripheral ulcerative keratitis (PUK) with scleritis in a patient with undiagnosed granulomatosis with polyangiitis (GPA), formerly known as Wegener's granulomatosis. GPA is a type of systemic vasculitides that affects small- and medium-sized vessels, with primary involvement of upper respiratory tract and kidney. Patients may suffer from recurrent nose bleeds, saddle-nose deformity, pulmonary haemorrhage, scleritis, PUK, glomerulonephritis, and arthritis. Antineutrophilic cytoplasmic antibodies (ANCA) are autoantibodies produced by a person's immune system that attack proteins within the person's neutrophil. Proteinase 3 (PR3) and myeloperoxidase (MPO) are the two most common subsets of ANCA. 85% of the samples with cytoplasmic (cANCA) will have anti-PR3 antibodies (which is highly associated with GPA) and 90% of the perinuclear (pANCA) will have anti-MPO antibodies (which is highly associated with microscopic polyangiitis). In uncontrolled GPA-related PUK, cyclophosphamide or rituximab has been shown to best control disease and induce remission.

Ebrahimiadib N, et al. Successful treatment strategies in granulomatosis with polyangiitis-associated peripheral ulcerative keratitis. *Cornea* 2016;35:1459–65.

10. Answer: B

Pterygium is a common degenerative conjunctival fibrovascular lesion extending from the conjunctiva to the cornea. It is characterized by elastotic degeneration of the substantia propria. UV light plays an important role in primary pterygium but not recurrent pterygium, which is more related to surgical trauma. Presence of Stocker's iron line at the head of pterygium is an indicative sign of chronicity of pterygium. The Hudson–Stahli line is an innocuous iron line commonly found at the inferior 1/3 of the cornea in older people. Evidence suggests that fibrin glue may result in lower risk of recurrence and lesser operating time than sutures for fixing the conjunctival graft during pterygium surgery.

American Academy of Ophthalmology. *Pterygium*, 2015. Available at: http://eyewiki.aao.org/Pterygium

Romano V, et al. Fibrin glue versus sutures for conjunctival autografting in primary pterygium surgery. *Cochrane Database Syst Rev* 2016;12:CD011308.

11. Answer: A

The *WT1* tumour suppressor gene lies next to the *PAX6* gene on 11p13, so can also be affected in sporadic aniridics. This is associated with Wilms tumour (nephroblastoma). The most commonly affected gene involved in trabeculodysgenesis, or primary congenital glaucoma is *CYP1B1* (Chr2p) and also *MYOC* (Chr1q). Peters anomaly is usually sporadic, with multiple genes isolated as the cause including *PAX6*, *PIT2X*, *FOXC1*, *CYP1B1*, and *MYOC*. Questions in the exam therefore are unlikely to focus on specific genes for Peters anomaly.

Gould DB, John SW. Anterior segment dysgenesis and the developmental glaucoma are complex traits. *Hum Mol Genet* 2002;11:1185–93.

12. Answer: A

This answer reflects the new NICE guidelines which suggest: 'Offer a generic prostaglandin analogue to people with suspected chronic open angle glaucoma and intraocular pressure of 24 mmHg or more, in line with the recommendations on treatment for people with ocular hypertension.' This is different to the previous iteration of the guidelines, which focussed on different primary medications based on corneal thicknesses and age.

Reproduced from National Institute for Health and Care Excellence. Glaucoma: Diagnosis and Management (NG81) November 2017. Available on: www.nice.org.uk/guidance/ng81

13. Answer: C

This is a complex scenario and is not without some controversies, but raises the importance of understanding implications of medicines on the pregnant patient and the developing fetus.

The US Food and Drug Administration (FDA) has classified glaucoma medications as follows:

- Class B (*medications have varying and /or contradictory human and animal data.*)—Brimonidine only
- The rest of the glaucoma medications are classified as class C (**side effects in animal models, or where inadequate animal and human studies are available**)—β-blockers, carbonic anhydrase inhibitors (topical or systemic), and prostaglandin analogues.

This classification is based on the little existing evidence. There is some varied clinical practice, but for the purposes of the exam, brimonidine is the safest medication during pregnancy. Importantly post-partum this should be stopped if the intention is to breastfeed, as it passed to the milk and can cause respiratory depression in the newborn. Prostaglandin is probably the least safe, as it is similar to the hormones that stimulate uterine contractions and has been shown to induce miscarriage in animals. Option D is not an option as the vignette describes glaucoma progression. It should be noted though that during pregnancy in those with ocular hypertension/primary open angle glaucoma the IOP tends to decrease, so if there was no progression monitoring could be an option.

Razeghinejad MR, et al. Pregnancy and glaucoma. *Surv Ophthalmol* 2011;56:324–5.

Salim S. Glaucoma in pregnancy. *Curr Opin Ophthalmol* 2014;25:93–7.

14. Answer: A

This is the main cause though the new vessels themselves cause some degree of mechanical blockage of the trabecular meshwork. Option B is incorrect—although VEGF and pigment epithelium derived factor (PEDF) may independently affect aqueous drainage, the extent of their effect is currently not known and is not supposed to contribute the elevation of intraocular pressure significantly. Option C is incorrect as there are no specific inflammatory particles that are produced; however, there is often some level of anterior segment inflammation. Option D is incorrect. There is no known glaucoma that occurs from overproduction of aqueous humour, although certain medications can increase the production to varying degrees.

McLaren JW, et al. Effect of ibopamine on aqueous humor production in normotensive humans. *Invest Ophthalmol Vis Sci* 2003;44:4853–8.

Rodrigues GB, et al. Neovascular glaucoma: a review. *Int J Retina Vitreous* 2016;2:26.

15. Answer: B

The vignette describes pigment dispersion syndrome (PDS) with elevated intraocular pressure. Trabeculectomy success rates are similar to that of primary open angle glaucoma, but with reported increased rates of hypotony maculopathy.

Glaucoma may develop in 33–50% of patients with PDS. It can be clinically similar to pseudoexfoliation (PXF), although in PXF the iris transillumination defects tend to be closer to the pupillary margin, and the pigmentation of the angle is more sporadic and heterogeneous. There may also be evidence of pseudoexfoliative materials in the anterior segment. Patients with PDS tend to be myopes, with some evidence suggesting the degree of myopia in those who develop glaucoma is higher than in those who do not. Laser trabeculoplasty tends to be effective; however, a greater incidence in post-laser IOP spikes has been reported. Peripheral iridotomy has been purported as a potential treatment for PDS to equalize the pressure between anterior and posterior chambers and reduce the posterior bowing of the iris but not to deepen the anterior chamber angle. However, a recent Cochrane collaboration review found insufficient evidence of high quality on the effectiveness of peripheral iridotomy for pigmentary glaucoma or PDS. The vignette describes an open angle, and PDS is an open angle glaucoma. If you see a patient with occludable or narrow but visibly pigmented angles, the diagnosis is likely to be different (e.g. primary angle closure or primary angle closure glaucoma).

Michelessi M, Lindsley K. Peripheral iridotomy for pigmentary glaucoma. *Cochrane Database Syst Rev* 2016;2:CD005655.

Niyadurupola N, Broadway DC. Pigment dispersion syndrome and pigmentary glaucoma—a major review. *Clin Exp Ophthalmol* 2008;36:868–82.

16. Answer: A

Square-edged IOLs are associated with lower rates of PCO. Silicone IOLs have a lower refractive index, but otherwise accurate. PMMA lens have a higher rate of PCO but otherwise accurate.

Denniston AKO, Murray PI. *Oxford Handbook of Ophthalmology*, 3rd edition. Oxford, UK: Oxford University Press, 2014; pp. 324–8.

17. Answer: D

Biometry readings are considered acceptable if a soft contact lens (CL) wearer has not worn the CLs for 1 week or more. For rigid gas permeable contact lenses, the requirement is 4 weeks.

The other findings suggesting repeat biometry are:

(a) Axial length >0.7 mm difference between the two eyes

(b) Mean corneal power difference greater than 0.9 D between the two eyes

(c) Axial length <21.2 mm or >26.6 mm in either eye

(d) Mean corneal power <41 D or >47 D in either eye

(e) Delta K (corneal astigmatism) >2.5 D in either eye

(f) If the patient has biometry performed after dilation or tonometry

Knox-Cartwright N, et al. The Cataract National Dataset electronic multicentre audit of 55,567 operations: when should optical biometric measurements be rechecked? *Eye (Lond)* 2010;24:894–900.

Royal College of Ophthalmologists. *Cataract Surgery Guidelines*, September 2010; p. 45. Available at: https://www.rcophth.ac.uk/wp-content/uploads/2014/12/2010-SCI-069-Cataract-Surgery-Guidelines-2010-SEPTEMBER-2010-1.pdf

18. Answer: A

Microspherophakia is the clinical term for a small, spherical lens but no criteria are used to determine specific size or curvature. It can be inherited as an isolated abnormality (autosomal dominant familial microspherophakia), associated with conditions Weill–Marchesani (AR), Marfan's syndrome (AD), homocystinuria (AR), Peters anomaly, hyperlysinaemia (AR), Alport syndrome (X-linked dominant), and congenital rubella. It is associated with an increased risk of acute or chronic angle closure glaucoma. Patients who develop this may benefit from lens extraction. A clinical triad of acute angle closure, shallow anterior chamber, and myopia is highly suggestive of microspherophakia.

American Academy of Ophthalmology. *Microspherophakia*, 2019. Available at: http://eyewiki.aao.org/Microspherophakia

19. Answer: A

Gold and chlorpromazine are also known to cause inconsequential lens opacities. Medication induced posterior subcapsular lenticular opacities are commonly seen in patients with long-term systemic or topical steroid use. Sunflower cataract is typically caused by Wilson's disease, a disorder of copper metabolism that can lead to abnormal deposits of copper in the lens and peripheral cornea (Kayser–Fleischer ring), as well as the liver, brain, and other parts of the body. Vossius ring is an anterior lens opacity, caused by compression of the iris onto the anterior lens surface due to blunt trauma.

Ikäheimo K, et al. Visual functions and adverse ocular effects in patients with amiodarone medication. *Acta Ophthalmol Scand* 2002;80:59–63.

20. Answer: C

Unilateral cataract causes higher risk of amblyopia than bilateral cataract. As a general guide unilateral cataract should be operated on prior to 6 weeks to avoid amblyopia, and bilateral cataract within 10 weeks. A very simple aide memoir is '**S**ingle eye **S**ix weeks, **T**wo eyes **T**en weeks'. As the structures of the eye are much more pliable in younger patients, leaving the corneal wound unsutured will result in higher amount of astigmatism.

Lim ME, et al. Update on congenital cataract surgery management. *Curr Opin Ophthalmol* 2017;28:87–92.

21. Answer: C

Proliferative vitreoretinopathy remains the leading cause for retinal re-detachment and can result in poor visual outcomes. The aim of revision surgery is to relieve the underlying retinal traction (either by peeling the membrane off or by using a relieving retinectomy). Silicone oil endotamponade is the most likely choice in a patient with Grade C proliferative vitreoretinopathy. Perfluoropropane (C3F8) is shown to be similarly effective as silicone oil in terms of achieving at least 5/200 vision and macular attachment at a minimum of one year. Perfluorocarbon can be used as a short-acting endotamponade (usually in the management of giant retinal tears with associated retinal detachment). Shorter-acting gas tamponade is unlikely to be used in this setting due to the higher risk of failure.

Schwartz SG, et al. Tamponade in surgery for retinal detachment associated with proliferative vitreoretinopathy. *Cochrane Database Syst Rev* 2014;(2):CD006126.

22. Answer: A

RSRD is a relatively rare form of retinal detachment (RD), accounting for 1–2% of all rhegmatogenous RD. They mostly occur in a temporal location and surgical outcomes are inferior when compared with conventional rhegmatogenous RD. They can occur when an outer leaf break is present only (fluid from the schitic cavity can move into the subretinal space). The associated proliferative vitreoretinopathy (PVR) rate at presentation is reported as 21% (Grade B and C).

Jeourdi AM, et al. Management of degenerative retinoschisis-associated retinal detachment. *Ophthalmology Retina* 2017;1:266–71.

Xue K, et al. Incidence, mechanism and outcomes of schisis retinal detachments revealed through a prospective population-based study. *Br J Ophthalmol* 2017;101:1022–6.

23. Answer: C
Postoperative bacterial endophthalmitis should be considered as an ophthalmic emergency and prompt treatment is required. The Endophthalmitis Vitrectomy Study (EVS) found that patients presenting with vision of perception of light only, had a significantly better visual outcome when randomized to the pars plana vitrectomy group. The European Society of Cataract & Refractive Surgeons (ESCRS) Guidelines for Prevention and Treatment of Endophthalmitis Following Cataract Surgery gives recommendations on the time scale for the management of this condition.

Endophthalmitis Vitrectomy Study Group. Results of the Endophthalmitis Vitrectomy Study. A randomized trial of immediate vitrectomy and of intravenous antibiotics for the treatment of postoperative bacterial endophthalmitis. *Arch Ophthalmol* 1995;113:1479–96.

24. Answer: D
Sympathetic ophthalmia (SO) is an uncommon bilateral granulomatous panuveitis. Ocular surgery, predominantly retinal surgery, is the commonest cause within the United Kingdom. The incidence has been reported as 0.03/100 000. Prompt diagnosis and treatment can lead to good visual outcomes. The role of enucleation in the management of SO is still debated.

Kilmartin DJ, et al. Prospective surveillance of sympathetic ophthalmia in the UK and Republic of Ireland. *Br J Ophthalmol* 2000;84:259–63.

25. Answer: B
FEVR is a heritable vitreoretinopathy characterized by anomalous retinal vascular development. The hallmark of the disease is the avascularity of the peripheral retina, which can lead to exudation, haemorrhage, neovascularization, and RD. The most common inheritance pattern is autosomal dominant, followed by autosomal recessive and X-linked recessive. Wide-field fluorescein angiography is the gold standard in diagnosing and monitoring patients with FEVR because more than half of asymptomatic family members of patients with FEVR can have subclinical findings that are not visible on slit-lamp examination. This is also the reason why a negative family history is not useful in excluding the diagnosis of FEVR. Early laser photocoagulation of the avascular peripheral retina has been shown to reduce the risk of disease progression.

Tauqeer Z, Yonekawa Y. Familial exudative vitreoretinopathy: pathophysiology, diagnosis, and management. *Asia Pac J Ophthalmol (Phila)* 2018;7:176–82.

26. Answer: A
RAM is an acquired saccular or fusiform dilatation of the large arterioles of the retina, usually within the first three orders of bifurcation. It is most commonly observed in elderly women and is associated with systemic vascular conditions such as hypertension. RAM can cause visual loss via exudation (exudative RAM) or preretinal, intraretinal, subretinal or trilaminar haemorrhages (haemorrhagic RAM). It is widely recognized that haemorrhagic RAM usually does not require treatment as it has a tendency to thrombose. Haemorrhagic RAM usually has a better visual prognosis than exudative RAM, especially when macular oedema and exudates persist for several months in exudative type. The most common treatment for RAM is laser photocoagulation either directly to or around the aneurysm to prevent bleeding or to exudative lesion to reduce macular oedema.

Pitkänen L, et al. Retinal arterial macroaneurysms. *Acta Ophthalmol* 2014;92:101–4.

27. Answer: B

It is recommended that all candidates sitting the Fellowship of the Royal College of Ophthalmologists (FRCOphth) exam are similar with this guideline. The document contains a section on both the epidemiology and natural history of retinal vein occlusions. The Royal College of Ophthalmologists (RCOphth) published guidelines on the retinal vein occlusion in July 2015; see following link.

Royal College of Ophthalmologists. *Clinical Guidelines: Retinal Vein Occlusion*, 2015. Available at: https://www.rcophth.ac.uk/wp-content/uploads/2015/07/Retinal-Vein-Occlusion-RVO-Guidelines-July-2015.pdf

28. Answer: A

Dexamethasone intravitreal implant has NICE approval for the management of macular oedema secondary to both branch and central retinal vein occlusions. Fluocinolone acetonide is licensed by NICE for the management of chronic diabetic macular oedema but not retinal vein occlusion.

Haller JA, et al. Dexamethasone intravitreal implant in patients with macular edema related to branch or central retinal vein occlusion twelve-month study results. *Ophthalmology* 2011;118:2453–60.

National Institute for Health and Care Excellence (NICE). *Dexamethasone Intravitreal Implant for the Treatment of Macular Oedema Secondary to Retinal Vein Occlusion. Technology Appraisal Guidance [TA229]*, 2011. Available at: https://www.nice.org.uk/guidance/ta229

National Institute for Health and Care Excellence (NICE). *Fluocinolone Acetonide Intravitreal Implant for Treating Chronic Diabetic Macular Oedema After an Inadequate Response to Prior Therapy. Technology Appraisal Guidance [TA301]*, 2013. Available at: https://www.nice.org.uk/guidance/ta301

29. Answer: D

Figure 6.1 shows a fundal appearance consistent with haemorrhagic occlusive retinal vasculitis (HORV). This is a rare, but devastating, complication of cataract surgery in which intracameral vancomycin has been used.

The American Society of Cataract and Refractive Surgery (ASCRS) and the American Society of Retina Specialists (ASRS) formed a joint task force to define the clinical characteristics of HORV and to study its prevalence, cause, treatment, and outcomes.

Witkin AJ, et al. Vancomycin-associated hemorrhagic occlusive retinal vasculitis: clinical characteristics of 36 eyes. *Ophthalmology* 2017;124:583–95.

30. Answer: B

This is a favourite topic in FRCOphth Part 2 exam. The most common general health problems associated with retinitis pigmentosa (RP) (so-called systemic) are obesity and hearing loss. An awareness of systemic associations is important as treatment can be initiated to prevent further progression, e.g. a high-calorie diet devoid of foods rich in phytanic acid (such as butter and animal fat) combined with plasmapheresis in Refsum syndrome. Common systemic syndromes and their distinguishing features are listed next:

   A. Syndromes with RP and hearing loss
- i. Usher syndrome
- ii. Refsum syndrome: ataxia, ichthyosis, anosmia
- iii. Alport syndrome: posterior polymorphous corneal dystrophy (PPCD), anterior lenticonus, fleck retinopathy, renal failure

iv. Waardenburg syndrome: heterochromia, dystopia canthorum, white forelock
B. Syndromes with RP without hearing loss
   i. Bassen–Kornzweig syndrome (abetalipoproteinaemia): steatorrhoea, fat-soluble vitamin deficiency and ataxia, progressive external ophthalmoplegia
   ii. Bardet–Biedl syndrome: truncal obesity, polydactyly, short stature, and renal failure
   iii. Lawrence–Moon syndrome: same as Bardet–Biedl but without obesity and polydactyly
   iv. Mucopolysaccharidoses: all types except 6 (Maroteaux–Lamy syndrome) and 7 (Sly)
   v. Neuronal ceroid lipofuscinosis: dementia, seizures, and pigment retinopathy
      (a) Infantile: Jansky–Bielschowsky
      (b) Juvenile: Vogt–Spielmeyer–Batten disease
      (c) Adult: Kufs syndrome
   vi. Kearn–Sayre syndrome: chronic progressive external ophthalmoplegia (CPEO), ataxia, heart block

National Organization for Rare Disorders (NORD). *Retinitis Pigmentosa*. Available at: https://rarediseases.org/rare-diseases/retinitis-pigmentosa/

31. Answer: B

The illustration describes a case of left horizontal gaze palsy, which is most likely caused by a left sixth nerve nucleus lesion. Understanding of the anatomy and physiology of the supranuclear pathway is essential in reaching the accurate diagnosis of this type of ocular motility problem. Here follows a summary of the important structures and functions of the supranuclear pathway (Table 6.2).

Table 6.2 Important structures and functions of the supranuclear pathway

Structures	Functions	Examples
6th nerve nucleus	Supplies ipsilateral LR and contralateral MR	Left 6th nucleus damage → Left horizontal gaze palsy
PPRF	Horizontal gaze centre, supplies 6th nerve nucleus	Left PPRF damage → Left horizontal gaze palsy
POT	Smooth pursuit centre, supplies ipsilateral 6th nerve nucleus	Left POT/parietal damage → Left smooth pursuit deficit
MLF	Connects ipsilateral MR and contralateral 6th nerve nucleus	Left MLF dysfunction → Left INO → Left adduction deficit and right abduction nystagmus

MR, medial rectus; LR, lateral rectus; PPRF, paramedian pontine reticular formation; POT, parietal-occipital-temporal; MLF, medial longitudinal fasciculus; INO, internuclear ophthalmoplegia.

Denniston AKO, Murry PI. *Oxford Handbook of Ophthalmology*, 3rd edition. Chapter 16: Neuro-ophthalmology, pp. 696–7. Oxford, UK: Oxford University Press, 2014.

32. Answer: B

In most adults over the age of 50 years the most likely cause of a sixth nerve palsy is a microvascular event. Many patients have associated risk factors such as diabetes and cardiovascular risk factors; however, this man had no obvious risks and there is a group of patients who have an isolated sixth nerve palsy where no cause is found. It is vital, however, to rule out any significant pathology that may cause a sixth nerve palsy, especially when there is no spontaneous recover of nerve palsy after 3 months from the onset of symptoms.

Kung NH, Van Stavern GP. Isolated ocular motor nerve palsies. *Semin Neurol* 2015;35:539–48.

33. Answer: D

MGJWS ptosis is a type of congenital ptosis caused by synkinetic movement of the external pterygoid (not internal pterygoid) muscle and the levator palpebrae superioris muscle. It represents 2–13% cases of congenital ptosis. It usually presents unilaterally, but may rarely present bilaterally. Amblyopia is usually caused by strabismus and anisometropia instead of ptosis.

Pearce FC, et al. Marcus-Gunn jaw-winking syndrome: a comprehensive review and report of four novel cases. *Ophthalmic Plast Reconstr Surg* 2017;33:325–8.

34. Answer: B

This patient has features of a Horner's syndrome with a unilateral ptosis and anisocoria. However, some of the changes in this case are subtle and need further investigations, and this is frequently the case in Horner's syndrome. The patient has already been treated with antibiotics for a supposed ear infection, which may be misleading but often a carotid artery dissection can present as ear or neck pain. Often there is a history of trauma, but dissection can be spontaneous and can occur even after minor trauma. Argyll Robertson and longstanding Adie's syndromes will cause miotic pupils but should not cause ptosis.

Patel RR, et al. Cervical carotid artery dissection: current review of diagnosis and treatment. *Cardiol Rev* 2012;20:145–52.

35. Answer: C

This is a clinical vignette suggestive of optic neuritis. The visual acuity is usually reduced in one eye and may worsen over a 2-week period then starts to improve after a further 4 weeks. There is often pain around or behind the eye and is often worse on eye movement. The patents usually have reduced vision in the affected eye ranging from 6/6 to no perception of light with reduced or absent colour vision. There is usually a RAPD and fundal examination may reveal a slightly swollen or normal optic nerve (>60% cases).

Patients with optic neuritis can develop many types of visual field defects including an altitudinal field defect or an arcuate field defect but the most common field defect is a central scotoma. A junctional scotoma would imply involvement of the optic nerve and chiasm, so would be very rare in optic neuritis. Optic neuritis means inflammation of the optic nerve, it does not imply any diagnosis.

Toosy AT, et al. Optic neuritis. *Lancet Neurol* 2014;13:83–99.

36. Answer: C

Various nuclear and fascicular sixth nerve syndromes have been described in the literature. The following is a summary of the syndromes (Table 6.3).

Silverman IE, et al. The crossed paralyses. The original brain-stem syndromes of Millard–Gubler, Foville, Weber, and Raymond–Cestan. *Arch Neurol* 1995;52:635–8.

37. Answer: A

NA-AION usually presents as unilateral visual disturbance and can present with a varying degree of visual loss. In addition to optic nerve head swelling, there is often an altitudinal visual field defect with crowded disc. A large cup:disc ratio in the fellow eye should raise the suspicion

Table 6.3 Syndromes associated with nerve palsies and contralateral hemiparesis

Syndromes	Clinical features	Lesion site
Eight-and-a-half	Ipsilateral gaze palsy, ipsilateral INO, and ipsilateral 7th nerve palsy	6th and 7th nerve nuclei, PPRF + MLF
Foville	Ipsilateral gaze palsy, ipsilateral 5th and 7th nerve palsies, and contralateral hemianaesthesia	Dorsolateral pons
Millard–Gubler	Ipsilateral 6th and 7th nerve palsies and contralateral hemiparesis	Ventral pons
Raymond–Cestan	Ipsilateral 6th nerve palsy and contralateral hemiparesis	Ventral pons

INO, internuclear ophthalmoplegia; PPRF, paramedian pontine reticular formation; MLF, medial longitudinal fasciculus.

of other causes. Many patents have a history of vascular disorders such as hypertension, hypercholesterolaemia, or diabetes, but some patients have no obvious risk factors at all. The use of steroid treatment in NA-AION at the early stages to prevent further visual loss remains a highly debatable and controversial topic.

Kerr NM, et al. Non-arteritic anterior ischaemic optic neuropathy: a review and update. *J Clin Neurosci* 2009;16:994–1000.

38. Answer: B

MD is an uncommon autosomal dominant disease caused by expanded CTG trinucleotide repeat, which can lead to earlier and more severe disease in successive generation. It is characterized by inability to relax the muscle (myotonia) and muscle wasting (dystrophy). It is most commonly reported in French Canadians. Respiratory failure is the most common cause (30%) of death in MD, followed by cardiac conduction abnormality (20%). The most common feature of ophthalmoplegia is the deficit in adduction, resulting in pseudointernuclear ophthalmoplegia. It is also associated with other ocular features such as Christmas tree cataract, miosis, low intraocular pressure (due to ciliary body detachment), and retinal degeneration.

American Academy of Ophthalmology. *Ocular Manifestations of Myotonic Dystrophy*. Available at: http://eyewiki.aao.org/Ocular_Manifestations_of_Myotonic_Dystrophy

39. Answer: A

Syphilis testing includes treponemal testing and non-treponemal testing (RPR and VDRL). Treponemal tests remain positive after acquisition of syphilis, whether treated or not. Non-treponemal tests are quantified and can distinguish between active disease (ratio >1:16) and inactive, treated disease. Quantitative VDRL/RPR helps stage the infection and can indicate the need for treatment in some cases, where the patients have been previously treated and may have been re-infected. The presence of positive treponemal testing alongside high RPR indicates active infection and need for systemic therapy. False positive results may occur with any of the serological tests and causes include lupus, RA, and Lyme disease; the titre is usually low in false positive results in comparison to most true positives (Table 6.4).

Table 6.4 Syphilis testing

	Treponemal test	
	Positive	Negative
Positive	Active, untreated syphilis	False positive
Negative	Previously treated syphilis or inactive untreated syphilis (confirm with history)	True negative
	False positive (confirm with second treponemal test)	

Kingston M, et al. UK national guidelines on the management of syphilis 2015. *Int J STD AIDS* 2016;27:421–46.

40. Answer: D

Syndromes with ophthalmic manifestations are popular topics. Susac's syndrome is a rare condition characterized by the clinical triad of encephalopathy, sensorineural hearing loss, and branch retinal artery occlusion(s) (BRAO). On FFA sectoral vessel hyperfluorescence is seen. MRI shows a distinctive pattern of corpus callosum lesions that differ from those seen in demyelination. Cogan syndrome is characterized by vertigo, hearing loss, and interstitial keratitis; BRAOs are not a feature. In demyelinating disease, intraocular involvement can include intermediate uveitis and vessel sheathing, due to perivascular leucocytes, but not BRAOs. Venous sinus thrombosis can cause headache, cranial nerve palsies, papilloedema, and neurological disturbance but is not characterized by the development of BRAO.

Susac JO, et al. MRI findings in Susac's syndrome. *Neurology* 2003;61:1783–7.

41. Answer: B

Löfgren's syndrome is an acute form of sarcoidosis characterized by polyarthritis or polyarthralgia, bilateral hilar lymphadenopathy, and erythema nodosum. Variant forms are sometimes observed. Serum ACE levels are elevated in approximately 60% of patients with sarcoidosis and can therefore be within normal limits. Rheumatoid arthritis is an important differential but negative autoantibodies and the presence of bilateral hilar lymphadenopathy (BHL) support the diagnosis of Löfgren's syndrome. Heerfordt's syndrome is a different manifestation of sarcoidosis characterized by facial nerve palsy, fever, anterior uveitis, and parotid enlargement.

Iannuzzi MC, et al. Sarcoidosis. *N Engl J Med* 2007;357:2153–65.

42. Answer: C

Alport syndrome is a disorder of basement membrane type IV collagen and features ocular, renal, and cochlear involvement manifesting as sensorineural deafness, progressive renal failure, and characteristic ocular signs. Renal disease progresses from microscopic haematuria to progressive proteinuria and insufficiency. Ocular examination can be very useful for the diagnosis of the condition, particularly the lens, for evidence of anterior/posterior lenticonus or cataract (anterior polar or cortical). Fleck retinal changes are also observed and sometimes posterior polymorphous dystrophy. A description of anterior lenticonus, fleck retina, and early onset renal failure is strongly suggestive of this condition. Posterior subcapsular cataract is not a feature of Alport syndrome and is observed in uveitis, corticosteroid, and radiation exposure, MD, and as age-related lens change.

Colville DJ, Savige J. Alport syndrome. A review of the ocular manifestations. *Ophthalmic Genet* 1997;18:161–73.

Savige J, et al. Ocular features in Alport syndrome: pathogenesis and clinical significance. *Clin J Am Soc Nephrol* 2015;10:703–9.

43. Answer: C

Headache and eye pain are a common presentation and cause diagnostic confusion for neurologists and ophthalmologists alike. The key to this question is knowledge of primary and secondary headache syndromes and being able to distinguish them from secondary headaches. High-flow oxygen can be effective for cluster headache (CH) and is used as a therapeutic trial to aid diagnosis. However, CH is defined as attacks of excruciating pain lasting 30–180 minutes with absence of pain between attacks. Hemicranial continua is a much rarer primary headache disorder defined as strictly unilateral, relentless headache or facial pain. The response to indomethacin is swift and exquisite. Sumatriptan is the treatment of choice for abortion of migraine attacks but the clinical features are more consistent with hemicranias than migraine. Herpes zoster can convincingly mimic primary headaches, but usually either abates or declares itself the typical skin lesions or at least one of its ocular manifestations.

Prakash S, Adroja B. Hemicrania continua. *Ann Indian Acad Neurol* 2018;21:S23–30.

44. Answer: D

The diagnosis of delayed visual maturation is really done retrospectively. It can be isolated in a child with no other anomalies, or associated with mental retardation and/or seizure. It can also include children with a primary visual abnormality and a superimposed visual maturation delay. This is an area where the ophthalmologist and the paediatrician should work together well. The other causes of normal eye exam and subnormal vision are cortical visual impairment in whom the visual evoked potential (VEP) will be abnormal but not in all children. There might be neurodevelopmental abnormalities.

In the early stages of inherited retinal dystrophies, the eye exam can be normal, however it is normally associated with high myopic or hypermetropic refractive error, positive family history, and abnormal ERG.

Pehere N, et al. Cerebral visual impairment in children: causes and associated ophthalmological problems. *Indian J Ophthalmol* 2018;66:812–5.

Weiss AH, et al. The infant who is visually unresponsive on a cortical basis. *Ophthalmology* 2001;108:2076–87.

45. Answer: B

Diagnosis of euryblepharon is based on several clinical features:
- Bilateral symmetrical enlargement of the horizontal palpebral apertures
- Elongated lid margins. The horizontal palpebral fissure length is increased to approximately 35 mm from the average length of 28–30 mm
- Vertical shortening of eyelid skin
- Downward and lateral displacement of outer canthi
- Other features include lateral ectropion, reduced blink rate, lagophthalmos, with exposure keratopathy

McCord CD Jr, et al. Congenital euryblepharon. *Ann Ophthalmol* 1979;11:1217–24.

46. Answer: B

The ophthalmologist should be concerned for PHACES syndrome when a haemangioma is segmental and over 5 cm. The acronym PHACE stands for:

P—Posterior fossa brain malformations

H—Haemangiomas

A—Arterial lesions (blood vessel abnormalities in the head or neck)

C—Cardiac abnormalities (aortic coarctation)

E—Eye abnormality

An echocardiogram to exclude cardiac anomalies such as coarctation of aorta, other aortic arch anomalies, and other vascular anomalies is necessary. An MRI/MRA scan of the head and neck is mandatory to exclude Dandy–Walker malformation and other posterior fossa malformations.

Haggstrom AN, et al. Risk for PHACE syndrome in infants with large facial hemangiomas. *Paediatrics* 2010;126:418–26.

Metry DW, et al. The many faces of PHACE syndrome. *J Pediatr* 2001;139:117–23.

47. Answer: D

Orbital cellulitis occurs as a secondary extension of acute or chronic bacterial sinusitis, especially the ethmoid sinusitis. Intravenous antibiotic treatment is the choice for children of <9 years of age with orbital subperiosteal abscess as it is commonly caused by single microbial organisms, whereas surgical intervention for orbital subperiosteal abscess is more likely to be required if the children are over 9 years of age. In addition, the latter group is more commonly associated with polymicrobial and anaerobic infection. Clinical improvement does not correlate well with repeat CT scan analysis as it can take up to 72 hours to see radiological improvement. Blindness occurs in up to 11% of cases.

Liao JC, Harris GJ. Subperiosteal abscess of the orbit: evolving pathogens and the therapeutic protocol. *Ophthalmology* 2015;122:639–47.

Nageswaran S, et al. Orbital cellulitis in children. *Pediatr Infect Dis J* 2006;25:695–9.

48. Answer: D

All four conditions are a form of craniosynostosis, which refers to partial or complete premature fusion of cranial sutures. Ocular hypertelorism, proptosis, beaking of the nose, and midfacial hypoplasia are common facial features of the craniosynostosis. These four conditions can be remembered with the mnemonic '**CAMP**'.

(a) <u>C</u>rouzon syndrome is associated with normal intelligence and normal hands and feet. The severity of facial deformity is milder than of Apert.

(b) <u>A</u>pert syndrome in addition has severe symmetrical syndactly of fingers and toes. Learning disability requiring special education is also a common accompaniment.

(c) <u>M</u>uenke syndrome features include unilateral or bilateral coronal synostosis, proptosis, downward slanting palpebral fissure, hearing loss, developmental delay, and specific bone anomalies of the hand and feet.

(d) <u>P</u>feiffer syndrome type 1 has the classic phenotype of brachycephaly, midface hypoplasia, broad, radially deviated thumbs, and/or big toes along with normal intelligence.

Kutkowska-Kaźmierczak A, et al. Craniosynostosis as a clinical and diagnostic problem: molecular pathology and genetic counseling. *J Appl Genet* 2018;59:133–47.

49. Answer: A

The features are suggestive of viral conjunctivitis. The diagnosis and management of ophthalmia neonatorum are based on the time of onset and characteristics of conjunctivitis. Some commonly used treatment regimes are given next, but always refer to the local microbiology/infectious disease guideline or discuss with the respective team (Table 6.5).

Table 6.5 Commonly used treatment regimes for viral conjunctivitis

Types of conjunctivitis	Onset	Features	Management
Chemical (1% silver nitrate)	At birth	Watery	1% silver nitrate solution is no longer in common use
Viral	1–14 days	Non-purulent discharge, hazy cornea due to dendritic ulcer/stromal keratitis	See Option A
Gonococcal	<5 days	Severe purulent discharge	See Option C
Bacterial, non-gonococcal	4–5 days	Purulent discharge	See Option B
Chlamydia	5–14 days	Mucopurulent discharge	See Option D

Data from Allen UD, Robinson JL. Prevention and management of neonatal herpes simplex virus infections. *Paediatr Child Health* 2014;19:201-6; and *Ophthalmia neonatorum*. BCSC series: Pediatric Ophthalmology and Strabismus. American Academy of Ophthalmology 2010.

50. Answer: B

Congenital megalocornea is a non-progressive, enlarged cornea with a horizontal diameter of more than 13 mm in the absence of congenital glaucoma. Myopia is the most common associated refractive error. It is rare and usually bilateral, inherited as a X-linked trait in most instances and 90% are males. The condition maps to Xq21–22. Autosomal dominant inheritance has also been reported. Management consists of careful observation for complications such as cataract formation, dislocated lens, and glaucoma.

Meire FM, et al. X-linked megalocornea. Ocular findings and linkage analysis. *Ophthalmic Paediatr Genet* 1991;12:153–7.

51. Answer: A

The Parks–Bielschowsky or Park's three-step test is used to isolate **single** paretic muscle in acquired vertical diplopia. The test works by observing the vertical deviation in primary gaze, left and right gaze, and right and left head tilt. Where the hyperdeviations are of the greatest magnitude indicate where the paretic muscle should be working maximally. The following is a diagram (Figure 6.4) for reference.

Step 1: If the right eye is the hyperdeviated eye, we know that the muscle that is failing is either responsible for pulling the right eye down or for pulling the left eye up. Our suspects in the right eye are the right superior oblique (RSO) or right inferior rectus (RIR). In the left eye, it is the left superior rectus (LSR) or LIO.

Step 2: When we look at the right gaze, the muscles most responsible for the eyes' vertical position are the right superior and inferior rectus muscles and the left superior and inferior oblique muscles.

Step 3: When the head is tilted to the left, the right eye needs to turn outwards (excyclotorsion) and the left eye needs to turn inwards (incyclotorsion). The muscles responsible for these movements are the RIO, RIR, and the LSO, LSR.

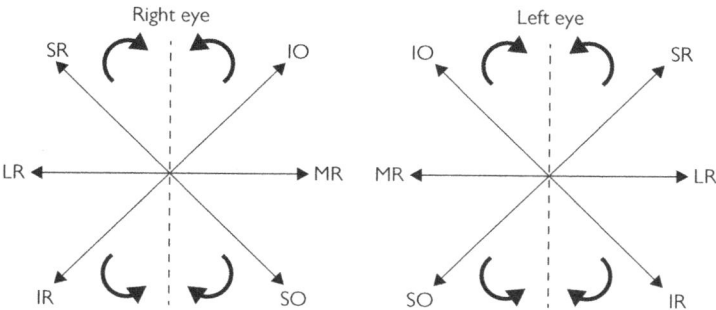

Figure 6.4

In this case by process of elimination the affected muscle is the RIR.

American Academy of Ophthalmology. *Three Step Test for Cyclovertical Muscle Palsy*, 2019. Available at: http://eyewiki.aao.org/Three_Step_Test_for_Cyclovertical_Muscle_Palsy

52. Answer: A

Greenstick orbital floor fractures occur in paediatric population where the fracture fragment can act as a 'trap door' entrapping the interior rectus muscle. This can elicit the oculocardiac reflex producing bradycardia, nausea, syncope, and rarely bradycardia on attempted eye movement against the entrapped muscle. It therefore requires urgent surgical release. All the other criteria are traditional indicators for surgical correction of an orbital fracture but not on an urgent basis.

Boyette JR, et al. Management of orbital fractures: challenges and solutions. *Clin Ophthalmology* 2015;9:2127–37.

53. Answer: D

Because of the extensive anastomoses of facial vessels, it is possible to inject intra-arterial embolus of filler inadvertently in almost any region of the face. Highest risk areas are injections around the glabellar, nasal dorsum, nasojugal, and nasolabial folds.

Humzah MD, et al. The treatment of hyaluronic acid aesthetic interventional induced visual loss (AIIVL): a consensus on practical guidance. *J Cosmet Dermatol* 2019; 18(1):71–6.

54. Answer: A

Severe thyroid eye disease is characterized by signs of sight-threatening pathology. The most common of these is dysthyroid optic neuropathy due to compression or stretch resulting in a RAPD, unless equally bilateral. Other presentations of severe disease are corneal exposure, sight-threatening raised intraocular pressure, and globe subluxation.

Chemosis, esotropia, and lid malposition can occur in moderate TED.

Perros P, et al. Thyroid eye disease. *BMJ* 2009;338:b560.

55. Answer: C

Fasanella Servat is a destructive and outdated operation that has a high rate of postoperative complications, so its use is in decline. Frontalis sling is required when the levator function is poor, usually below 4 mm. Levator advancement can be achieved via an anterior or posterior approach, and can be adjusted according to the degree of ptosis and levator function. Conservative amblyopia management will not have long-term success when the visual axis is occluded.

Finsterer J. Ptosis: causes, presentation and management. *Aesthetic Plast Surg* 2003;27:193–204.

56. Answer: C

Cicatricial ectropion is the turning out of the lid due to shortage within the anterior lamella, usually contracture of the skin. This can be caused by trauma, burns, scarring from infection (e.g. HZO), skin tumours (e.g. BCC), and medications. Lid laxity can be a risk factor for developing a non-cicatricial entropion or ectropion. OCP can cause a cicatricial entropion due to contracture of the conjunctiva turning the lid in. Dacryoadenitis can cause a mechanical ptosis.

Bedran EG, et al. Ectropion. *Semin Ophthalmol* 2010;25:59–65.

57. Answer: D

The causes of enophthalmos can be broadly divided into three categories: (1) structural alternation in bony orbit; (2) orbit fat atrophy; and (3) retraction. Small eye may cause apparent enophthalmos. All the options listed in this question are causes of enophthalmos, but silent sinus syndrome (SSS) is the most common where there is no history of trauma. As the name suggested, SSS usually presents in a silent/asymptomatic manner. Although it is supposedly linked with a history of sinusitis, there is often very little history. Sclerosing metastases usually arise from breast primary and, like scleroderma, it can cause muscle fibrosis and orbital fat atrophy, resulting in enophthalmos.

Athanasiov PA, et al. Non-traumatic enophthalmos: a review. *Acta Ophthalmol* 2008;86:356–64.

58. Answer: B

All except pain can be features of both SCC and BCC. SCC is an aggressive tumour, has a propensity to spread via perineural invasion so can cause pain, dysaesthesia, or anaesthesia. The overall rate of regional lymph node metastases ranges from 10% to 25%.

Thosani MK, et al. Periocular squamous cell carcinoma. *Dermatol Surg* 2008;34:585–99.

59. Answer: A

Various clinical, histopathologic, cytogenetic features and gene expressions have been implicated in the prognosis of uveal melanoma, in terms of risk of metastasis and mortality. These include older age at presentation, male gender, larger tumour basal diameter and thickness, ciliary body location, epithelioid cell type, high mitotic activity, monosomy 3, loss of chromosomes 1p, 6q, or 8p, and gain of 8q. The following review paper provides a very good summary on this subject.

Kaliki S, et al. Uveal melanoma: Estimating prognosis. *Indian J Ophthalmol* 2015;63:93–102.

60. Answer: B

Non-Hodgkin's lymphomas constitute one-half of the malignancies arising in the orbit and the ocular adnexae. Mucosa-associated lymphoid tissue (MALT)-type lymphoma is the most common histological category in this anatomic region. The following is a useful summary table of the most common intraocular and orbital tumours in children and adults (Table 6.6):

Castillo BV Jr, Kaufman L. Pediatric tumors of the eye and orbit. *Pediatr Clin North Am* 2003;50:149–72.

Margo CE, Mulla ZD. Malignant tumors of the orbit. Analysis of the Florida cancer registry. *Ophthalmology* 1998;19:835–46.

Ting DS, et al. A 10-year review of orbital biopsy: the Newcastle Eye Centre Study. *Eye (Lond)* 2015;29:1162–6.

Table 6.6 The most common intraocular and orbital tumours in children and adults

		Children	Adult
Benign	Intraocular	Very rare	Choroidal naevus
	Orbital	Dermoid/epidermoid cyst; capillary haemangioma (2nd)	Cavernous haemangioma
Malignant	Intraocular	Retinoblastoma	*Primary:* Choroidal melanoma *Secondary:* Choroidal metastases
	Orbital	*Primary:* Rhabdomyosarcoma *Secondary:* Neuroblastoma	Lymphoproliferative tumour

61. Answer: C

This is a question examining the candidate's knowledge on the systemic association of retinal astrocytoma, which is a rare benign glioma that typically presents in childhood and adolescence. It is related to tuberous sclerosis and neurofibromatosis. Tuberous sclerosis is associated with cardiac rhabdomyoma, pulmonary lymphangioleiomyoma, renal angiomyolipoma, subependymal giant cell astrocytoma, and adenoma sebaceum. Pheochromocytoma is linked to Von Hippel–Lindau syndrome.

O'Shea WF, Powers JE. Solitary retinal astrocytoma. *J Am Optom Assoc* 1991;62:519–24.

Rowley SA, O'Callaghan FJ, Osborne JP. Ophthalmic manifestations of tuberous sclerosis: a population-based study. *Br J Ophthalmol* 2001;85:420–3.

62. Answer: C

Schwartz–Matsuo syndrome is elevated IOP and mild anterior uveitis (AU) associated with rhegmatogenous RD. The RD is typically shallow, with peripheral retinal breaks particularly retinal dialysis. The only evidence of uveitis is anterior chamber (AC) cells; posterior synechiae, flare, keratotic precipitates or posterior uveitis indicate an inflammatory condition. The IOP is typically high with fluctuations. AC photoreceptor outer segments and aqueous outflow obstruction is a proposed mechanism for raised IOP. Exudative RD can complicate uveitis involving the posterior segment—there is only AU here so Option A is incorrect. The presence of a tear indicates this is a rhegmatogenous rather than an exudative detachment. Posner–Schlossman syndrome is a form of recurrent unilateral AU, with very few cells, fine KPs, and very high IOP but is not associated with RD. Ocular trauma is a risk factor for sympathetic ophthalmia—this is excluded because the fellow eye is normal.

Matsuo T. Photoreceptor outer segments in aqueous humor: key to understanding a new syndrome. *Surv Ophthalmol* 1994;39:211–33.

Mitry D, et al. Photoreceptor outer segment glaucoma in rhegmatogenous retinal detachment. *Arch Ophthalmol* 2009;127:1053–4.

63. Answer: A

Juvenile idiopathic arthritis (JIA) is the commonest rheumatic disease in children and JIA-related uveitis is the most common extra-articular manifestation. The risk factors for chronic AU in JIA patients include presence of antinuclear antibody (ANA), young age at diagnosis, female gender, and oligoarticular disease (involvement of up to four joints). In contrast, male gender, HLA-B27 positivity, and enthesitis-related arthritis are risk factors for acute AU.

Sen ES, Ramanan AV. Juvenile idiopathic arthritis-associated uveitis. *Best Pract Res Clin Rheumatol* 2017;31:517–34.

64. Answer: C

Syphilis can reactivate in the eye many years after initial primary infection. Manifestations of ocular syphilis are many but the pale macular lesion with disruption at the level of the photoreceptors is typical of posterior placoid syphilitic uveitis. A metastatic deposit would cause a raised, fundus lesion, its colour dependent on composition and the state of the retinal pigment epithelium. Cancer-associated retinopathy may cause outer retinal damage but there will not be any macular lesion. Tuberculosis can manifest in a variety of ways but would not be expected to cause the described OCT changes. The absence of haemorrhage and inner retinal disturbance goes against zoster-associated acute retinal necrosis.

Wells J, et al. Ocular syphilis: the re-establishment of an old disease. *Eye (Lond)* 2018;32:99–103.

65. Answer: B

Adalimumab (Humira®) is a biologic agent. It is humanized antitumour necrosis factor alpha (TNF-α) monoclonal antibody. TNF-alpha is an important target in non-infectious uveitis and infliximab is another anti-TNF agent. Pivotal trials for the efficacy of adalimumab in the treatment of uveitis are the SYCAMORE and VISUAL I and II studies. Rituximab is a different biologic agent and is monoclonal antibody against CD20, a B-cell marker, used for treatment of systemic vasculitides. Anti-VEGF therapy is used for treatment of AMD, RVO, and diabetic maculopathy. Interferon therapy is indicated for the treatment of Behçet's disease, including uveitis.

Ramanan AV, et al. Adalimumab plus methotrexate for uveitis in juvenile idiopathic arthritis. *N Engl J Med* 2017;376:1637–46.

66. Answer: A

The Jarisch–Herxheimer reaction is an acute febrile illness with headache, myalgia, chills, and rigours which resolves within 24 hours. This is common in early syphilis and is usually not clinically significant unless there is neurological or ophthalmic involvement. The UK syphilis guidelines recommend steroid therapy when treating neurological (includes ophthalmic) syphilis with **prednisolone 40–60 mg for 3 days starting 24 hours before antitreponemal antibiotics**. A longer course of oral steroid may be necessary for severe ophthalmic involvement but it is important that the timing of initiation is carefully coordinated with antibiotic therapy because steroid exposure without appropriate antitreponemal treatment can cause worsening of syphilitic disease.

Kingston M, et al. UK national guidelines on the management of syphilis 2015. *Int J STD AIDS* 2016;27:421–46.

67. Answer: A

Following is the summary of the pharmacology of topical intraocular pressure-lowering medication (Table 6.7).

Table 6.7 Pharmacology of topical intraocular pressure-lowering medications

Medications	Mechanisms	Examples
Prostaglandin analogue	↑ uveoscleral outflow	Latanoprost, bimatoprost
β-blocker*	↓ aqueous production	Betaxolol, timolol, carteolol
Carbonic anhydrase inhibitor	↓ aqueous production	Brinzolamide, dorzolamide
Alpha-2 agonist	↑ uveoscleral outflow + ↓ aqueous production	Apraclonidine, brimonidine
Cholinergic	↑ trabecular outflow	Pilocarpine

*Betaxolol is a β-1 agonist (cardioselective), which has less pulmonary side effects. Carteolol is a non-selective β-agonist but has intrinsic sympathomimetic activity, which increases the systolic blood pressure, heart rate, and cardiac contractility.

Data from Tataru CP, Purcarea VL. Antiglaucoma pharmacotherapy. *J Med Life* 2012;5:247–51.

68. Answer: C

Fluoroquinolone (FQ) is an antibiotic that inhibits bacterial DNA synthesis via interaction with DNA gyrase and topoisomerase. It has been reported to induce tendinitis and tendon rupture. Ciprofloxacin was found to be the causal agent in 90% of the cases. Risk factors for FQ-induced tendon rupture include age >60 years, steroid use, renal impairment, diabetes mellitus, and a history of musculoskeletal (MSK) disorders. The tendinopathy may occur between a few hours and few months after the start of FQ treatment, with a median onset of 6 days, and the effect is dose dependent. The pathophysiology remains elusive; however, various concepts have been introduced. These include FQ-related direct cytotoxic effect on enzymes found in MSK tissues, the chelating properties against several metal ions, which can cause direct toxicity to type 1 collagen synthesis and promote collagen degradation. Ciclosporin can cause a range of side effects, including hypertension, hyperglycaemia, hyperlipidaemia, gingival hyperplasia, and hirsutism among others. Cyclophosphamide can cause myelosuppression, cardiac, pulmonary, and liver toxicity, haemorrhagic cystitis, and neoplasms.

Kim GK. The risk of fluoroquinolone-induced tendinopathy and tendon rupture: What does the clinician need to know? *J Clin Aesthet Dermatol* 2010;3:49–54.

69. Answer: C

IFIS was first described by Chang and Campbell in 2005. The current use of tamsulosin, alfuzosin, terazosin, benzodiazepines, quetiapine, and finasteride are all associated with IFIS. The duration of α-blocker use was not found to be associated with IFIS. The recent review also highlighted the elevated risk of IFIS in patients taking rivastigmine with a short axial length. Quetiapine may also increase the risk of acute primary angle closure due to its anticholinergic effect.

Chatziralli IP, et al. Risk factors for intraoperative floppy iris syndrome: a prospective study. *Eye (Lond)* 2016;30:1039–44.

70. Answer: A

Botulinum toxin is a neurotoxin that is derived from *Clostridium botulinum*, a Gram-positive anaerobic bacterium. It primarily acts by binding to the presynaptic high-affinity recognition sites on the cholinergic nerve terminals and thereby decreasing the presynaptic release of ACh. Myasthenia gravis is caused by autoantibodies blocking the postsynaptic ACh receptors whereas Lambert–Eaton myasthenic syndrome is caused by autoantibodies blocking the presynaptic voltage-gated calcium channels at the neuromuscular junction, reducing the release of presynaptic

ACh. Organophosphate inhibits acetylcholinesterase, leading to accumulation of ACh at the neuromuscular junction.

Barnes M. Botulinum toxin—mechanisms of action and clinical use in spasticity. *J Rehabil Med* 2003;(41 Suppl):56–9.

71. Answer: B

Bacteria that take up crystal violet dye are Gram positive and those that allow crystal violet dye to wash off are Gram negative. The following are the common staining techniques used for corneal samples (Table 6.8).

Table 6.8 Common staining techniques for corneal samples

Staining techniques	Intended microorganisms
Gram	Bacteria, fungi, and acanthamoeba
Giemsa	Bacteria, fungi, and acanthamoeba
Gomori methenamine silver (GMS)	Fungi
Calcofluor white	Fungi and acanthamoeba
Periodic acid Schiff	Fungi and acanthamoeba
Ziehl–Neelsen	Fungi, acanthamoeba, mycobacteria, and nocardia

Denniston AKO, Murray PI. *Oxford Handbook of Ophthalmology*, 3rd edition. Chapter 7: Cornea; p. 223. Oxford, UK: Oxford University Press, 2014.

Sharma S. Diagnosis of infectious diseases of the eye. *Eye (Lond)* 2012;26:177–84.

72. Answer: D

FFA incorporates a blue excitation filter and a yellow green barrier filter. The sodium fluorescein used is 70–80% bound to plasma albumin. It is metabolized by the liver and excreted by the kidney in 24 hours. FFA is not found to cause a high rate of birth anomalies or complications during pregnancy; however, it is generally avoided unless its use is deemed absolute necessary. With the current advancing techniques in retinal imaging such as OCT and OCT angiography, the use of FFA in pregnancy can usually be avoided.

Halperin LS, et al. Safety of fluorescein angiography during pregnancy. *Am J Ophthalmol* 1990;109:563–6.

73. Answer: B

On fluorescein angiography, APMPPE has a characteristic appearance with lesion hypofluorescence in the early stages, due to blockage, followed by lesion staining in the late stages of the angiogram. On indocyanine green angiography (ICGA) the lesions remain hypocyanescent throughout the angiogram and lesions may be more numerous than detected clinically. APMPPE is typically a bilateral disease, preceded by a prodromal illness, and has no sex predilection (Table 6.9).

Salvatore S, et al. Multimodal imaging in acute posterior multifocal placoid pigment epitheliopathy demonstrating obstruction of the choriocapillaris. *Ophthalmic Surg Lasers Imaging Retina* 2016;47:677–81.

Table 6.9 Appearance and presentation characteristics of APMPPE

	History	Clinical	FAF	FFA	ICG
MEWDS	Young females; flu type illness	Unilateral; No-little vitritis; grey/white dots-spots 100–200 μm lesions, macular to mid periphery optic disc swelling; foveal granularity	Multiple hyper-AF spots	Early hyperfluorescence (hyper-F) spots; Late hyper-F Wreath like macular change	Hypo-F lesions
APMPPE	Young patients; flu type illness	Bilateral white-yellow placoid lesions (can be large) posterior pole to mid periphery. Vitritis may be present	Hypo-AF lesions	Early: hypo-F lesions Late: hypo-F lesions	Hypo-F lesions. More numerous than seen on FFA
PIC	Young myopic; typically female. May present with CNV	No-mild vitritis. Multiple white lesions (50–200 μm), become atrophic scars +/– pigmentation in time. Peripapillary atrophy. Linear lesions in periphery. CNV as complication	Hypo-AF lesions, edge hyper-FAF if active. Edge fades as becomes inactive. Atrophic lesions hypo-FAF	Hyper-F lesions Window defects if scars	Hypo-F More numerous than seen on FFA
MFC	Young patients	Multiple lesions, can be large 100–300 μm or bigger in posterior pole and periphery. Vitritis present. CNV is complication	Hypo-AF lesions corresponding to chorioretinal atrophy. Hyper-FAF can be seen within active lesions	Hyper-F lesions	Hypo-F

CNV, choroidal neovascularization.

74. Answer: B

pERG assesses macular function. P50 assesses macular cone function and N95 assesses macular ganglion cells function. Amplitudes, peak times, and N95/P50 ratio (typically >1.1) are key components in interpreting the pattern electroretinogram (PERG).

Holder GE. Pattern electroretinography (PERG) and an integrated approach to visual pathway diagnosis. *Prog Retin Eye Res* 2001;20:531–61.

75. Answer: A

W4D test is a useful orthoptic test that can be used with both distance and near fixation to differentiate between suppression, abnormal retinal correspondence, and BSV. However, it can only be interpreted if a manifest squint is present or absent. The patient is asked to wear a green lens in front of the right eye to filter out all colours except green, and a red lens in front of the left eye to filter out all colours except red. He or she will be asked to view a box with four lights: one red (top), two green (middle) and one white (bottom).

Following is the interpretation of the results:
(A) All four lights = presence of BSV or harmonious abnormal retinal correspondence (ARC) (if manifest deviation is present)
(B) Three green lights = suppression of left eye (because the right eye sees the green light only)
(C) Two red lights = suppression of right eye
(D) Three green and two red lights = diplopia

Kanski JJ, Bowling B. *Clinical Ophthalmology: A Systematic Approach*, 7th edition. Chapter 18: Strabismus: Clinical evaluation; pp. 750–4. Edinburgh, UK/New York, NY: Elsevier/Saunders, 2011.

76. Answer: A

The binocular status such as stereopsis can be measured with several types of orthoptic tests, including Frisby, Lang, Titmus, and TNO. Frisby and Lang tests do not require any glasses whereas Titmus and TNO require polaroid glasses and red-green glasses, respectively. It is also important to remember that some of these tests such as Frisby, Lang, and Titmus tests may give monocular clues. Hess chart also requires red-green glasses for dissociating the eyes for measurement of ocular deviation.

Lee J, McIntyre A. Clinical tests for binocular vision. *Eye (Lond)* 1996;10:282–5.

77. Answer: D

The image shown in Figure 6.3 is an MRI T2-weighted scan with FLAIR sequence. On the first glance, the candidate might confuse this with a T1-weighted scan as the vitreous and cerebrospinal fluid (CSF) appear dark. However, in the T2-weighted scan, with or without FLAIR sequence, the grey matter should appear in lighter grey (or relatively hyperintense) as compared to the white matter, which should appear in darker grey (or relatively hypointense). This is the opposite for T1-weighted scan. MRI FLAIR sequence is similar to a T2-weighted image but the former has the ability to suppress signals from cerebrospinal fluid (CSF).

Simha A, et al. Magnetic resonance imaging for the ophthalmologist: a primer. *Indian J Ophthalmol* 2012;60:301–10.

Yau GS, et al. Neuromyelitis optica spectrum disorder in a Chinese woman with ocular myasthenia gravis: first reported case in the Chinese population. *Neuroophthalmology* 2014;38:140–4.

78. Answer: B

Serological measurements of antiacetylcholine receptor (AChR) antibody are highly sensitive for generalized myasthenia gravis (MG; around 80%) but lower in ocular myasthenia gravis (around 45%). In 20% of patients with MG that have negative anti-AChR antibody, 30–40% were found to have antityrosine kinase MuSK antibody. These patients may have symptoms very similar to AChR-positive MG, but some patients may have a bulbar form with few ocular symptoms. Anti-low-density lipoprotein receptor-related protein (LRP4) antibody has recently been found in patients with double antibodies (AChR and MuSK) negative MG. Anticyclic citrullinated peptide (CCP) is useful in diagnosing rheumatoid arthritis, with high specificity, present early in the disease process, and has the ability to identify severe cases.

Niewold TB, et al. Anti-CCP antibody testing as a diagnostic and prognostic tool in rheumatoid arthritis. *QJM* 2007;100:193–201.

Rivner MH, et al. Muscle-specific tyrosine kinase and myasthenia gravis owing to other antibodies. *Neurol Clin* 2018;36:293–310.

79. Answer: B

About day 22, two small grooves develop either side of the developing forebrain in the neural folds. These are called the optic sulci. As the neural tube closed, the grooves become out pockets known as optic vesicles. They are formed from the diencephalon at approximately day 25 of gestation.

The following is the timeline of ocular embryology (in gestation):
- 23 days: optic pits appearance
- 25 days: invagination of optic vesicle
- 28 days: induction of lens
- 33 days: closure of embryonic fissure (starts between optic nerve and iris, then progresses anteriorly and posteriorly)

Barishak YR. Embryology of the eye and its adnexae. *Dev Ophthalmol* 1992;24:1–142.

80. Answer: A

There are typically four cell types in choroidal melanoma, namely type A, type B, epithelioid cells, and a mixture of all three cell types. It has been shown that epithelioid cell type is associated with the worst prognosis compared to other cell types.

Sedoon JM, et al. Death from uveal melanoma. Number of epithelioid cells and inverse SD of nucleolar area as prognostic factors. *Arch Ophthalmol* 1987;105;801–6.

81. Answer: A

OAT deficiency is also known as gyrate atrophy (GA) of the choroid and retina. This is an autosomal recessive dystrophy caused by mutations in the gene for ornithine aminotransferase (OAT), located on chromosome 10. This presents with progressive chorioretinal degeneration, myopia, night blindness, and eventually complete blindness in the fourth or fifth decade. OAT normally maintains a stable ornithine level in mitochondria. In OAT deficiency, hyperornithinaemia inhibits arginine:glycine amidinotransferase (AGAT), causing creatine deficiency. Dietary restriction of arginine has been used to treat some GA patients, the diet is very difficult to maintain and must be monitored by paediatricians with experience in metabolic disease. Vitamin B_6 (or pyridoxine) treatment lowers the plasma ornithine levels in a small percentage of GA patients.

Kaiser-Kupfer MI, et al. Gyrate atrophy of the choroid and retina: long-term reduction of ornithine slows retinal degeneration. *Arch Ophthalmol* 1991;109:1539–48.

82. Answer: B

Slit-lamp fundus lenses and indirect ophthalmoscopy with condensing lenses produce inverted, magnified, and real images.

American Academy of Ophthalmology. *BCSC Series, 2011–2012*: Chapter 8: Telescopes and optical instruments, pp. 243–82. San Francisco, CA: American Academy of Ophthalmology, 2012.

83. Answer: A

ANOVA test is used to compare the mean of three or more groups. Mann–Whitney U test (or Wilcoxon rank-sum test) is a non-parametric test for examining the mean between two groups and T-test is the parametric test for examining the mean between two groups. Contingency tables, including chi-squared test and Fisher's exact test, is used for examining categorical variables between two or more groups. The following reference provides a good summary table of the commonly used statistical tests.

Nayak BK, Hazra A. How to choose the right statistical test? *Indian J Ophthalmol* 2011;59:85–6.

84. Answer: A

The original TVT study looked at the 5-year outcome of Tube Versus Trabeculectomy surgery in patients with uncontrolled glaucoma who had previous ocular surgery. The main findings were:

- Tube shunt surgery had a higher success rate compared to trabeculectomy with mitomycin C (MMC) during 5 years of follow-up
- Both procedures were associated with similar IOP reduction and use of medical therapy at 5 years
- Additional glaucoma surgery was needed more frequently after trabeculectomy with MMC than tube shunt placement

Following the TVT study, the PTVT (Primary Tube Versus Trabeculectomy) study was published looking at patients with uncontrolled glaucoma with no previous ocular surgery. The study found that patients in the trabeculectomy group had a higher success rate.

Gedde SJ, et al. Treatment outcomes in the Tube Versus Trabeculectomy (TVT) study after five years of follow-up. *Am J Ophthalmol* 2012;153:789–803.

85. Answer: B

One cup of fresh sliced apricots has 0.33 mg of zinc, one cup of cubed avocado has 0.96 mg of zinc, three dates contain 0.32 mg of zinc, and one cup of sliced kiwi has 0.25 mg of zinc. The original Age-Related Eye Disease Study (AREDS) formulation contained 80 mg as zinc oxide and AREDS2 contained 25 mg.

National Eye Institute (NIH). Available at: https://nei.nih.gov/faqs/macular-degeneration-areds-and-areds2

86. Answer: A

The DVLA driving standards is a popular question in both Part 2 written and oral exams. Candidates are advised to familiarize with these standards. For a class 1 driver (car and motorcycle), patient does not have to inform DVLA when only one eye is affected, unless vision of the affected eye is non-perceptive to light (NPL). In addition, patient will need to inform DVLA if the eye with ocular hypertension (OHT) progresses to glaucoma.

Driver and Vehicle Licensing Agency (DVLA). *Assessing Fitness to Drive: A Guide for Medical Professionals*, September 2019. Available at: https://www.gov.uk/government/uploads/system/uploads/attachment_data/file/596959/assessing-fitness-to-drive-a-guide-for-medical-professionals.pdf

87. Answer: B

Capacity evaluation is a two-step process. Does the patient have mild cognitive impairment or dementia (mini-mental state examination and test letter and word fluency)? Regarding the decision, can the patient understand, appreciate, give reasons, and communicate their decision? The patient should have adequate and relevant information about the issue under discussion (disease, treatment options, and so on). The clinician should use open-ended questions. Capacity can be rated as adequate, inadequate, and marginal.

Hegde S, Ellajosyula R. Capacity issues and decision-making in dementia. *Ann Indian Acad Neurol* 2016;19:S34–9.

Wong JG, et al. Capacity to make health care decisions: Its importance in clinical practice. *Psychol Med* 1999;29:437–46.

88. Answer: C

The QALY is a measure of the value of health outcomes which makes the assumption that health is a function of life and quality of life. A perfect health year is calculated as following: 1 year of life × 1 utility value. The value is normally expressed 0–1 (0 is dead and perfect health 1). For example, bed ridden has a utility value of 0.5. Therefore, 1 × 0.5 = 0.5 QALY. NICE have used QALYs to evaluate health since 2013.

Weinstein MC, et al. QALYs: the basics. *Value Health* 2009;12:S5–9.

89. Answer: D

Scleral buckling has the highest risk of transmission due to the likelihood of drainage of subretinal fluid. CJD is a fatal human form of transmissible spongiform encephalopathy associated with an accumulation of prion proteins in brain tissue. In humans, the disease can be familial (autosomal dominant) or sporadic (usually in older patients). Variant CJD (vCJD), thought to be related to ingestion of contaminated beef, usually occurs in younger patients. All are rare. Because the disease can be very slowly progressive and can have a prolonged preclinical phase, there is a concern about potential transmission in patients without any symptoms or signs of the disease. Posterior segment and some orbital procedures are considered high risk; anterior segment operations are considered low risk.

Gov.UK. *Minimise Transmission Risk of CJD and vCJD in Healthcare Settings: Managing CJD/vCJD Risk in Ophthalmology. Annex L*, 2011. Available at: https://assets.publishing.service.gov.uk/government/uploads/system/uploads/attachment_data/file/209770/Annex_L_-_Managing_CJD_vCJD_risk_in_ophthalmology.pdf

90. Answer: A

Patients planning to take hydroxychloroquine long term (i.e. over 5 years) should have a baseline examination in a hospital eye department ideally within 6 months, but definitely within 12 months, of starting therapy with a colour retinal photograph and SD-OCT scans of the macula. Patients should be referred for annual screening after 5 years of therapy and be reviewed annually thereafter while on therapy. At each screening visit, patients should undergo 10–2 Humphrey visual field testing, followed by pupillary dilation and imaging with both SD-OCT and wide-field fundus autofluorescence imaging (FAF). If wide-field FAF is not available, FAF can be acquired in several photographic fields to encompass the macula and extramacular areas. Patients with abnormalities on wide-field FAF with normal 10–2 visual field test results should undergo 30–2 visual field testing on another date. Patients with persistent and significant visual field defects consistent with hydroxychloroquine retinopathy, but without evidence of structural defects on SD-OCT or FAF may be considered for multifocal electroretinography. Screening before 5 years should only be considered if additional factors exist (high-dose prescribed, concomitant tamoxifen therapy, or renal insufficiency). A useful aide memoir for guidelines is 5 × 5 rule (ideally keep dosage <5 mg/kg/day and screen after 5 years of drug use).

The Royal College of Ophthalmologists. *Hydroxychloroquine and Chloroquine Retinopathy: Recommendations on Screening*, 2018. Available at: https://www.rcophth.ac.uk/wp-content/uploads/2018/07/Hydroxychloroquine-and-Chloroquine-Retinopathy-Screening-Guideline-Recommendations.pdf

INDEX

Notes
Tables and figures are indicated by t or f following the page number.
Page numbers in q refer to Question and a refer to Answer
vs. indicates a comparison or differential diagnosis

A

abetalipoproteinaemia (Bassen–Kornzweig syndrome) 186a
abusive head trauma (shaken baby syndrome) 82q, 104a
acanthamoeba keratitis (AK) 158q, 179a
accommodative convergence/accommodation (AC/A) ratio 123q, 133a
accommodative esotropia 81q, 101–102a
ACCORD Eye study 149a
ACE (angiotensin-converting enzyme) 166q
acetazolamide 9q, 26a
acquired Brown syndrome 80q, 100a
acquired third nerve palsies 48q, 70t
acute anterior uveitis 116q, 126a
acute compressive optic neuropathy 85q, 107a
acute iatrogenic secondary angle glaucoma 10q, 28a
acute inferior macula, retinal detachment 36q, 54a
acute posterior multifocal pigment placoid epitheliopathy (APMPPE) 111a, 173q, 198a, 199t
acute postoperative endophthalmitis 11q, 30a
acute retinal necrosis (ARN) 72a
acyclovir 150a
adalimumab (Humira®) 171q, 196a
Adie's syndrome 67a, 187a
Adie's tonic pupil 44q, 65a
adipose tissue, glucose receptor 138q, 146a
Advanced Glaucoma Intervention Study (AGIS) 8q, 25a
aflibercept (Eylea/VEGF Trap) 58a, 116q, 126–127a
  diabetic macular oedema 154a
AGAT (arginine:glycine amidinotransferase) 201a
Age-Related Eye Disease Study (AREDS) 151a, 202a
Age-Related Eye Disease Study 2 (AREDS2) 128a
age-related macular degeneration (AMD) 117q, 128a, 140q, 148a, 175q, 202a
  nutritional supplements 141q, 151a
AGIS (Advanced Glaucoma Intervention Study) 8q, 25a
AK (acanthamoeba keratitis) 158q, 179a
Alagille syndrome 59a
albinism 52q, 76a
α-2 adrenergic agonists 197t
  side effects 10q, 28t

alpha-galactosidase deficiency, Fabry's disease 75a
Alport syndrome 167q, 183a, 185a, 189a
  anterior lenticonus 33a
alveolar rhabdomyosarcoma 99–100a
amaurosis fugax 143q, 152a
amblyopia, unilateral cataracts 183a
AMD (age-related macular degeneration) 117q, 128a, 175q, 202a
American Society of Cataract and Refractive Surgery (ASCRS) 185a
American Society of Retina Specialists (ASRS) 185a
amniotic membrane 6q, 23a
ANA (antinuclear antibody) 195a
analytic methods 143q, 153a
anaphylactic shock, fluorescein angiography 51q, 74a
ANCA (antineutrophil cytoplasmic antibodies) 112a, 159q
aneurysm, intracranial 123q, 133a
angiography
  fluorescein see fluorescein angiography
  indocyanine green see indocyanine green angiography (ICGA)
angioid streaks 37q, 58a
angiotensin-converting enzyme (ACE) 166q
aniridia 7q, 25a
anisocoria 165q, 187a
  Horner's syndrome 187a
ANOVA test 201a
anterior ischaemic optic neuropathy, bilateral sequential optic neuropathy vs. 68a
anterior lenticonus 33a
anterior segment dysgenesis (Axenfeld–Rieger syndrome) 7q, 21a, 25a
  chromosomal analysis 159q, 180a
anterior segment optical coherence tomography (AS-OCT) 121q, 132a
anterior uveitis syndrome 88q, 111a
  acute 116q, 126a
anti-acetylcholine receptor (AChR) antibody 200a
antibiotics 127t
anti-neutrophil cytoplasmic antibodies (ANCA) 112a, 159q

anti-nuclear antibody (ANA) 195a
anti-treponemal antibodies, syphilis treatment 196a
anti-tumour necrosis factor agent 114a
anti-vascular endothelial growth factor (VEGF) treatment 128a
Anton syndrome 52q, 76a
Apert syndrome 191a
APMPPE (acute posterior multifocal pigment placoid epitheliopathy) 111a, 173q, 198a, 199t
aponeurotic dehiscence 83q, 105a
aponeurotic ptosis 105t
apraclonidine 43q, 197t
apricots, zinc 202a
aqueous misdirection (malignant glaucoma) 10q, 28a
AREDS (Age-Related Eye Disease Study) 151a, 202a
AREDS2 (Age-Related Eye Disease Study 2) 128a
arginine:glycine amidinotransferase (AGAT) 201a
Argyll Robertson pupil 187a
arm-eye time, FFA 120q, 130a
ARN (acute retinal necrosis) 72a
Arnold–Chiari syndrome, Budd–Chiari syndrome vs. 73–74a
A-scan 122q, 132a
ASCRS (American Society of Cataract and Refractive Surgery) 185a
AS-OCT (anterior segment optical coherence tomography) 121q, 132a
ASRS (American Society of Retina Specialists) 185a
autosomal dominant familial microspherophakia 182a
Avellino cortical dystrophy 1a, 15–16q
avocado, zinc 202a
Axenfeld–Rieger anomaly 7q, 25a
Axenfeld–Rieger syndrome see anterior segment dysgenesis (Axenfeld–Rieger syndrome)
axial proptosis, unilateral 86q, 109a
azathioprine (AZA) 125a

B

bacterial endophthalmitis 143q, 153a
bacterial keratitis 5q, 21–22a
Bagolini glasses, torsion measurement 133a
Bardet–Biedl syndrome 186a
Bartonella henselae infection
    cat-scratch disease 73a
    Parinaud's oculo-glandular syndrome 6q, 23a
basal cell carcinoma (BCC)
    squamous cell carcinoma vs. 170q, 194a
    upper lid 86q, 109a
    vismodegib 117q, 128a
basic exotropia (BE) 98a
Bassen–Kornzweig syndrome (abetalipoproteinaemia) 186a
Bazex syndrome 85q, 107a
BCC see basal cell carcinoma (BCC)
BE (basic exotropia) 98a
Beauchamp, Tom 152a
Behçet's disease 88q, 112a
    Crohn's disease vs. 113a
    HLA associations 112a

Benedikt syndrome 70t
β-blockers 197t
    contraindications 125a
    side effects 10q, 28t
betaxolol 197t
BETT (Birmingham Eye Trauma terminology) 83q, 104a, 104f
bevacizumab, dexamethasone vs. 61a
BEVORDEX study 61a
BHL see bilateral hilar lymphadenopathy (BHL)
BIGH3 gene
    Meesmann dystrophy 18a
    Meretoia's syndrome 178a
bilateral capillary abnormalities 40q, 62a
bilateral granulomatous panuveitis 184a
bilateral hilar lymphadenopathy (BHL) 189a
    new-onset polyarthralgia 166q
bilateral inferonasal lens subluxation 12q, 31a
bilateral periorbital ecchymosis (raccoon eyes) 105a
bilateral red eye 168q, 191–192a
bilateral retinal striae 116q, 127a
bilateral sequential optic neuropathy, anterior ischaemic optic neuropathy vs. 68a
bilateral superior oblique palsies 49q, 71a
bimatoprost 197t
biometry repetition 161q, 182a
biomicroscopic classification 55a, 55t
birdshot chorioretinopathy 111a
    HLA 88q, 112a
    HLA-A29 112a
Birmingham Eye Trauma terminology (BETT) 83q, 104a, 104f
bitemporal hemianopia 123q, 134q
blepharophimosis, ptosis and epicanthus inversus syndrome (BPES) 106a
blepharophimosis syndrome type 2 84q, 106a
blindness
    cortical blindness 52q, 76a
    see also vision loss
blood agar 131t
Blue Mountain Eye Study, age-related macular degeneration 140q, 148a
blunt trauma, double vision 169q, 193a
blurred vision 166q, 171q, 189a, 196a
Borrelia burgdorferi infection, erythema chronicum migrans 73a
botulinum toxin 172q, 197–198a
Bowen's disease (conjunctival epithelial neoplasia) 16a
Bowman's layer, curly fibres 4q, 20a
BPES (blepharophimosis, ptosis and epicanthus inversus syndrome) 106a
brain heart infusion 131t
branch retinal artery occlusion (BRAO) 189a
brimonidine 197t
    side effects 125a
brinzolamide 197t
British National Formulary (BNF), acetazolamide contraindications 125a

Brown syndrome
  acquired 80q, 100a
  congenital 100a
Bruch's membrane 137q, 145a
Budd–Chiari syndrome 51q, 73–74a
  Arnold–Chiari syndrome vs. 73–74a
bulbar conjunctiva, primary acquired melanoma 22a

C

calcification, retinoblastoma 146a
calcineurin inhibitors 114a
calcofluor white stain 198t
CAMP mnemonic 191a
cancer-associated retinopathy (CAR) 43q, 64a, 196a
canthaxanthin 64a
capacity 176q, 202a
capillary abnormalities, bilateral 40q, 62a
capillary haemangioma 43q, 64a
carbonic anhydrase inhibitors 197t
  side effects 10q, 28t
carotene 151a
carotid endarterectomy (CEA) 141q, 151a
carteolol 197t
cataracts
  congenital cataracts 78q, 95a, 161q, 183a
  hypermature cataracts 11q, 29a
  posterior subcapsular cataracts see posterior subcapsular cataract
  sunflower cataracts 183a
  unilateral, amblyopia and 183a
  unilateral cataracts 183a
cataract surgery
  femtosecond laser-assisted cataract surgery 14q, 33a
  intraocular lenses 160q, 182a
  posterior capsule rupture 11q, 29–30a
  postoperative bacterial endophthalmitis 162, 184a
  problems after 13q, 32a
  problems in 13q, 32a
CAT-FANGS mnemonic 179a
cat-scratch disease 73a
cavernous haemangioma 64a, 109a
CCF (cortico-cavernous fistula) 82q, 103a
CCTS (Collaborative Corneal Transplant Studies) 7q, 24a
central nervous system (CNS), anterior segment dysgenesis 7q, 25a
central retinal vein occlusion 37q, 57a
central serous chorioretinopathy (CSCR) 42q, 62–63a, 118q, 119f, 129a
central vision deterioration 43q, 64a
CFEOM (congenital fibrosis of extraocular muscles) 81q, 101a
CHALeLS mnemonic 17a
chaperon 142q, 152a
Charles Bonnet syndrome 52q, 76a
Chédiak–Higashi syndrome 52q, 76a
chemical eye injury 2q, 17a, 157q, 177a, 177t
  classification 16a, 16t
  prognosis 1q, 16a

chemodenervation, acute onset of concomitant esotropia 97a
chest X-ray, thymoma 67a
children
  parental worries about vision 167q, 190a
  vision impairment 77q, 92a
Childress, James 152a
Chi-squared test 148a, 201a
chlorpromazine 183a
chocolate agar 131t
cholinergic medications 197t
chorioretinopathy, birdshot see birdshot chorioretinopathy
choroidal melanoma 201a
  metastases 170q, 194a
  prognosis 174q, 201a
choroidal naevus 87q, 110–111a
choroidal neovascularization (CNV) 42q, 63a
  choroidal neovascular membrane 130a
choroidal neovascular membrane (CNVM) 118q, 128a
  CT 37q, 38f, 58a
chromosomal analysis, anterior segment dysgenesis 159q, 180a
chronic anterior uveitis 171q, 195–196a
chronic conjunctivitis 118q, 129a
Churg–Strauss syndrome (CSS) eosinophilic granulomatosis with polyangiitis (EGPA)
CI (convergent insufficiency) 98a
cicatricial ectropion 169q, 194a
ciclosporin 197a
  mechanism of action 128a
  pregnancy and 125a
CJD (Creutzfeldt–Jakob disease) 176q, 203a
Claude syndrome 70t
clinically detectable retinal thickness 60a
clinically significant diabetic maculopathy 60a
closed globe injury, gun wounds 104a
cluster headache (CH) 190a
CMO (cystoid macular oedema) 111–112a
CNTGS (Collaborative Normal Tension Glaucoma Study) 8q, 25a
CNV see choroidal neovascularization (CNV)
CNVM see choroidal neovascular membrane (CNVM)
coagulase-negative staphylococci, bacterial endophthalmitis 54a
Cochrane collaboration, pigment dispersal syndrome 182a
Collaborative Corneal Transplant Studies (CCTS) 7q, 24a
Collaborative Normal Tension Glaucoma Study (CNTGS) 8q, 25a
Collaborative Ocular Melanoma Study (COMS) 140q, 149a, 149t
compressive optic neuropathy, acute 85q, 107a
computed tomographic angiography (CTA), Horner's syndrome 134a
computed tomography (CT)
  choroidal neovascular membrane 37q, 38f, 58a
  Horner's syndrome 134a
  infective orbital cellulitis 104–105a
  intracranial aneurysm 133a
  neurofibromatosis type 1 106a

COMS (Collaborative Ocular Melanoma Study) 140q, 149a, 149t
congenital Brown syndrome 100a
congenital cataracts 78q, 95a, 161q, 183a
congenital (infantile) esotropia 77q, 94a
congenital fibrosis of extraocular muscles (CFEOM) 81q, 101a
congenital glaucoma 115q, 125a
congenital megalocornea 168q, 192a
congenital optic pit maculopathy 57a
congenital ptosis 105t
congenital upper eyelid ptosis 169q, 193a
congenital Zika syndrome (CZS) 75a
  tyrosinase 75a
Congo red stain 15q
conjunctiva
  bulbar, primary acquired melanoma 22a
  fibrovascular lesions 159q
  melanosis 21a
  naevus 21a
  papilloma 21a
  pigmented lesions 4q, 21a
conjunctival epithelial neoplasia (Bowen's disease) 16a
conjunctivitis
  chronic conjunctivitis 118q, 129a
  mydricaine 126a
  viral infection see viral conjunctivitis
consent
  age issues 141q, 151–152a
  foreign language 142q, 152a
contralateral eye, muscle supply 145a
contralateral hemiparesis 188t
contralateral oculomotor nucleus 137q, 145a
convergence retraction nystagmus 71a
convergent insufficiency (CI) 98a
convergent squint, sudden onset 79q, 97a
cooked meat broth 131t
copper 151a
cornea
  congenital megalocornea 168q, 192a
  dystrophies, gene mutations 2q, 18a
  epithelium penetrating infections 2q, 17a
  hazy cornea 168q, 191–192a
  leukaemia, anterior segment dysgenesis 7q, 25a
  scraping, culture media 120q, 131a, 131t
corneal arcus 3q, 19a
corneal collagen cross-linking (CXL) 157q, 177–178a
corneal grafts
  disease recurrence 148q, 178a
  rejection of 19t
  subepithelial/stromal corneal graft rejection 3q, 19a
corneal impression cytology 2q, 17–18a
cornea verticillata (vortex keratopathy) 158q, 179–180a
coronal magnetic resonance imaging, septo-optic dysplasia 123q, 124f, 134a
corpus callosum lesions 166q, 189a
cortical blindness 52q, 76a

cortico-cavernous fistula (CCF) 82q, 103a
corticosteroids 114a
  central serous chorioretinopathy 62–63a
  Jarisch–Herxheimer reaction 172q, 196a
  see also steroids
cosmetic squints 141q, 151–152a
cost-benefit analysis 153a
cost-effectiveness 153a
cost-minimization 153a
cost-utility 153a
co-trimoxazole 125a
craniofacial abnormalities 7q, 25a
craniosynostosis 191a
CRAVE mnemonic 71a
Creutzfeldt–Jakob disease (CJD) 176q, 203a
Crohn's disease, Behçet's disease vs. 113a
Crouzon syndrome 191a
cryotherapy
  retinal detachment treatment 54a
  retinoblastoma 99a
Cryotherapy for Retinopathy of Prematurity (CRYO-ROP) study 93a
CSCR (central serous chorioretinopathy) 42q, 62–63a, 118q, 119f, 129a
CT see computed tomography (CT)
CTA (computed tomographic angiography), Horner's syndrome 134a
culture media 131t
  corneal scraping 120q, 131a, 131t
curly fibres, Bowman's layer 4q, 20a
CXL (corneal collagen cross-linking) 157q, 177–178a
cyclophosphamide 197a
cyclosporine
  mechanism of action 117q, 127a
  side effects 117q, 128a
CYP1B1 gene 159q
cystoid macular oedema (CMO) 111–112a
cytomegalovirus infection 50q, 72a
CZS see congenital Zika syndrome (CZS)

D

dacryocystocele 81q, 102a
dacryoscintigram (DSG) 124q, 135a
DALK (deep anterior lamellar keratoplasty) 6q, 23–24a
Dandy–Walker malformation 191a
dapsone 129a
data analysis, glaucoma 139q, 147a
DCCT (Diabetic Control and Complications Trial) 60a
decompensated (partially accommodative) exotropia 101a
decontamination of instruments 144q, 154a
deep anterior lamellar keratoplasty (DALK) 6q, 23–24a
delayed visual maturation 190a
dendritic keratitis management 1a, 15q
depression, topiramate 127a
dexamethasone
  bevacizumab vs. 61a
  intravitreal implant 61–62a

macular oedema management 185a
retinal implants 185a
DEXA (dual energy X-ray absorptiometry) scan 50q, 72–73a
diabetes mellitus type I
 diabetic retinopathy 39q, 60a
 proliferative retinopathy 56a
 vitreous haemorrhage 9q, 27a
diabetes mellitus type 2
 cholesterol management 140q, 148a
 diabetic retinopathy 50q, 72a
 diagonal diplopia 47q, 68a
 macular oedema 40q, 61–62a
Diabetic Control and Complications Trial (DCCT) 60a
diabetic macular oedema
 dexamethasone vs. bevacizumab 61a
 diabetes mellitus type 2 40q, 61–62a
 fluocinolone acetonide 40q, 61a
 management 144q, 154a
diabetic maculopathy 60a
diabetic retinopathy
 diabetes mellitus type 1 39q, 60a
 diabetes mellitus type 2 50q, 72a
 three port pars plana vitrectomy 36q, 55–56a
Diabetic Retinopathy Vitrectomy Study (DRVS) 55–56a
diagonal diplopia 47q, 68a
DIF test 15q
diplopia
 acquired Brown syndrome 100a
 diagonal diplopia 47q, 68a
 new-onset 164q, 186a
 vertical diplopia 45q, 45t, 67a, 168q, 192–193a
disease-modifying antirheumatic drug (DMARD) guidelines 125–126a
distance exotropia (DE) 98a
DON (dysthyroid optic neuropathy) management 84q, 106a
dorzolamide 197t
double elevator palsy (monocular elevation deficiency) 79q, 97–98a
double Maddox rod, torsion measurement 133a
double vision, blunt trauma 169q, 193a
Driver and vehicle Licensing Agency (DVLA) 142q, 152a, 176q, 202a
driving
 transient vision loss 143q, 152a
 vision requirements 176q, 202a
 visual field loss 142q, 152a
droopy eyelids 43q, 43t, 65a
DRS study 60–61a
dry age-related macular degeneration treatment 42q, 63–64a
dry eyes 157q, 178a
DSG (dacryoscintigram) 124q, 135a
dual energy X-ray absorptiometry (DEXA) scan 50q, 72–73a
Duane syndrome type II 78q, 95–96a
DULL-PC mnemonic 70a
dysthyroid optic neuropathy (DON) management 84q, 106a

E

Early Manifest Glaucoma Study (EMGS) 8q, 25a
Early Treatment for Diabetic Retinopathy Study (ETDRS) 39q, 60–61a, 60a
Early Treatment of Retinopathy of Prematurity (ETROP) study 93a
ear pain 165q, 187a
economic evaluation 153a, 153t
Effectiveness of early lens extraction for the treatment of primary angle closure glaucoma (EAGLE) 25a
EGFR (epidermal growth factor receptor) inhibitors 119f, 129a
EGPA (eosinophilic granulomatosis with polyangiitis) 84q, 105–106a
Ehlers–Danlos syndrome, keratoconus and 20a
electrodiagnostic tests 58a
electronegative electroretinogram (ERG) 38q, 58–59a
embryonal rhabdomyosarcoma 100a
EMGS (Early Manifest Glaucoma Study) 8q, 25a
endogenous endophthalmitis 90q, 114a
endophthalmitis
 bacterial 143q, 153a
 endogenous 90q, 114a
 management 153a
Endophthalmitis Vitrectomy Study (EVS) 32a, 184a
endotamponade 161q, 183a
endothelial corneal graft rejection 19t
enophthalmos, causes 194a
enzyme deficiency 52q, 75a
EON (ethambutol optic neuropathy) 69a
eosinophilic granulomatosis with polyangiitis (EGPA) 84q, 105–106a
epidermal growth factor receptor (EGFR) inhibitors 119f, 129a
epilepsy, topiramate 127a
epithelial corneal graft rejection 19t
epithelial disturbance, retinal pigment 42q, 63a
eplerenone 62–63a
ERG (electronegative electroretinogram) 38q, 58–59a
erythema chronicum migrans 50q, 73t
ESCRS see European Society of Cataract & Refractive Surgeons (ESCRS)
esotropia
 accommodative esotropia 81q, 101–102a
 infantile (congenital) esotropia 77q, 94a
ETDRS (Early Treatment for Diabetic Retinopathy Study) 39q, 60–61a, 60a
ethambutol optic neuropathy (EON) 69a
ETROP (Early Treatment of Retinopathy of Prematurity) study 93a
European Society of Cataract & Refractive Surgeons (ESCRS)
 Guidelines for Prevention and Treatment of Endophthalmitis Following Cataract Surgery 55t, 184a
 postoperative endophthalmitis prophylaxis 36q, 55a
euryblepharon 167q, 190a
EVS (Endophthalmitis Vitrectomy Study) 32a, 184a

exotropia
  basic exotropia 98a
  distance exotropia 98a
  non-refractive exotropia 101a
  partially accommodative (decompensated) exotropia 101a
  refractive exotropia 101a
extraocular muscle surgery 97a
exudative retinal artery macroaneurysm 184a
eyelids
  congenital upper eyelid ptosis 169q, 193a
  droopy eyelids 43q, 43t, 65a
  full-thickness defect reconstruction 86q, 108a, 108t
  upper eyelid basal cell carcinoma 86q, 109a
eye pain
  headache 167q, 190a
  hypermature cataract 11q, 29a
Eylea see aflibercept (Eylea/VEGF Trap)

F

Fabry's disease 179a
  alpha-galactosidase deficiency 75a
  posterior subcapsular cataract 33a
facial asymmetry 169q, 194a
facial injection sites 169q, 193a
FAF see fundus autofluorescence (FAF)
FAME trials 61a
familial exudative vitreoretinopathy (FEVR) 162q, 184a
familial microspherophakia, autosomal dominant 182a
Fasanella Servat 193–194a
fascicular third nerve syndromes 48q, 70a, 70t
FBC (full blood count), infective orbital cellulitis 104a
femtosecond laser-assisted cataract surgery (FLACS) 14q, 33a
Fenofibrate Intervention and Event Lowering in Diabetes Study (FIELD) 149a
FEVR (familial exudative vitreoretinopathy) 162q, 184a
FFA see fundus fluorescein angiography (FFA)
FHC (Fuchs heterochromatic cyclitis) 9q, 26–27a, 89q, 113a
FIELD (Fenofibrate Intervention and Event Lowering in Diabetes Study) 149a
Fisher's exact test 201a
FK506 see tacrolimus (fujimycin/FK506)
FLACS (femtosecond laser-assisted cataract surgery) 14q, 33a
Flexner–Wintersteiner rosettes, retinoblastoma 146a
floaters 171q, 196a
fluocinolone acetonide
  diabetic macular oedema 40q, 61a
  macular oedema management 185a
fluorescein angiography
  acute posterior multifocal pigment placoid epitheliopathy 198a
  anaphylactic shock 51q, 74a
fluoroquinolone 197a
flying saucer sign 130–131a
Food and Drug Administration (FDA, US), glaucoma medication 181a
Forbes–Albright syndrome 75a

foreign language, consent and 142q, 152a
forniceal conjunctiva, primary acquired melanoma 22a
Förster–Fuchs' spot 63a
FOXC1 gene 21a
Francisella tularensis infection 6q, 23a
Fraser competence 151a
FRAX® 73a
Friedman criteria, idiopathic intracranial hypertension 66a
Frisby test 200a
Fuchs heterochromatic cyclitis (FHC) 9q, 26–27a, 89q, 113a
fujimycin see tacrolimus (fujimycin/FK506)
full blood count (FBC), infective orbital cellulitis 104a
full-thickness lid defect, reconstruction 86q, 108a, 108t
fundus autofluorescence (FAF) 121f, 121q, 131a
  long-term with hydroxychloroquine 203a
fundus fluorescein angiography (FFA) 173q, 198a
  arm-eye time 120q, 130a
  CNVM 119q, 130a
fusidic acid 117q, 127a, 127t

G

galactosaemia 75a
galactose-1-phosphate uridyltransferase deficiency 75a
gamma-interferon assay (G-IFN/Quantiferon®) 130a
  tuberculosis diagnosis 113a
Gardner syndrome 85q, 107a
GCA see giant-cell arteritis (GCA)
gefitinib 118q, 129a
gene mutations, corneal dystrophies 2q, 18a
Gerstmann syndrome 69a
gestational diabetes 74a
giant-cell arteritis (GCA) 44q, 66–67a
  tocilizumab 126a
  tonic pupils 65a
giant retinal tears, retinal detachment 39q, 59a
Giemsa staining 198t
G-IFN see gamma-interferon assay (G-IFN/Quantiferon®)
Gillick competence 151a
glaucoma
  acute iatrogenic secondary angle glaucoma 10q, 28a
  congenital glaucoma 115q, 125a
  data analysis 139q, 147a
  laser trabeculoplasty 10q, 29a
  latanoprost therapy 160q, 181a
  lens-induced glaucoma 11q, 29a
  lens particle glaucoma 29a
  malignant glaucoma 10q, 28a
  neovascular glaucoma 160q, 181a
  open angle glaucoma 9q, 27a
  phacoanaphylactic glaucoma 29a
  phacolytic glaucoma 29a
  phacomorphic glaucoma 29a
  primary angle closure glaucoma 8q, 25a
  primary congenital glaucoma see primary congenital glaucoma (PCG)
  primary open angle glaucoma see primary open angle glaucoma

red cell glaucoma 9q, 27a
  treatment 159q, 181a
glucocorticoids
  dysthyroid optic neuropathy management 106a
  induced osteoporosis 50q, 72–73a
  ptosis 84q, 107a
glucose-6-phosphate dehydrogenase (G6PD) deficiency 118q, 129a
glucose receptor, adipose tissue/striated muscle 138q, 146a
GMS (Gomori methenamine silver) stains 198t
gold, lens opacities 183a
Goldman–Favre syndrome 63a
Gomori methenamine silver (GMS) stains 198t
gonioscopy, peripheral anterior synechiae 5q, 22a
Gorlin–Golz syndrome (naevoid BCG syndrome) 85q, 107a
gradient accommodative convergence/accommodation (AC/A) ratio 133a
Gram staining 198t
granulomatosis with polyangiitis (GPA) (Wegener's granulomatosis)
  peripheral alternative keratitis 159q
  scleritis 112a
granulomatous panuveitis, bilateral 184a
Grave's disease see thyroid eye disease (TED) (Grave's disease)
greenstick floor fracture (white eye blow-out fracture) 102–103a
greenstick orbital fractures 193a
Griscelli syndrome 52q, 76a
Guillain–Barré syndrome, Zika virus infection 75a
gun wounds 83q, 104a
gyrate atrophy 175q, 201a

H

haemangioma
  cavernous haemangioma 64a, 109a
  racemose haemangioma 64a
  segmental capillary haemangioma 167q, 190a
haemorrhage, vitreous in diabetes type 1 9q, 27a
haemorrhage occlusive retinal vasculitis (HORV) 163f, 163q, 185a
haemorrhagic retinal artery macroaneurysm 184a
hazy cornea 168q, 191–192a
HbA1C levels 50q, 72a
headache
  cluster headache 190a
  ocular pain 167q, 190a
  temporal headache 66a
hearing loss 166q, 189a
Hedgehog pathway, vismodegib 128a
HEDS (Herpetic Eye Disease Study) 15q, 141q, 149–150a
hemianopia, bitemporal 123q, 134q
hemifacial spasm 51q, 74a
hemiparesis, contralateral 188t
hepatitis C infection 22a
Hermansky–Pudlak syndrome 52q, 76a
herpes simplex keratitis (HSK) 149–150a
  acanthamoeba keratitis vs. 179a

herpes simplex virus iridocyclitis 150a
herpes zoster-associated acute retinal necrosis 196a
herpes zoster ophthalmicus (HZO) 148q, 178a
herpes zoster ophthalmoplegia 3q, 18–19a
  tonic pupils 65a
herpes zoster vaccination 6q, 24a
Herpetic Eye Disease Study (HEDS) 15q, 141q, 149–150a
herpetic simplex keratitis (HSK) 15q
Hess chart, torsion measurement 133a
Hess tests 132a
Histoplasma capsulatum 128a
HIV infection, ocular surface squamous neoplasia 16a
HLA
  birdshot chorioretinopathy 88q
  disease associations 112a
Holmes–Adie syndrome 67a
Homer–Wright pseudo-rosettes, retinoblastoma 146a
homocystinuria 12q, 31a, 183a
hookworm, Mooren's ulcer 22a
Horner's syndrome 124q
  MRI FLAIR 134a
  unilateral ptosis and anisocoria 187a
HORV (haemorrhage occlusive retinal vasculitis) 163f, 163q, 185a
HSK (herpetic simplex keratitis) 15q
Hudson–Stahl line 159q
Humira® (adalimumab) 171q, 196a
hydroxychloroquine 176, 203a
hydroxychloroquine maculopathy, OCT 120f, 120q, 130–131a
hypercholesterolaemia, corneal arcus 19a
hyperlysinaemia 183a
hypermature cataract 11q, 29a
hypermetropia 10q, 28a
hyper-reflective deposits, optic disc drusen 38q, 59a
hypertension
  ocular see ocular hypertension (OHT)
  RAPD 46q, 68a
hypoplasia, midfacial 168q, 191a
HZO (herpes zoster ophthalmicus) 148q, 178a

I

iatrogenic secondary angle glaucoma, acute 10q, 28a
ice pack test, ocular myasthenia 67a
ICE (iridocorneal) syndrome 5q, 22a
ICGA see indocyanine green angiography (ICGA)
IDEX 133a
idiopathic intracranial hypertension (IIH) 44q, 66a
IFIS (intraoperative floppy iris syndrome) 32a, 197a
IIH (idiopathic intracranial hypertension) 44q, 66a
illuvien 154a
imiquimod 129a
immunosuppression
  cytomegalovirus infection 50q, 72a
  pregnancy contraindications 115q, 125a
impotence 9q, 26a
incorrect rejection, null hypothesis 140q, 148a

indocyanine green angiography (ICGA) 96a, 121q, 131–132a
  acute posterior multifocal pigment placoid epitheliopathy 198a
infantile (congenital) esotropia 77q, 94a
infective orbital cellulitis 104–105a
inferior proliferative vitreoretinopathy 161q, 183a
inferior rectus muscle 145a
inferonasal lens subluxation, bilateral 12q, 31a
inflammatory diseases, tonic pupils 65a
inheritance patterns 138q, 147a
instrument decontamination 144q, 154a
interferon-alpha 64a
intermittent esotropia (IXT) 98a
International Society for Clinical Electrophysiology of Vision (ISCEV) 58a
intra-arteria embolus of filler 193a
intracranial aneurysm 123q, 133a
intraocular lenses (IOLs)
  cataract surgery 160q, 182a
  posterior capsule opacification (PCO) 160q, 182a
intraocular pressure (IOP)
  elevation of 160q, 181–182a
  medications for 10q, 27–28a, 28t
  primary congenital glaucoma 96a
  treatments 115q, 125a
  Urrets–Zavalia syndrome (UZS) 3q, 18a
intraoperative floppy iris syndrome (IFIS) 32a, 197a
intravitreal injection
  lampalizumab 42q, 63–64a
  silicone oil for pseudophakic eye 13q, 33a
IOLs see intraocular lenses (IOLs)
IOP see intraocular pressure (IOP)
ipsilateral eye, muscle supply 145a
ipsilateral sixth and seventh nerve palsies 165q, 187a, 188t
iridocorneal (ICE) syndrome 5q, 22a
ISCEV (International Society for Clinical Electrophysiology of Vision) 58a
ischaemia, third nerve palsy 46q, 68a
IXT (intermittent esotropia) 98a

J

Jansky–Bielschowsky syndrome 186a
Jarisch–Herxheimer reaction, corticosteroids 172q, 196a
jaw claudication, giant-cell arteritis 66a
juvenile idiopathic arthritis (JIA) 171q, 195–196a
juvenile X-linked retinoschisis (XLR) 63a, 78q, 96a

K

Kay Picture 169q, 193–194a
Kayser–Fleischer rings 183a
  Wilson's disease 20a
Kearns–Sayre syndrome (KSS) 80q, 100a
keratitis 117q, 128a
  bacterial 5q, 21–22a
  herpetic simplex keratitis 15q
  microbial keratitis 17a
keratoconjunctivitis, vernal 7q, 24a

keratoconus 4q, 20a
  penetrating keratoplasty 3q, 18a
keratoplasty, deep anterior lamellar keratoplasty 6q, 23–24a
Kifs syndrome 186a
kiwi fruit, zinc 202a
Klebsiella pneumonia infection, endogenous endophthalmitis 90q, 114a
Knudson's two-hit hypothesis 110a
Kruskal–Wallis test 149a

L

LAMA1 gene 147a
Lambert–Eaton syndrome 197–198a
lampalizumab 63–64a
Lang test 200a
LARGE mnemonic 18a
laser photocoagulation, retinoblastoma 99a
laser trabeculoplasty, glaucoma 10q, 29a
latanoprost 197t
  glaucoma 160q, 181a
  mechanism of action 172q, 196–197a
  pregnancy 181a
Lawrence–Moon syndrome 186a
Leber's hereditary optic neuropathy (LHON) 46q, 49q, 67–68a, 71a
  acute phase 81q, 101a
Lees test, ocular deviation 122q, 132–133a
lenses 137q, 146a
  intraocular see intraocular lenses (IOLs)
  opacity 161q, 183a
lens-induced glaucoma 11q, 29a
lens particle glaucoma 29a
Leptospira interrogans 73a
LHON see Leber's hereditary optic neuropathy (LHON)
Lifitegrast 7q, 24–25a
LIGHT trial 29a
limbal conjunctiva 22a
limbal ischaemia 1q, 16q
limbal stem cell deficiency (LSCD) 2q, 17a
  corneal impression cytology 2q, 17–18a
lipofuscinosis, neuronal ceroid 186a
Löfgren's syndrome 189a
Lowe's syndrome 179a
  anterior lenticonus 33a
LSCD see limbal stem cell deficiency (LSCD)
Lyme disease
  erythema chronicum migrans 73a
  tonic pupils 65a
lymphoma, orbital inflammatory disease vs. 86q, 109a

M

macular cystic changes, vitamins 42q, 63a
macular degeneration, dry age-related
  treatment 42q, 63–64a
macular holes, sttage2 full-thickness 36q, 55a
macular oedema, diabetic see diabetic macular oedema
macular pucker 41f, 41q, 62a

macular telangiectasia 40q, 62a
macular telangiectasia type 2 63a
MacuShield 117q, 128a
magnetic resonance angiography (MRA), intracranial aneurysm 133a
magnetic resonance imaging (MRI)
　coronal in septo-optic dysplasia 123q, 124f, 134a
　coronal, septo-optic dysplasia 123q, 124f, 134a
　FLAIR, Horner's syndrome 134a
　infective orbital cellulitis 104–105a
　neurofibromatosis type 1 106a
　T2-weighted scan with FLAIR sequence 174f, 200a
　Wilson's disease 20a
malignant glaucoma (aqueous misdirection) 10q, 28a
malnutrition 47q, 68–69a
MALT (mucosa-associated lymphoid tissue) lymphoma 194a
Mann–Whitney tests 148a, 201a
Mantoux skin testing 130a
MAR (melanoma-associated retinopathy) 43q, 64a
Marcus–Gunn jaw-winking syndrome (MGJWS) 164q, 187a
marfanoid stature 12q, 31a
Marfan syndrome 182–183a
　keratoconus and 20a
MD (myotonic dystrophy) 166q, 188a
mean 139q, 148a
　comparison of 175q, 201q
mean refractive spherical equivalent (MRSE) 147a
MED (monocular elevation deficiency/double elevator palsy) 79q, 97–98a
medial canthus, swelling below 81q, 102a
medial rectus muscle 145a
median 139q, 148a
medical ethics 142q, 152a
Meesmann dystrophy 2q, 4q, 18a, 20a
megalocornea, congenital 168q, 192a
melanoma
　choroidal see choroidal melanoma
　ocular melanoma 87q, 110a
　primary acquired melanoma 5q, 22a
　uveal melanoma 194a
melanoma-associated retinopathy (MAR) 43q, 64a
Meretoja's syndrome 178a
mesoderm 146a
meso-xanthine 117q, 128a
methotrexate 125a
MEWDS (multinucleate evanescent white dot syndrome) 87q, 111a, 199t
MFC 199t
MGJWS (Marcus–Gunn jaw-winking syndrome) 164q, 187a
microadenoma 75a
microbial keratitis 17a
microbiological staining 172q, 198a, 198t
Microplasmin for Intravitreal Injection–Traction Release without Surgical Treatment (MIVI-TRUST) 56a
microspherophakia 161q, 182–183a
microspherophakia, autosomal dominant familial 182a
microtropia 96a

microvascular sixth nerve palsy 186–187a
midfacial hypoplasia 168q, 191a
migraine 53q, 76a
　topiramate 127a
mitomycin C 128a
MIVI-TRUST (Microplasmin for Intravitreal Injection–Traction Release without Surgical Treatment) 56a
MMAGHMLACSLO mnemonic 15–16q
mode 139q, 148a
modified Dandy criteria, idiopathic intracranial hypertension 66a
modified Hughes classification 157q
monocular elevation deficiency (MED/double elevator palsy) 79q, 97–98a
Mooren's ulcer 5q, 22a
MPO (myeloperoxidase) 159q
MRA (magnetic resonance angiography), intracranial aneurysm 133a
MRI see magnetic resonance imaging (MRI)
MRSE (mean refractive spherical equivalent) 147a
mucopolysaccharidoses 186a
mucosa-associated lymphoid tissue (MALT) lymphoma 194a
Muenke syndrome, craniosynostosis 191a
Muir–Torre syndrome 85q, 107a
multinucleate evanescent white dot syndrome (MEWDS) 87q, 111a, 199t
multiple sclerosis 47q, 69a
musculoskeletal (MSK) disorders 197a
myasthenia gravis 197–198a
　autoantibodies 174q, 200a
　diagnostic tests 67a
myasthenic ptosis 105t
Mycobacterium tuberculosis infection 119q, 130a
mycophenolate mofetil 125a
mydricaine 116q, 126a
myeloperoxidase (MPO) 159q
MYOC gene 159q
myogenic ptosis 105t
myopia, congenital megalocornea 192a
myopic refractive surprise 12q, 30–31a, 31t
myotonic dystrophy (MD) 166q, 188a

N

NA-AION (non-arteritic anterior ischaemic optic neuropathy) 44q, 65–66a, 68a, 165q, 187–188a
naevoid BCG syndrome (Gorlin–Golz syndrome) 85q, 107a
nanophthalmia 32a
NASCET (North America Symptomatic Carotid Endarterectomy) study 141q, 151a
National Osteoporosis Guideline Group (NOG) 73q, 73t
NDSEP (NHS Diabetic Eye Screening Programme) 143q, 153–154a
neovascular glaucoma 160q, 181a
nerve palsies 188t
　acquired third nerve palsies 48q, 70t
　ipsilateral sixth and seventh nerve palsies 165q, 187a, 188t
　microvascular sixth nerve palsy 186–187a
　third nerve palsies see third nerve palsy

neural crest cells 138q, 146a
  embryologic origins 146a
neuroectoderm 146a
neurofibromatosis type 1 80q, 100–101a
  investigations pre-surgery 84q, 106–107a
neuroimaging 173q, 174f, 200a
  intracranial aneurysm 123q, 133a
neuromyelitis optica (NMO), bilateral sequential optic
    neuropathy vs. 68a
neuronal ceroid lipofuscinosis 186a
NFAT (nuclear factor of activated T cells) 127t
NHS Diabetic Eye Screening Programme (NDSEP) 143q,
    153–154a
niacin (vitamin B_3/nicotinic acid) 42q, 63a
NICE (National Institute for Health and Care Excellence)
  choroidal neovascular membrane guidelines 58a
  corneal collagen cross-linking 177a
  dexamethasone intravitreal implant 61–62a
  diabetic control guidelines 72a
  glaucoma treatment 181a
  macular oedema management 163q, 185a
  ocriplasmin 36q, 56a
  tuberculosis treatment 130a
nicotinic acid (vitamin B_3/niacin) 42q, 63a
NMO (neuromyelitis optica), bilateral sequential optic
    neuropathy vs. 68a
NOG (National Osteoporosis Guideline Group) 73a, 73t
non-arteritic anterior ischaemic optic neuropathy
    (NA-AION) 44q, 65–66a, 68a, 165q, 187–188a
non-Hodgkin's lymphoma 194a
non-nutrient agar with E coli overlay 131t
non-parametric tests 148a
non-purulent discharge 168q, 191–192a
non-refractive exotropia 101a
North America Symptomatic Carotid Endarterectomy
    (NASCET) study 141q, 151a
Nothnagel syndrome 70t
nuclear factor of activated T cells (NFAT) 127t
null hypothesis, incorrect rejection 140q, 148a
nutritional supplements, AMD 141q, 151a
nystagmus
  convergence retraction 71a
  see-saw nystagmus 48q, 69–70a

O

OAT (ornithine aminotransferase) deficiency 201a
occult membrane classification 130a
OCP (ocular cicatricial pemphigoid) 1a, 15q
ocriplasmin 36q, 56a, 56t
Ocriplasmin for treatment for Symptomatic Vitreomacular
    Adhesion Including Macular Hole (OASIS) 56a
OCS (ocular trauma score) 82q, 103a, 103t
OCT see optical coherence tomography (OCT)
ocular albinism, X-linked 81q, 102a
ocular cicatricial pemphigoid (OCP) 1a, 15q
ocular deviation, Lees test 122q, 132–133a
ocular embryolog6y 201a

ocular fundus, abusive head trauma (shaken baby
    syndrome) 104a
ocular hypertension (OHT) 10q, 28a
  reviews 28t
Ocular Hypertension Study (OHTS) 8q, 25a
ocular melanoma 87q, 110a
ocular motility problems 164q, 186a
ocular myasthenia 45q, 67a
ocular pain see eye pain
ocular surface squamous neoplasia (OSSN) 2q, 16–17a
ocular trauma score (OCS) 82q, 103a, 103t
oculomotor nucleus, contralateral 137q, 145a
oedema
  cystoid macular oedema 111–112a
  diabetic macular see diabetic macular oedema
  post-cataract surgery macular oedema 11q, 30a
  post-phacoemulsification cystoid macular
    oedema 11q, 30a
OHT see ocular hypertension (OHT)
OHTS (Ocular Hypertension Study) 8q, 25a
OID (orbital inflammatory disease), lymphoma vs. 86q, 109a
omega-3 fatty acids 151a
one-way analysis of variance 148a
ONTT (Optic Neuritis Treatment Trials) 141q, 150a, 150t
open angle glaucoma 9q, 27a
ophthalmic artery embolism 169q, 193a
ophthalmic ultrasonography 120q, 131a
optical coherence tomography (OCT) 40f, 40q, 41f, 62a,
    116q, 127a, 133a, 134a
  anterior segment optical coherence tomography
    (AS-OCT) 121q, 132a
  conditions 118q, 119f, 129a
  hydroxychloroquine maculopathy 120f, 120q, 130–131a
  long-term with hydroxychloroquine 203a
  retinal dearrangement 171q, 196a
optic disc drusen 38q, 59a
optic disc maculopathy 36q, 57a
optic neuritis 187a
  imaging 123q, 134a
  multiple sclerosis 47q, 69a
Optic Neuritis Treatment Trials (ONTT) 141q, 150a, 150t
optic neuropathy
  acute compressive 85q, 107a
  bilateral sequential vs. anterior ischaemic 68a
optic pit maculopathy, congenital 57a
optic sulci 201a
optic vesicle 174q, 201a
orbital cellulitis 168q, 191a
  infective 104–105a
orbital floor fracture 82q, 102–103a
orbital inflammatory disease (OID), lymphoma vs. 86q, 109a
orbital lesions 86q, 109a
orbital malignancy diagnosis 170q, 194–195a, 195t
orbital metastases 109a
ornithine aminotransferase (OAT) deficiency 201a
orthoptic tests 173q, 200a
OSSN (ocular surface squamous neoplasia) 2q, 16–17a

osteogenesis imperfecta, keratoconus and 20a
osteoporosis 72–73a
Ozurdex 154a

P

PACK (photoactivated chromophore for keratitis)-CXL 177a
Paediatric Eye Disease Investigator Group, congenital (infantile) esotropia 94a
pain
  ear pain 165q, 187a
  eyes see eye pain
palinopsia 71a
PAM (primary acquired melanoma) 5q, 22a
panretinal photocoagulation (PRP)
  Early Treatment for Diabetic Retinopathy Study (ETDRS) 39q, 60a
  proliferative diabetic retinopathy 39q, 60a
panuveitis
  bilateral granulomatous 184a
  severe active bilateral 115q, 125a
PAPER-CLIP mnemonic 58a
papilloedema 51q, 73–74a
parametric tests 148a
paretic extraocular muscles 168q, 192–193a, 193f
parietal lobe infarction 48q, 69a
Parinaud dorsal midbrain syndrome 48q, 70–71a
Parinaud's oculo-glandular syndrome (POGS) 6q, 23a
Parks–Bielschowsky test 192a
Park's three-step test 192a
partially accommodative (decompensated) exotropia 101a
partial third nerve palsy 47q, 68a
PAT (prism adaptation test) 122q, 133a
pattern electroretinogram (pERG) 173q, 199a
PAX6 gene 21a
PCG see primary congenital glaucoma (PCG)
PCMO (post-cataract surgery macular oedema) 11q, 30a
PCO see posterior capsule opacification (PCO)
PDR see proliferative diabetic retinopathy (PDR)
PDS (pigment dispersal syndrome) 160q, 181–182a
PDT see photodynamic therapy (PDT)
PEDF (pigment epithelium derived factor) 181a
pellucid marginal degeneration (PMD) 5q, 23a
penetrating infections, corneal epithelium 2q, 17a
penetrating keratoplasty (PKP) 3q, 6q, 19a, 23–24a
  keratoconus 3q, 18a
Pentacam machine 122q, 132a
perfluorocarbon 183a
pERG (pattern electroretinogram) 173q, 199a
periocular swelling, unilateral 93q, 104–105a
periodic acid-Schiff stain 198t
periorbital ecchymosis, bilateral (raccoon eyes) 105a
peripheral alternative keratitis (PUK) 159q, 180a
peripheral anterior synechiae, gonioscopy 5q, 22a
peripheral neurofibromatosis see neurofibromatosis type 1
Peter's anomaly 4q, 21a, 183a
Pfeiffer syndrome, craniosynostosis 191a
PHACES syndrome 190–191a

Phacoanaphylactic glaucoma 29a
phacoemulsifications 11q, 30a
phacolytic glaucoma 29a
phacomorphic glaucoma 29a
phakomatoses 138q, 146a
pheochromocytoma 195a
PHN (post-herpetic neuralgia) 178a
photoactivated chromophore for keratitis (PACK)-CXL 177a
photodynamic therapy (PDT)
  vascular abnormalities 63a
  verteporfin and 42q, 63a
photophobia 2q, 17a, 157q, 188a
phytanic acid alpha hydrolase deficiency 75a
PIC 199t
pigment dispersal syndrome (PDS) 160q, 181–182a
pigmented lesions, conjunctiva 4q, 21a
pigment epithelium derived factor (PEDF) 181a
pilocarpine 197t
pituitary adenoma 123q, 134q
pituitary tumours
  adenoma 123q, 134q
  prolactin production 52q, 75a
PITX2 gene 21a
PITZ3 gene 96a
PIV (punctate inner choroidopathy) 111a
PKP see penetrating keratoplasty (PKP)
plaque radiotherapy, retinoblastoma 99a
pleomorphic adenomas 109a
plexiform neurofibroma 106a
PMD (pellucid marginal degeneration) 5q, 23a
pneumatic retinopexy 54a
POGS (Parinaud's oculo-glandular syndrome) 6q, 23a
POHS (presumed optical histoplasmosis syndrome) 118q, 128a
polyarthralgia, new-onset 166q, 189a
Poretti–Boltshauser syndrome 147a
Posner–Schlossman syndrome 9q, 27a, 195a
post-cataract surgery macular oedema (PCMO) 11q, 30a
posterior capsule opacification (PCO) 13q, 33a
  intraocular lenses (IOLs) type 160q, 182a
posterior capsule rupture, cataract surgery 11q, 29–30a
posterior lenticonus 96a
posterior reversible encephalopathy syndrome 74a
posterior segment ischaemia 160q, 181a
posterior subcapsular cataract 96a
  associated diseases 14q, 33a
post-herpetic neuralgia (PHN) 178a
postoperative endophthalmitis (POE), acute 11q, 30a
post-phacoemulsification bacterial endophthalmitis 36q, 54–55a, 55t
post-phacoemulsification cystoid macular oedema (CMO/Irvine–Gass syndrome) 11q, 30a
PR see proliferative retinopathy (PR)
prednisolone
  peripheral alternative keratitis 159q
  syphilis treatment 196a
pre-eclamptic toxaemia 51q, 74a

pregnancy
  drug contraindications 115q, 125a
  latanoprost 181a
preoperative prism correction 133a
presumed optical histoplasmosis syndrome
  (POHS) 118q, 128a
primary acquired melanoma (PAM) 5q, 22a
primary angle closure glaucoma 8q, 25a
primary angle closures, terminology 10q, 27a, 27t
primary biliary cirrhosis 179a
primary congenital glaucoma (PCG) 7q, 25a, 79q, 96a
  genetics 159q
primary open angle glaucoma 138q, 147a
  topical β-blockers 9q, 26a
primary Sjögren's syndrome (PSS) 158q, 179a
Primary Tube Versus Trabeculectomy (PTVT) study 202a
Principles of Biomedical Ethics (Beauchamp and
  Childress) 152a
prism adaptation test (PAT) 122q, 133a
prolactin, pituitary tumours 52q, 75a
prolactinoma 75a
proliferative diabetic retinopathy (PDR)
  high-risk definition 39q, 60–61a
  panretinal photocoagulation 39q, 60a
proliferative retinopathy (PR)
  classification 54a
  retinal detachment 36q, 54a
proliferative vitreoretinopathy (PVR) 183a
  retinoschisis-related retinal detachment 183–184a
proptosis
  steroid therapy 85q, 107a
  unilateral axial 86q, 109a
prostaglandin analogues 197t
  side effects 10q, 28t
proteinase 3 (PR3) 159q
PRP see panretinal photocoagulation (PRP)
psammoma bodies, retinoblastoma 146a
pseudoexfoliation (PXE) 182a
pseudoexfoliation syndrome (PXS) 12q, 32a
pseudophakic eye, intravitreal silicone oil 13q, 33a
PSS (primary Sjogren's syndrome) 158q, 179a
pterygium 159q, 180a
ptosis 165q, 187a
  aponeurotic dehiscence 83q, 105a
  congenital 105t
  congenital upper eyelid 169q, 193a
  features 105a, 105t
  glucocorticoids 84q, 107a
  unilateral 187a
PTVT (Primary Tube Versus Trabeculectomy) study 202a
PUK (peripheral alternative keratitis) 159q, 180a
Pulfrich phenomenon 52q, 76a
punctate inner choroidopathy (PIV) 111a
pupils
  Adie's tonic pupil 44q, 65a
  Argyll Robertson pupil 187a
  reverse pupil block 32a

  size difference between eyes 44q, 65a
  tonic pupils see tonic pupils
Purtscher-like retinopathy 74a
Purtscher retinopathy 74a
PVR see proliferative vitreoretinopathy (PVR)
PXE (pseudoexfoliation) 182a
PXS (pseudoexfoliation syndrome) 12q, 32a

Q

quality-adjusted-life-year (QALY) 176q, 203a
Quantiferon® see gamma-interferon assay (G-IFN/
  Quantiferon®)
quetiapine 172q, 197a

R

raccoon eyes (bilateral periorbital ecchymosis) 105a
racemose haemangioma 64a
RADIANCE trials 63a
RAM (retinal artery macroaneurysm) 162q, 184–185a
ranibizumab 154a
RAPD see relative afferent pupillary defect (RAPD)
RCOphth see Royal College of Ophthalmologists (RCOphth)
red cell glaucoma 9q, 27a
red eye, bilateral 168q, 191–192a
Reese–Ellsworth group, unilateral retinoblastoma 99a
refractive exotropia 101a
Refsum disease/syndrome 185a
  phytanic acid alpha hydrolase deficiency 75a
Reis–Buckler dystrophy 20a
relative afferent pupillary defect (RAPD) 87q, 111a,
  165q, 187a
  hypertension 46q, 68a
REPAIR trials 63a
retina
  astrocytoma 170q, 195a
  bilateral striae 116q, 127a
  breaks 57a
  optical coherence tomography 171q, 196a
  tears 37q, 57a
  unilateral lesions 80q, 99a
  vascular tumours 43q, 64a
retinal artery macroaneurysm (RAM) 162q, 184–185a
retinal detachment 119q, 129–130a, 161q, 183a
  acute inferior macular 36q, 54a
  differential diagnoses 129a
  giant retinal tears 39q, 59a
  proliferative retinopathy 36q, 54a
  treatment 36q, 54a, 90q, 91t, 114a
retinal pigment epithelium (RPE) 145a
  disturbance 42q, 63a
retinal vein occlusion (RVO) 37q, 57a, 163q, 185a
Retina Society, proliferative retinopathy classification 54a
retinitis 50q, 71a
retinitis pigmentosa (RP) 63a
  associated conditions 164q, 185–186a
retinoblastoma 99a
  genetics 110a

pathology 137q, 146a
  unilateral 99a
retinoblastoma protein (pRb) 138q, 146–147a
retinopathy
  diabetic see diabetic retinopathy
  of prematurity 77q, 93–94a
  proliferative see proliferative retinopathy (PR)
retinoschisis-related retinal detachment (RSRD) 162q, 183–184a
reverse pupil block 32a
rhabdomyosarcoma (RMS) 80q, 87q, 99–100a, 109–110a
  alveolar 99–100a
  embryonal 100a
rheumatoid arthritis 189a
  HLA associations 112a
  scleritis 112a
  tocilizumab 126a
  tonic pupils 65a
riboflavin 177a
Riddoch phenomenon 52q, 76a
rifampicin 62–63a
right divergent squints 79q, 98–99a
right Horner's syndrome 43q
right inferior rectus weakness 45q, 67a
Roper–Hall classification, chemical eye injury 16a, 157q
Royal College of Ophthalmologists (RCOphth)
  diabetic maculopathy guidelines 60a
  diabetic retinopathy risk 60a
  instrument decontamination 144q, 154a
  retinal vein occlusion guidelines 57a
RP see retinitis pigmentosa (RP)
RPE see retinal pigment epithelium (RPE)
RSRD (retinoschisis-related retinal detachment) 162q, 183–184a
Rude Little Green man mnemonic 178a
RVO (retinal vein occlusion) 37q, 57a, 163q, 185a

S

Sabouraud dextrose agar 131t
Sabril see vigabatrin (Sabril)
saddle nose deformity 52q, 74–75a
sample T-tests 148a
SANSIKA study 128a
sarcoidosis, tonic pupils 65a
SC see squamous cell carcinoma (SCC)
Schirmer's test 179a
Schwalbe's line 22a
Schwartz–Matsuo syndrome 9q, 27a, 195a
scleral buckle, retinal detachment treatment 54a
scleritis 89q
  diagnosis 89q, 112–113a
see-saw nystagmus 48q, 69–70a
segmental capillary haemangioma 167q, 190a
Seidel test, trabeculectomy 25–26a
septo-optic dysplasia (SOD) 123q, 124f, 134a
severe active bilateral panuveitis 115q, 125a
sexual harassment 142q, 152a

shaken baby syndrome (abusive head trauma) 82q, 104a
shingles vaccination 6q, 24a
SICCANOVE study 128a
silicon oil tamponade 183a
simulated IDEX 133a
SINA_LFTs mnemonic 145a
skew 139q, 148a
slit-lamp fundus lenses 175q, 201q
SO (sympathetic ophthalmia) 90q, 91t, 114a, 162, 184a
SOD (septo-optic dysplasia) 123q, 124f, 134a
SOF (superior orbital fissure) 137q, 145a
soft contact lenses, biometry repetition 182a
SOM (superior oblique myokymia) 47q, 69a
Sorsby fundus dystrophy 21a
spherical equivalents 139q, 147a
spiramycin 113a
spironolactone 62–63a
Sporotrichum schenckii infection 6q, 23a
squamous cell carcinoma (SCC) 194a
  basal cell carcinoma vs. 170q, 194a
squints 81q, 101–102a
  cosmetic squints 141q, 151–152a
  right divergent 79q, 98–99a
  sudden onset convergent squint 79q, 97a
SSTT mnemonic 183a
STAIB-LONG mnemonic 66a
Standardization of Uveitis Nomenclature (SUN) 88q, 111–112a
Staphylococcus infections
  acute postoperative endophthalmitis 30a
  bacterial endophthalmitis 54a
statistical tests 140q, 148–149a
steatorrhoea 164q, 185–186a
stereopsis 200a
steroids
  macular oedema management 163q, 185a
  proptosis 85q, 107a
  see also corticosteroids
Sticker's syndrome 78q, 94a
Stickler syndrome 59t
  retinal detachment 59a
Stocker's iron line 159q
strabismus 78q, 95a
  acute onset of concomitant esotropia 97a
  sudden-onset 80q, 99a
  thyroid eye disease 79q, 98a
Streptococcus infections 30a
striated muscle, glucose receptors 138q, 146a
stromal corneal graft rejection 19t
Sturge–Weber syndrome (SWS) 77q, 92a, 146a
subepithelial/stromal corneal graft rejection 3q, 19a
subperiosteal abscess 168q, 191a
sulphonamide 115q, 125a
SUN (Standardization of Uveitis Nomenclature) 88q, 111–112a
sunflower cataracts, Wilson's disease 183a
superficial basal cell carcinoma 118q, 129a

superior oblique myokymia (SOM) 47q, 69a
superior oblique palsies, bilateral 49q, 71a
superior orbital fissure (SOF) 137q, 145a
superotemporal quadrant swelling 85q, 108a
suprachoroidal buckling 54a
supranuclear pathway 186a
surface ectoderm 146a
Susac's syndrome 189a
sutures 146a
SWS (Sturge–Weber syndrome) 77q, 92a, 146a
sympathetic ophthalmia (SO) 90q, 91t, 114a, 162, 184a
synoptophore, torsion measurement 133a
syphilis (*Treponema pallidum* infection) 73a
    Parinaud's oculo-glandular syndrome 6q, 23a
    reactivation 196a
    testing for 166q, 188a, 189t
    treatment 172q, 196a

T

tacrolimus (fujimycin/FK506)
    mechanism of action 117q, 127a, 128a
    pregnancy and 125a
tamoxifen 43q, 64a
TED see thyroid eye disease (TED) (Grave's disease)
temporal artery biopsy, giant-cell arteritis 66–67a
temporal headache 66a
TFSOMUHHD mnemonic 110–111a
TGFB1 gene 178a
thermotherapy, retinoblastoma 99a
thiopurine methyltransferase (TPMT) 115q, 125–126a
third nerve palsy
    acquired 48q, 70t
    ischaemia 46q, 68a
    partial 47q, 68a
three port pars plana vitrectomy 36q, 55–56a
thymoma 67a
thyroidectomy 43q, 43t, 65a
thyroid eye disease (TED) (Grave's disease) 85q, 86q, 107–108a, 109a, 169q, 193a
    strabismus 79q, 98a
thyroiditis 179a
timolol 197t
TIMP3 gene 21a
Titmus test 200a
TNO 200a
tocilizumab 116q, 126a
TON (traumatic optic neuropathy) 82q, 103a
tonic pupils
    associated diseases 65a
    pharmacological tests 45q, 67a
topical β-blockers, side effects 9q, 26a
topical ciclosporin (Ikervis) 128a
topical intraocular pressure-lowering medication 196–197a, 197t
topical steroids, bacterial keratitis 5q, 21–22a
topiramate, bilateral retinal striae 127a
torsional nystagmoid movement 47q, 69a

torsion, measurement of 122q, 133a
total retinal detachment 171q, 195a
toxic anterior segment syndrome (TASS) 13q, 33a
toxoplasma uveitis, management 89q, 113a
TPMT (thiopurine methyltransferase) 115q, 125–126a
trabeculectomy 8q, 25–26a, 26a
trabeculotomy
    Fuchs heterochromatic cystitis (FHC) 26–27a
    pigment dispersal syndrome (PDS) 181–182a
trachoma, trichiasis 105t
transient vision loss, driving 143q, 152a
transpupillary diode laser 93–94a, 93t
traumatic optic neuropathy (TON) 82q, 103a
treponemal antibody testing 166q, 188a, 189t
Treponema pallidum infection see syphilis (*Treponema pallidum* infection)
triamcinolone
    choroidal neovascular membrane 58a
    presumed optical histoplasmosis syndrome 128a
trichiasis 83q, 105a
trigeminal neuralgia 127a
t-tests 201a
tuberculosis 196a
    diagnosis 113a
Tube Versus Trabeculectomy (TVT) study 175q, 202a
TVT (Tube Versus Trabeculectomy) study 175q, 202a
tyrosinase 75a

U

UK eye retrieval and eye bank services 144q, 155a
ultrasonography, ophthalmic ultrasonography 120q, 131a
ultrasound biomicroscopy (UBM) 131t
unilateral axial proptosis 86q, 109a
unilateral cataracts, amblyopia 183a
unilateral periocular swelling 93q, 104–105a
unilateral ptosis 187a
unilateral retinal lesion 80q, 99a
unilateral retinoblastoma 99a
unit of analysis issue 147a
upper eyelid basal cell carcinoma 86q, 109a
upper eyelid ptosis, congenital 169q, 193a
Urrets–Zavalia syndrome (UZS) 3q, 18a
Usher syndrome 185a
uveal melanoma 194a
uveitis
    acute anterior 116q, 126a
    adalimumab 171q, 196a
    chronic anterior 171q, 195–196a
    classification 88q, 111–112a
    differential diagnosis 89q, 113a

V

variant Creutzfeldt–Jakob disease (vCJD) 203a
vasoproliferative tumours 41f, 41q, 62a, 64a
VAVFC (visual field constriction attributable to vigabatrin) 153a
VEGF (vascular endothelial growth factor) 181a

VEGF Trap see aflibercept (Eylea/VEGF Trap)
VEIN mnemonic, thyroid eye disease 109a
VEP (visual evoked potential) 122q, 132a, 190a
vernal keratoconjunctivitis (VKC) 7q, 24a
verteporfin 42q, 63a
vertical diplopia 45q, 45t, 67a, 168q, 192–193a
vigabatrin (Sabril) 143q, 153a
   mechanism of action 116q, 126a
   side effects 64a
viral conjunctivitis 191–192a
   treatment 192t
vision
   blurred 166q, 171q, 189a, 196a
   central vision deterioration 43q, 64a
   delayed visual maturation 190a
   double, blunt trauma 169q, 193a
vision loss 67–68a
   sudden 44q, 49q, 66–67a, 72a
   transient vision loss in driving 143q, 152a
   see also blindness
vismodegib 117q, 128a
VISTA trial 61a
visual acuity reduction 47q, 68–69a
visual disturbances, intermittent 47q, 49q, 69a, 71a
visual evoked potential (VEP) 122q, 132a, 190a
visual field constriction attributable to vigabatrin (VAVFC) 153a
visual field loss, driving license 142q, 152a
vitamin B_3 (niacin/nicotinic acid) 42q, 63a
vitamin(s), macular cystic changes 42q, 63a
vitamin B_2 177a
vitamin C 151a
vitamin E 151a
vitrectomy
   tamponade with 54a
   three port pars plana vitrectomy 36q, 55–56a
vitreoretinal clinics, biomicroscopic classification 55a, 55t
vitreous haemorrhage, diabetes type 1 9q, 27a

VIVID trial 61a
VJC (vernal keratoconjunctivitis) 7q, 24a
Vogt–Koyanagi–Harada (VKH) disease 119q, 129a
Vogt–Spielmeyer–Batten disease 186a
Von-Hippel–Lindsay syndrome 195a
von Recklinghausen neurofibromatosis see neurofibromatosis type 1
vortex keratopathy (cornea verticillata) 158q, 179–180a
Vossius ring 183a
V-RRR mnemonic 150a

W

Waardenburg syndrome 52q, 76a, 186a
   anterior lenticonus 33a
Weber syndrome 70t
Wegener's granulomatosis see granulomatosis with polyangiitis (GPA) (Wegener's granulomatosis)
Weill–Marchesani syndrome 182–183a
wide-field fluorescence angiography, familial exudative vitreoretinopathy 184a
Wilcoxon rank-sum tests 201a
Wilcoxon signed-rank tests 148a
Wilson's disease 4q, 20a
   sunflower cataracts 183a
World Health Organization (WHO), cataract surgery 12q, 31a
Worth four-dot (W4D) test 173q, 199–200a
WT1 tumour suppressor gene 159q
Wyburn–Mason syndrome 64a, 146a

X

X-linked ocular albinism 81q, 102a
X-linked recessive juvenile retinoschisis (XLRS) 96a

Z

Ziehl–Nielsen staining 198t
zinc 151a
   supplements 175q, 202a
zoster-associated acute retinal necrosis 196a

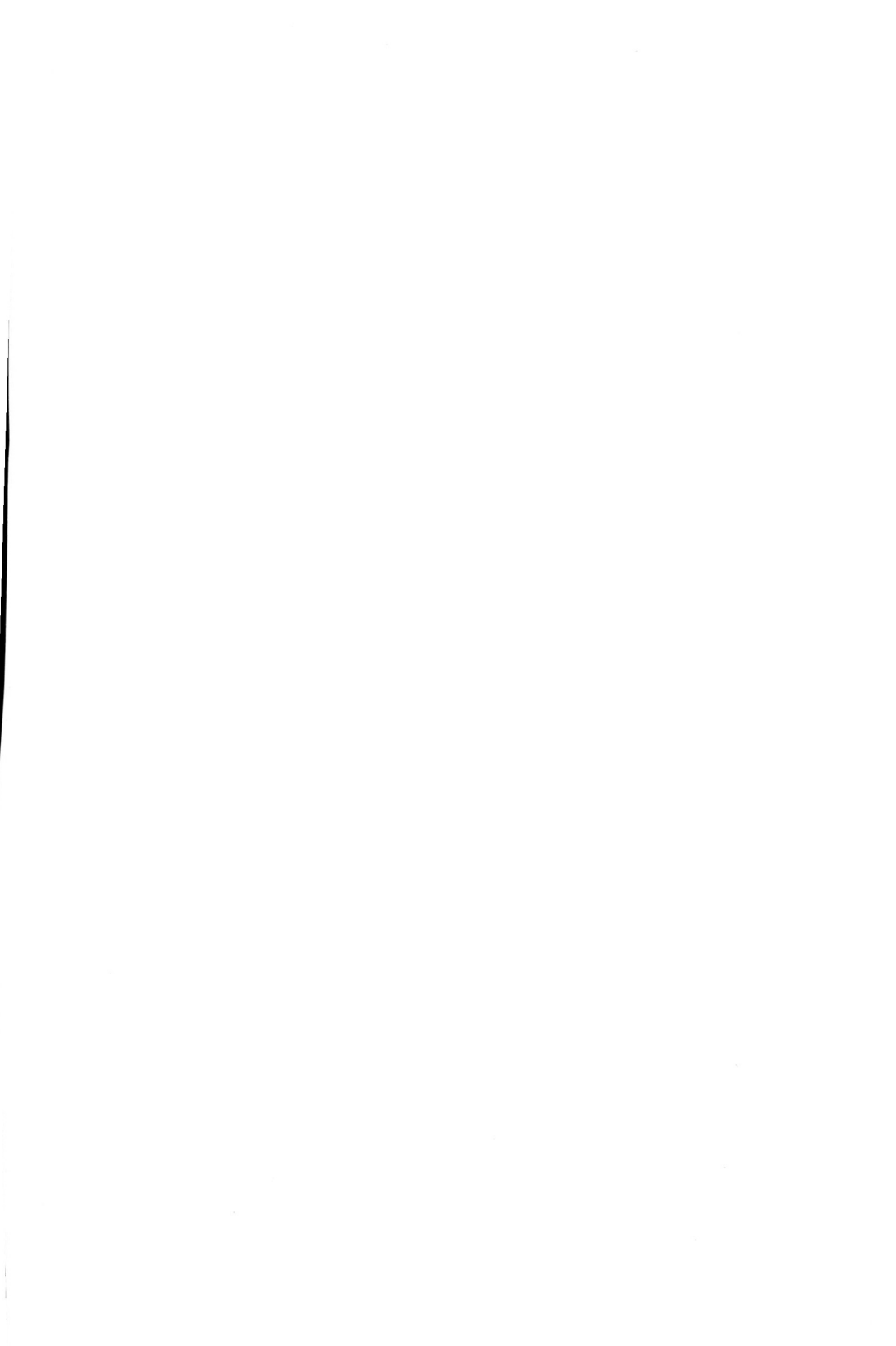

Made in the USA
Monee, IL
03 May 2026

49437400R00136